Contemporary Approaches to Neuropsychological Assessment

CRITICAL ISSUES IN NEUROPSYCHOLOGY

Series Editors

Antonio E. Puente
University of North Carolina, Wilmington

Cecil R. Reynolds
Texas A&M University

A Continuation Order Plan is available for this series. A continuation order will bring delivery of each new volume immediately upon publication. Volumes are billed only upon actual shipment. For further information please contact the publisher.

Contemporary Approaches to Neuropsychological Assessment

Edited by

Gerald Goldstein

Pittsburgh Veterans Affairs Healthcare System and
University of Pittsburgh
Pittsburgh, Pennsylvania

and

Theresa M. Incagnoli

School of Medicine
State University of New York at Stony Brook
Stony Brook, New York

Plenum Press • New York and London

Library of Congress Cataloging-in-Publication Data

On file

ISBN 0-306-45521-8

© 1997 Plenum Press, New York
A Division of Plenum Publishing Corporation
233 Spring Street, New York, N. Y. 10013

http://www.plenum.com

10 9 8 7 6 5 4 3 2 1

Printed in the United States of America

Contributors

Daniel Allen • Department of Veterans Affairs Medical Center, Pittsburgh, Pennsylvania 15206

Thomas J. Boll • Department of Surgery, Division of Neurological Surgery, Section of Neuropsychology, University of Alabama at Birmingham, Birmingham, Alabama 35294-4551

Gerald Goldstein • Pittsburgh VA Health Care System, and University of Pittsburgh, Pittsburgh, Pennsylvania 15260

Theresa Incagnoli • School of Medicine, State University of New York, Stony Brook, New York 11790

Robert L. Kane • Baltimore Department of Veterans Affairs Medical Center, Baltimore, Maryland 21201

Gary G. Kay • Department of Neurology, Georgetown University Hospital, Washington, DC 20007

Lisa Morrow • Western Psychiatric Institute and Clinic, Pittsburgh, Pennsylvania 15213

James A. Moses, Jr. • Department of Veterans Affairs Medical Center, Stanford University, Palo Alto, California 94304-1207

Paul D. Nussbaum • Aging Research and Education Center, Lutheran Affiliated Services, Mars, Pennsylvania 15044; and University of Pittsburgh, School of Medicine, Pittsburgh, Pennsylvania 15260

Arnold D. Purisch • Irvine, California 92718

v

Homer B. C. Reed • Neuropsychology Laboratory, New England Medical Center, Boston, Massachusetts 02111

James C. Reed • Wayland, Massachusetts 01778

Marcie Wallace Ritter • Department of Psychology, Carnegie-Mellon University, Pittsburgh, Pennsylvania 15213

Fredric E. Rose • Department of Veterans Affairs, Decatur, Georgia 30033

Elbert W. Russell • Veterans Administration Medical Center, Miami, Florida 33143

Jerry J. Sweet • Evanston Hospital, Evanston, Illinois 60201

Cynthia Westergaard • Evanston Hospital, Evanston, Illinois 60201

Roberta F. White • Department of Neurology, Boston University School of Medicine, and Department of Veterans Affairs Medical Center, Boston, Massachusetts 02130

Mark A. Williams • Department of Surgery, Division of Neurological Surgery, Section of Neuropsychology, University of Alabama at Birmingham, Birmingham, Alabama 35294-4551

Preface

This volume reflects, in part, an update of *Clinical Application of Neuropsychological Test Batteries,* edited by Theresa Incagnoli, Gerald Goldstein, and Charles Golden some 10 years ago. While the initial concept of the present editors involved doing a straightforward update of each chapter, it soon became apparent that the field of clinical neuropsychology had changed so dramatically and rapidly that substantial changes in the outline had to be made.

It was our view that sufficient interest remained in the standard comprehensive neuropsychological test batteries to make an update worthwhile. We asked four senior people to take on this assignment, James Moses, Jr., and Arnold Purisch in the case of the Luria–Nebraska Battery, and James Reed and Homer Reed for the Halstead–Reitan Battery. These individuals all have long-term associations with these procedures and can be viewed as pioneers in their development. However, it also seemed to us that there was an increasing interest in the psychometric aspects of the standard procedures and in assessment issues related to the relative merits of using standard or individualized assessment strategies. Thus, we have chapters by Elbert Russell and Gerald Goldstein that provide discussions of these current methodological and clinical issues.

During the past 10 years, the cognitive revolution has made a strong impact on neuropsychology. The interest of cognitive psychologists in brain function has increased dramatically, and we now have an active field of cognitive neuropsychology, something that was only beginning 10 years ago. The chapter by Marcie Wallace Ritter and Lisa Morrow provides an orientation to these new developments, as well as some major illustrations of the relevance of experimental cognitive research and theory to clinical neuropsychology. In a sense, this chapter replaces the previous chapters on language, memory, and visual–spatial abilities, since these areas are now heavily permeated by cognitive theory.

In the previous volume, Harold Goodglass wrote a chapter on flexible batteries in assessment that probably represents one of the first formal and coherent presentations of what is now known as the process approach. There seems little question that there have been major advances in the development of this method of assessment, with numerous oral and written presentations of its methods and philosophy and with the appearance of new tests and scoring methods based on process approach theory. The chapter by Roberta White and Fredric Rose provides an overview and update of this important movement in clinical neuropsychology. Apparently, Harold Goodglass's seminal presentation has not fallen on blind eyes or deaf ears.

We felt that the field of clinical neuropsychology has become increasingly specialized but not fragmented. That is, there is still a core discipline, but we know a great deal more now about neuropsychological aspects of specific populations, notably children, the elderly, and individuals suffering from various forms of psychopathology. We therefore include chapters on child assessment by Mark Williams and Thomas Boll, on assessment of the elderly by Paul Nussbaum and Daniel Allen, and on psychopathology by Jerry Sweet and Cynthia Westergaard. These chapters reflect the existence of important emerging subspecialties within clinical neuropsychology and the growth of substantial research literatures in each of them. The inclusion of psychopathology is of great interest because it is a clear reflection of the biological revolution in psychiatry and psychopathology, and particularly because of the exciting prospect of learning more about how the brain functions in such puzzling disorders as schizophrenia and autism.

One future scenario for clinical neuropsychological assessment, and perhaps psychological assessment in general, is the increasing replacement by computer technologies of standard testing, scoring, and perhaps interpretive procedures. While we have not gotten very far with interpretation, the administration and scoring of tests with computer assistance have become a common practice. Robert Kane and Gary Kay, two of the major figures in this area, review recent developments in their chapter.

The editors would like to acknowledge Mariclaire Cloutier, Eliot Werner, and Tony Puente for their continued support. The contributors are congratulated for the scholarship and thoroughness of their work. The editors acknowledge the substantial support of this work by the Department of Veterans Affairs.

Gerald Goldstein
Theresa Incagnoli

Contents

Recent Trends in Neuropsychological Assessment
An Overview and Update

THERESA INCAGNOLI

UTILIZATION OF STANDARD AND FLEXIBLE BATTERIES IN CLINICAL EVALUATION

The discussion of fixed versus flexible neuropsychological batteries presented by Goldstein (Chapter 3) differs from other treatments of this topic in that the theoretical foundation underlying the fixed and flexible dimension is emphasized. It is Goldstein's contention that the central difference underlying this dimension rests upon the theoretical foundation of what one believes rather than upon the practical consideration of what one does. The dimensional–categorical approach to neuropsychological evaluation is contingent on a dimensional as opposed to a modular brain model (Moscovitch & Nachson, 1995). Moscovitch and Nachson state that

> The idea that the brain is modular is an old one, dating back at least to Gall who believed that different faculties were represented in different regions of the cortex. The opposing view, that the cortex functions as a unified whole, at least with regard to higher mental functions, has always challenged the modular one. At a deep level, the struggle between these two ideas about brain organization and function continues today. (p. 167)

THERESA INCAGNOLI • School of Medicine, State University of New York, Stony Brook, New York 11790

FIXED BATTERIES IN NEUROPSYCHOLOGICAL ASSESSMENT

Halstead–Reitan Neuropsychology Test Battery

Recent developments in the two most frequently utilized fixed neuropsychological batteries, the Halstead–Reitan and the Luria–Nebraska Neuropsychological batteries, are discussed by Reed and Reed (Chapter 4) and by Moses and Purisch (Chapter 5). Noteworthy developments for the Halstead–Reitan battery in the last decade include the development of new summary scores: the General Neuropsychological Deficit Scale (GNDS), the Left Neuropsychological Deficit Scale (LNDS), and the Right Neuropsychological Deficit Scale (RNDS) (Reitan & Wolfson, 1988, 1993). The GNDS is a summary index based on 42 variables from the Halstead–Reitan battery that characterizes the degree of overall impairment of neuropsychological functioning. This summary score ranges in classification from normal through mild, moderate, and severe degrees of impairment. Norm guidelines for the GNDS are presented by Reitan and Wolfson (1993, pp. 347–397). A sample computerized GNDS is also contained in that volume (pp. 825–832).

The GNDS was subject to an initial cross-validation study on a sample consisting of 73 brain-damaged individuals and 41 pseudoneurological controls (Sherer & Adams, 1993). When Reitan and Wolfson's (1988) cutoff scores were utilized as the basis of group assignment, 53.6% of the pseudoneurological controls were classified as brain-damaged on the GNDS, while 84.9% of the brain-damaged individuals were classified as such. Sherer and Adams note that such a poor classification of the pseudoneurological control group may well be due to a limitation when utilizing such subjects.

In a subsequent cross-validation study of the GNDS (Wolfson & Reitan, 1995), the mean GNDS of the brain-damaged group (55.02) was significantly worse than the mean GNDS for the control group (19.66). The sample for the study consisted of 50 brain-damaged and 50 intact controls matched for mean age and education who were not previously utilized as part of the Reitan and Wolfson (1988) study. While the 41 control subjects in the Sherer and Adams (1993) investigation reported neurological symptoms, 30 of the individuals also had psychiatric diagnoses. In contrast, the control sample of the Wolfson and Reitan (1995) investigation consisted of individuals with no such complaints, of whom only five were noted to have a psychiatric diagnosis. Wolfson and Reitan (1995) note that

> In order to obtain completely "clean" comparisons, we feel that the initial validation studies should compare groups of subjects who fall unequivocally into either a brain-damaged or non-brain-damaged group. Following such a determination, other comparison groups, comprised according to clinically relevant criteria, may be evaluated, and a pseudoneurologic comparison group would certainly be clinically relevant. (p. 130)

Few research attempts have been directed at cross-validation of the LNDS and the RNDS. The 73 brain-damaged subjects in the Sherer and Adams (1993) study were classified as being left, right, or diffusely brain-damaged based on neurodiagnostic studies alone. Even though 13 individuals were categorized as having lateralized brain-damage based on computed tomography (CT) scan or magnetic resonance imaging (MRI) findings, such individuals were in all likelihood diffusely impaired. When the 13 controls were eliminated, 64.3% of the left hemisphere, 23.5% of the right hemisphere, and 82.8% of the diffusely brain-damaged individuals were correctly classified utilizing Reitan and Wolfson's (1988) recommended cutoff scores. The authors note " . . . that the LNDS and RNDS are sensitive to group differences, but must be interpreted cautiously when assessing individual patients" (p. 434).

Russell (Chapter 2) reviews and compares three computerized scoring programs for the Halstead–Reitan Battery (HRB). These include the Neuropsychological Deficit Scale (NDS) (Reitan, 1991), the Comprehensive Norms for an Extended Halstead–Reitan Battery (CNEHRB) (Heaton, Grant, & Matthews, 1991), and the Halstead–Russell Neuropsychological Evaluation System (HRNES) (Russell, 1993). Although the core of all three batteries consists of the HRB and the Wechsler Adult Intelligence Scale (WAIS) or the Wechsler Adult Intelligence Scale—Revised (WAIS-R), the CNEHRB and HRNES include other supplemental tests.

Reitan's (1991) computer program consists of several indices, the GNDS, a new summary index of neuropsychological impairment and two lateralization scales, the LNDS and the RNDS. The CNEHRB (Heaton et al., 1991) had as its original intent comprehensive norms for the HRB and other supplemental tests for which a computer scoring program was later developed. Corrections for age, education, and gender are applied, while the metric unit consists of T-scores. Fuerst's (1993) critique of the computer component of the CNEHRB did not address either the norming procedure or the norms themselves. The HRNES is derived from the methods of Rennick (Russell, Neuringer, & Goldstein, 1970; Russell & Starkey, 1993) rather than Reitan. This extended HRB utilizes raw scores corrected for age, gender, and education, which are transformed into C scores. C scores utilize a mean of 100 and a standard deviation of 10. Although reviews of the HRNES have generally been favorable (Lynch, 1995; Mahurin, 1995; Retzlaff, 1995), Lezak (1995) was critical of the program.

Russell's evaluation of the three computerized scoring systems concludes that each system is valid in its own right. The NDS is suitable for those individuals who utilize a strict Reitan approach, while the CNEHRB and HRNES are appropriate for those whose assessment consists of an expanded HRB. Generally the similarities between the CNEHRB and HRNES were greater than the differences. Although differences were quite variable, exceptions occurred in relation to the Tapping Test and the Purdue Pegboard, where lower scale scores on the HRNES were required for impairment.

The Luria–Nebraska Neuropsychological Battery

The Luria–Nebraska Neuropsychological Battery (LNNB-I) has undergone changes and additions since 1980 when it was first commercially published. These include addition of the Delayed Memory Scale, which is discussed in the 1985 manual (Golden, Purisch, & Hammeke, 1985, pp. 300–303). Short forms of the LNNB-I have been proposed for the elderly and those in frail health. An odd–even short form has been developed by Horton, Anilane, Puente, and Berg (1988). A decision tree administration procedure has been developed by Golden (1989) to abbreviate examination time in individuals who are significantly cognitively impaired.

Other developments pertaining to the LNNB-I include the development of a Greek language version—LNNB-G (Donias, 1985; Donias, Vassilopoulou, Golden, & Lovell, 1989). High discriminant validity, high interrater reliability, and moderate to high interrater reliability have been reported. An alternative form of the Luria, the LNNB-Form II (LNNB-2), has been characterized by Moses and Purisch (Chapter 5) as "Perhaps the most significant single addition to the LNNB literature." The alternate form is noteworthy for the inclusion of the new clinical scale C12 or Intermediate Memory Scale. Unlike the Delayed Memory Scale of the LNNB-I, which was subsequently standardized on a different sample than that on which the clinical scales were originally developed, the Intermediate Memory Scale has the advantage of being normed on the same reference group as were the clinical scales.

Uniform T-score norms have been developed for the LNNB-2 (Moses, Schefft, Wong, & Berg, 1992) and are reported in normative tables that translate raw scores for the 12 clinical scales (see pp. 256–257). These uniform T-score norms for the LNNB-2 are the only ones that Moses and Purisch (Chapter 5) recommend utilizing, since they are both widely representative while containing a common scaling metric.

Although it was originally claimed that Forms I and II of the LNNB were equivalent (Golden et al., 1985), it has subsequently been determined that the two forms are not interchangeable (Moses & Chiu, 1993). The unfortunate consequences that can ensue when one assumes equivalence of these two forms have been delineated by Klein (1993) in reference to a forensic case.

Recent research in syndrome analyses of diverse disorders has been presented for both the HRB and the LNNB. Current studies in neurological disease and schizophrenia are reviewed for each of the batteries. In addition, research on systemic disease is discussed for the HRB, while studies addressing depression, learning disabilities, mental retardation, and normal aging effects are presented for the LNNB.

THEORETICAL APPROACHES TO NEUROPSYCHOLOGICAL EXAMINATION

The major new developments in the theoretical aspects of neuropsychological assessment have been in the applications of principles derived from the process approach (White & Rose, Chapter 7) and cognitive psychology (Ritter & Morrow, Chapter 8). The process approach was developed by Edith Kaplan during her tenure at the Boston VA. Central to the approach is the differentiation between "process and achievement" in development (Werner, 1937) "to understanding the dissolution of function in patients with brain damage" (Milberg, Hebben, & Kaplan, 1986, p. 66).

The process approach represents a systematic method to the evaluation of qualitative neuropsychological data. White and Rose (Chapter 7) discuss

> . . . the strategy or style of processing employed by the patient for task completion, the dissection of common tests into processing components that can be successfully or unsuccessfully carried out in completing the task, "pushing the limits" of patient processing capacities, the qualitative evaluation of error types, and systematic clinical observation and characterization of patient behavior during assessment. (pp. 174–175)

Proponents of the process approach, rather than utilizing a fixed set of neuropsychological tests that are administered to every individual, choose those instruments specifically chosen to address the evaluation needs of a particular patient. In contrast to the restricted focus on neurobehavioral syndromes posited by some process-oriented advocates, White (1992) proposes a more representative sampling of cognitive domains in individuals undergoing evaluation.

Process-oriented neuropsychologists utilize tests that have been either specifically developed by them or that are existing tests that have been adapted in some way to reflect the process approach. Tests developed by process-oriented neuropsychologists include the current 60-item version of the Boston Naming Test (Kaplan, Goodglass, & Weintraub, 1983); the Boston Diagnostic Aphasia Examination (Goodglass & Kaplan, 1976, 1983); the Cancellation Test (Weintraub & Mesulam, 1988); the California Verbal Learning Test, which is available in adult (Delis, Kramer, Kaplan, & Ober, 1987) and children's versions (Delis, Kramer, Kaplan, & Ober, 1994); the Delayed Recognition Span Test (Moss, Albert, Butters, & Payne, 1986); and nonverbal mood scales (Diamond, White & Moheban, 1990; Stern, Arruda, Hooper, Wolfner & Morey, 1997).

Existing tests that are administered in a manner reflecting the process approach include the WAIS-R as a Neuropsychological Instrument (Kaplan, Fein, Morris, & Delis, 1991), the Wechsler Memory Scale (Wechsler & Stone, 1945), the Wechsler Memory Scale—Revised (Wechsler, 1987), the Hooper Visual Organization Test (Hooper, 1958), the Rey–Osterreith Complex Figure (Rey, 1941), and the Recurrent Series Writing and Multiple Loops (White, 1992).

White and Rose (Chapter 6) review select research studies in various cognitive domains considered to best exemplify the qualitative analysis of the process approach. Interesting innovations include the development of the computerized assessment system MicroCog (Powell et al., 1993) and the validation of measures combining process-oriented tasks together with novel computer techniques in select types of brain-damaged individuals (Letz & Baker, 1988; White, Diamond, Krengel, Lindem, & Feldman, 1996).

Cognitive Psychology

Cognitive psychology is concerned with the functional integration of the various brain subsystems in the intact individual and the failure of such subsystems when brain damage occurs. Ritter and Morrow (Chapter 7) address the contribution of cognitive psychology to clinical neuropsychology and patient examination. The authors provide a selective review of studies in the fields of visual cognition, attention, and serial versus parallel processing in brain-damaged individuals. An example of how visual cognition experiments delineate such subsystems is provided in the work of Mishkin, Ungerleider, and Macko (1983), which documents how a dorsal (parietal) lesion produces only a spatial localization deficit, while a ventral (temporal) lesion produces only an object identification disorder. Because cognitive neuropsychology has advanced our comprehension of visual cognitive disorders, a comprehensive review of imagery in visual cognition, mental representation, and mental representation and neglect is provided.

Applications of cognitive psychology to clinical populations are of particular interest. Nebes, Brady, and Reynolds (1992) studied the differentiation in time between comparing each probe stimulus to a list versus time required to initiate a response. Subjects consisted of Alzheimer's patients, normal elderly, depressed elderly, and normal young. The greater slowness demonstrated by the Alzheimer's individual to check each item was reflected in a slope that was significantly greater than the other three groups. The slopes of the normal elderly, depressed elderly, and normal young did not differ from each other. The intercept (the time to perceive the probe and execute a response) did not differ between the Alzheimer's and the other two elderly groups. Clinical utilization of such findings warrants continued replication.

In summary, Ritter and Morrow demonstrate

> ... how the application of experiments developed in the cognitive psychology laboratory can help to identify specific underlying operations that are disrupted by focal brain lesions. Not only do these studies confirm the existence of cortical and subcortical areas that are specialized for cognitive operations, they also help to confirm or disconfirm underlying theories of mental processing. Moreover, the findings have far-reaching implications for rehabilitation. (p. 228)

NEUROPSYCHOLOGICAL EXAMINATION OF SELECT POPULATIONS

Child Neuropsychological Assessment

A major focus of the chapter on child neuropsychological assessment (Chapter 8) is a selective review of the cognitive tests developed some time in the past that continue to be utilized frequently, as well as those measures that have been more recently developed. Tests within cognitive domains of intelligence, achievement, language, visual–spatial and construction, somatosensory, and motor functions, attention, memory and learning, and problem solving are discussed. It is suggested that language functions be evaluated utilizing presently existing measures that are compatible with the neurodevelopmental model of linguistic development proposed by Crary, Voeller, and Haak (1988). The five components of attention proposed by Barkley (1988) are delineated along with corresponding measures to evaluate each sector. New measures specifically designed to evaluate memory and learning in children are surveyed. A description of the nine subtests comprising the Wide Range Assessment of Memory and Learning (Sheslow & Adams, 1990) are provided in Table 3 (Chapter 8).

Assessment of psychosocial, behavioral, and environmental factors is an integral component of the evaluation process. Williams and Boll note that "Variables such as motivation, impulsivity, and anxiety/depression are important to consider with respect to performance on neuropsychological tests" (p.). A list of standardized interviews, broadband rating scales, and self-report inventories to evaluate these factors is noted in Table 4. Williams and Boll also review the neuropsychological correlates of the syndromes of traumatic brain injury, learning disabilities, and attention deficit hyperactivity disorder. Neuropsychological outcome studies of traumatic brain injury in specified cognitive domains are also surveyed.

Neuropsychological Evaluation of the Elderly and Those with Severe Dementia

Nussbaum and Allen (Chapter 9) note that 12% of the population is now considered elderly when that term is defined as age 65 or over. Table 1 notes the three general categories—client characteristics, instrument and test environment characteristics, and examiner characteristics—that need to be considered when evaluating elderly demented individuals. Although neuropsychologists consider many of these client variables in any examination (e.g., sensory impairments, medication effects, psychiatric disorders), the significance of such factors markedly increases in a geriatric population.

Recently, there has been a much-needed proliferation of norms for the elderly. Heaton et al. (1991) have provided comprehensive norms for the HRB plus several additional tests extending to age 80. The *Clinical Neuropsychologist Supplement* (1992) presents results of the MAYO's older American normative studies for the WAIS-R for ages 56 through 97 (Ivnik et al., 1992a), the Wechsler Memory Scale—Revised for ages 56 through 94 (Ivnik et al., 1992b), and the updated Auditory Verbal Learning Test (AVLT) norms (Ivnik et al., 1992c) for ages 56 through 97.

Nussbaum and Allen survey the most widely utilized brief (10 minutes or less administration time) (see Table 2) and intermediate (up to 45 minutes) screening instruments for mild and moderate dementia (see Table 3). Of the brief screening instruments the most popular measure which has also been the most extensively studied is the Mini-Mental State Examination (Folstein, Folstein, & McHugh, 1975). A more recent study (Marshall & Mungas, 1995) has improved the overall sensitivity of this measure by statistically correcting for age and education. Of the intermediate-length screening instruments, the Dementia Rating Scale (Mattis, 1976, 1988) is the most well-established instrument.

Instruments that evaluate cognition in severely demented individuals just recently have been made available. Such tests fulfill the unmet need to evaluate cognitive functions in such individuals in a standardized fashion. Nussbaum and Allen located five neuropsychological measures for this specific population with some reported validity and reliability information. The majority of their discussion focuses on the Severe Impairment Battery (Saxton, McGonigle-Gibson, Swihart, Miller, & Boller, 1990; 1993), since it is the most widely reported instrument in the literature in terms of validity and reliability data.

Nussbaum and Allen present a survey of behavior rating scales utilized to evaluate dementia patients based on scales that were (1) either recently developed or applied to a dementia population, and (2) where recent validity and reliability data have been obtained. Information on the psychometric properties, test characteristics, and domains assessed for the London Psychogeriatric Rating Scale (Hersh, Kral, & Palmer, 1978), the Echelle Comportment et Adaptation (Ritchie & Ledersert, 1991), Neurobehavioral Rating Scale (Levin et al., 1987), and the Nurses' Observation Scale for Geriatric Patients (Spiegal et al., 1991) is provided.

EXAMINING PSYCHOPATHOLOGY AS PART OF NEUROPSYCHOLOGICAL ASSESSMENT

Evaluation of emotional function and possible psychopathology are integral components of the neuropsychological examination. Sweet and Westergaard (Chapter 10) provide a comprehensive review of common psychopathological disorders from both a neuropathological and neuropsychological perspective. Although most attention is focused on schizophrenia because of the vast research literature on this topic, unipolar depression and obsessive–compulsive disorders are also addressed. The authors note (p. 327) that such a discussion should "at the very least give pause when confronted with the outdated, but still commonplace, referral question asking for a distinction between functional versus organic (i.e., psychological versus brain-based) etiology."

When evaluating an individual for the presence or absence of brain damage, it is incumbent upon the clinician to consider explanations other than brain dysfunction when presented with impaired neuropsychological performance. A partial listing of such moderator variables frequently considered in neuropsychological interpretation is presented in Chapter 10, Table 1 (Sweet, in press). Emotional states (e.g., depression, anxiety), significant psychiatric disorders (e.g., schizophrenia, bipolar disorder), substance abuse, and deliberate attempts to feign symptoms are all alternative hypotheses that need to be ruled out prior to rendering a diagnosis of brain dysfunction.

The authors provide an overview of the measures used by neuropsychologists to evaluate emotional/personality functioning. It is of interest that in a recent survey of 279 neuropsychologists, 74% stated that they utilized objective personality measures "often" or "always" (Sweet, Moberg, & Westergaard, 1996). Although the diagnosis of brain damage solely based on emotional/personality measures is an inappropriate use of such instruments, evaluation of emotional functioning is an essential component of the neuropsychological examination.

The Minnesota Multiphasic Personality Inventory—2 (MMPI-2) continues to be the most frequently utilized objective personality measurement instrument. Other recent objective personality test revisions include the Millon Clinical Multiaxial Inventory—III (MCMI-III) (Millon, Millon, & Davis, 1994). Both the MMPI-2 and the MCMI-III are based on predecessors with a wealth of published information.

THE ROLE OF COMPUTERS IN NEUROPSYCHOLOGICAL EVALUATION

The use of computers to administer, score, and interpret neuropsychological tests is rapidly expanding and merits consideration in any review on extant developments in evaluation. After reviewing the advantages and limitations of computerized assessment, Kane and Kay (Chapter 11) present a review of computerized test batteries which include CogScreen–Aeromedical Edition (Kay, 1995), MicroCog (Powell et al., 1993), Automated Neuropsychological Assessment Metrics (Reeves, Kane, Winter, & Goldstone, 1995), the Neurobehavioral Evaluation System—2 (Letz & Baker, 1988), the Automated Portable Test System; Delta (Levander, 1987), and the California Computerized Assessment Package (Miller, 1996). Individualized computer tests such as the Nonverbal Selective Reminding Test (Kane & Perrine, 1988) and Synwork (Elsmore, 1994) as well as computer-based continuous performance tests such as the Test of Variables of Attention (McCarney & Greenburg, 1990) and the Conner's Continuous Performance Test (Conners, 1995) are also discussed.

Computer assessment allows for the assessment of performance efficiency, response time, and variability. Despite such potential advantages there has been a reluctance on the part of neuropsychologists to incorporate automated assessment in the evaluation process. Kane and Kay (Chapter 11) posit that the reasons for such include the lack of age, education, and culturally based norms; the limitations of evaluating cognitive domains such as language and memory; the cost of automated assessment; and the unfamiliarity of clinicians with computerized assessment procedures.

These limitations notwithstanding, it appears quite tenable to presume that such automated evaluations will represent the future direction in which neuropsychological examinations will proceed. Kane and Kay state

However, even today, computers provide a potent adjunct to traditional techniques by permitting the assessment of performance efficiency and consistency in a way not possible with standard measures, increasing the range of tasks which can be implemented during an examination and permitting an assessment of domains (e.g., divided attention) not possible with standard metrics. (p. 389)

ACKNOWLEDGMENT

I wish to thank Dr. Gerald Goodstein for his careful review of this manuscript.

REFERENCES

Barkley, R. A. (1988). Attention. In M. G. Tramontana & S. R. Hooper (Eds.), *Assessment issues in child neuropsychology. Critical issues in neuropsychology* (pp. 145–176). New York: Plenum Press.

Conners, K. C. (1995). *Conners' Continuous Performance Test computer program 3.0: User's manual.* Toronto: Multi-Health Systems.

Crary, M. A., Voeller, K. K. S., & Haak, N. J. (1988). Questions of developmental neurolinguistic assessment. In M. G. Tramontana & S. R. Hooper (Eds.), *Assessment issues in child neuropsychology. Critical issues in neuropsychology* (pp. 242–279). New York: Plenum Press.

Delis, D. C., Kramer, J. H., Kaplan, E., & Ober, B. A. (1987). *The California Verbal Learning Test— Research Edition.* San Antonio, TX: The Psychological Corp.

Diamond, R., White, R. F., & Moheban, C. (1990). *Nonverbal Analogue Profile of Mood States.* Unpublished test.

Donias, S. H. (1985). *The Luria–Nebraska Neuropsychological Battery: Standardized in a Greek population and transcultural observations.* Unpublished doctoral dissertation, Aristotelian University, Thessaloniki, Greece.

Donias, S. H., Vassilopoulou, E. O., Golden, C. J., & Lovell, M. R. (1989). Reliability and clinical effectiveness of the standardized Greek version of the Luria–Nebraska Neuropsychological Battery. *The International Journal of Clinical Neuropsychology, IX,* 129–133.

Elsmore, T. (1994). SYNWORK I: A PC-based tool for assessment of performance in a simulated work environment. *Behavioral Research Methods, Instruments, and Computers, 26,* 421–426.

Folstein, M. F., Folstein, S. E., & McHugh, P. R. (1975). Mini-mental State. A practical method for grading the cognitive state of patients for the clinician. *Journal of Psychiatric Research, 12,* 189–198.

Fuerst, D. R. (1993). A review of the Halstead–Reitan Neuropsychological Battery norms program. *The Clinical Neuropsychologist, 7,* 96–103.

Golden, C. J. (1989). Abbreviating administration of the LNNB in significantly impaired patients. *The International Journal of Clinical Neuropsychology, XI,* 177–181.

Golden, C. J., Purisch, A. D., & Hammeke, T. A. (1985). *The Luria–Nebraska Neuropsychological Battery Forms I and II manual.* Los Angeles: Western Psychological Services.

Goodglass, H., & Kaplan, E. (1976). *The assessment of aphasia and related disorders.* Philadelphia: Lea & Febiger.

Goodglass, H., & Kaplan, E. (1983). *The assessment of aphasia and related disorders* (2nd ed.). Philadelphia: Lea & Febiger.

Heaton, R. K., Grant, I., & Matthews, C. G. (1991). *Comprehensive norms for an expanded Halstead–Reitan Battery: Demographic corrections, research findings, and clinical applications.* Odessa, FL: Psychological Assessment Resources.

Hersch, E. L., Kral, V. A., & Palmer, R. B. (1978). Clinical value of the London Psychogeriatric Rating Scale. *Journal of the American Geriatrics Society, 26,* 348–354.

Hooper, H. E. (1958). *The Hooper Visual Organization Test Manual.* Los Angeles: Western Psychological Services.

Horton, A. M., Anilane, J., Puente, A. E., & Berg, R. A. (1988). Diagnostic parameters of an odd–even item short-form of the Luria–Nebraska Neuropsychological Battery. *Archives of Clinical Neuropsychology, 3,* 375–381.

Ivnik, R. J., Malec, J. F., Smith, G. E., Tangalos, E. G., Peterson, R. C., Kokmen, E., & Kurland, L. T. (1992a). Mayo's older Americans normative studies. WAIS-R norms for ages 56–97. *The Clinical Neuropsychologist, 6 (Supp.),* 1–30.

Ivnik, R. J., Malec, J. F., Smith, G. E., Tangalos, E. G., Peterson, R. C., Kokmen, E., & Kurland, L. T. (1992b). Mayo's older Americans normative studies: WMS-R norms for ages 56–97. *The Clinical Neuropsychologist, 6 (Supp.),* 49–82.

Ivnik, R. J., Malec, J. F., Smith, G. E., Tangalos, E. G., Peterson, R. C., Kokmen, E., & Kurland, L. T. (1992c). Mayo's older Americans normative studies: Updated AVLT norms for ages 56–97. *The Clinical Neuropsychologist, 6 (Suppl.),* 83–104.

Kane, R. L., & Perrine, K. R. (1988, February). Construct validity of a nonverbal analogue to the selective reminding verbal learning test. Paper presented as the meeting of the International Neuropsychological Society, New Orleans.

Kaplan, E., Fein, D., Morris, R., & Delis, D. C. (1991). *WAIS-R as a Neuropsychological Instrument.* San Antonio: The Psychological Corporation.

Kaplan, E., Goodglass, H., & Weintraub, S. (1983). *The Boston Naming Test* (2nd ed.). Philadelphia: Lea & Febiger.

Kay, G. G. (1995). *CogScreen Aeromedical Edition: Professional Manual.* Odessa, FL: Psychological Assessment Resources.

Klein, S. H. (1993). Misuse of the Luria–Nebraska localization scales—Comments on a criminal case study. *The Clinical Neuropsychologist, 7,* 297–299.

Letz, R., & Baker, E. Z. (1988). *Neurobehavioral Evaluation System: User's manual.* Winchester, MA: Neurobehavioral Systems, Inc.

Levander, S. (1987). Evaluation of cognitive impairment using a computerized neuropsychological test battery. *Nordic Journal of Psychiatry, 41,* 417–422.

Levin, H. S., High, W. M., Goeth, K. E., Sisson, R. A., Overall, J. E., Rhoades, H. M., Eisenberg, H. M., Kalisky, Z., & Gary, H. E. (1987). The Neurobehavioral Rating Scale: Assessment of the behavioral sequelae of head injury by the clinician. *Journal of Neurology, Neurosurgery, and Psychiatry, 50,* 183–193.

Lezak, M. D. (1995). *Neuropsychological Assessment* (3rd ed.). New York: Oxford University Press.

Lynch, W. J. (1995). Microcomputer-assisted neuropsychological test analysis. *Journal of Head Trauma Rehabilitation, 10,* 97–100.

Mahurin, R. K. (1995). Halstead–Russell Neuropsychological Evaluation System (HRNES). In J. C. Conley & J. C. Impara (Eds.), *12th Mental Measurements Yearbook* (pp. 448–451). Lincoln: University of Nebraska Press.

Marshall, S. C., & Mungas, D. (1995). Age and education correction for the Mini-Mental State Exam. *Journal of the International Neuropsychological Society, 1,* 166.

Mattis, S. (1976). Mental status examination for organic mental syndrome in the elderly patient. In R. Bellak & B. Karasa (Eds.), *Geriatric psychology* (pp. 77–121). New York: Grune & Stratton.

Mattis, S. (1988). *DRS: Dementia Rating Scale professional manual.* New York: Psychological Assessment.

McCarney, D., & Greenburg, L. M. (1990). *Tests of variables of attention computer program, version 5.01 for IBM PC or IBM compatibles: TOVA manual.* Minneapolis: University of Minnesota.

Millberg, W. P., Hebben, N., & Kaplan, E. (1986). The Boston process approach to neuropsychological assessment. In I. Grant & K. Adams (Eds.), *Neuropsychological assessment of neuropsychiatric disorders* (pp. 65–86). New York: Oxford University Press.

Miller, E. N. (1996). *California Computerized Assessment Package: Manual.* Los Angeles: Norland Software.

Millon, T., Millon, C., & Davis, R. (1994). *Millon Clinical Multiaxial Inventory—III manual.* Minneapolis, MN: National Computer Systems.

Mishkin, M., Ungerleider, L. G., & Macko, K. A. (1983). Object vision and spatial vision: Two cortical pathways. *Trends in Neurosciences, 6,* 414–417.

Moscovitch, M., & Nachson, I. (1995). Modularity and the brain: Introduction. *Journal of Clinical and Experimental Neuropsychology, 17,* 167–170.

Moses, J. A., Jr., & Chiu, M. L. (1993, October). *Nonequivalence of Forms I and II of the Luria–Nebraska Neuropsychological Battery for Adults.* Paper presented at the meeting of the National Academy of Neuropsychology, Phoenix, AZ.

Moses, J. A., Jr., Schefft, B. K., Wong, J. L., & Berg, R. A. (1992). Revised norms and decision rules for the Luria–Nebraska Neuropsychological Battery, Form II. *Archives of Clinical Neuropsychology, 7,* 251–269.

Moss, M. B., Albert, M. S., Butters, N., & Payne, M. (1986). Differential patterns of memory loss among patients with Alzheimer's disease, Huntington's disease, and alcoholic Korsakoff's syndrome. *Archives of Neurology, 43,* 239–246.

Nebes, R. D., Brady, C. G., & Reynolds, C. F. (1992). Cognitive slowing in Alzheimer's disease and geriatric depression. *Journal of Gerontology: Psychological Sciences, 47*(5), 331–336.

Powell, D. H., Kaplan, E. F., Whitla, D., Weintraub, S., Catlin, R., & Funkenstein, H. H. (1993). *MicroCog: Assessment of cognitive functioning—Manual.* San Antonio, TX: The Psychological Corporation.

Reeves, D., Kane, R. L., Winter, K. P., & Goldstone, A. (1995). *Automated Neuropsychological Assessment Metrics (ANAM V3.11): Clinical and neurotoxicology subsets.* (Scientific Report NCRF-SR-95-01). San Diego, CA: National Cognitive Recovery Foundation.

Reitan, R. M. (1991). *The Neuropsychological Deficit Scale for Adults computer program, users manual.* Tucson, AZ: Neuropsychology Press.

Reitan, R. M., & Wolfson, D. (1988). *Traumatic brain injury. Vol. II. Recovery and rehabilitation.* Tucson, AZ: Neuropsychology Press.

Reitan, R. M., & Wolfson, D. (1993). *The Halstead–Reitan Neuropsychological Test Battery, Theory and clinical interpretation* (2nd ed.). Tucson, AZ: Neuropsychology Press.

Retzlaff, P. (1995). Halstead–Russell Neuropsychological Evaluation System (HRNES). In J. C. Conley & J. C. Impara (Eds.), *12th Mental Measurements Yearbook* (pp. 451–453). Lincoln: University of Nebraska Press.

Rey, A. (1941). Psychological examination of traumatic encephalopathy. *Archives de Psychologie, 28,* 286–340 (Sections translated by J. Corwin & F. W. Bylsma, *The Clinical Neuropsychologist,* 1993, 4–9).

Ritchie, K., & Ledersert, B. (1991). The measurement of incapacity in the severely demented elderly. The validation of a behavioral assessment scale. *International Journal of Geriatric Psychiatry, 6,* 217–226.

Russell, E. W. (1993). *Halstead–Russell Neuropsychological Evaluation System, norms and conversion tables.* Unpublished data tables available from Elbert W. Russell, 6262 Sunset Dr., Suite PH 228, Miami, FL, 33143.

Russell, W. W., Neuringer, C., & Goldstein, G. (1970). *Assessment of brain damage. A neuropsychological approach.* New York: Wiley.

Russell, E. W., & Starkey, R. I. (1993). *Halstead–Russell Neuropsychological Evaluation System* [manual and computer program]. Los Angeles: Western Psychological Services.

Saxton, J., McGonigle-Gibson, K., Swihart, A., & Boller, F. (1993). *The Severe Impairment Battery (SIB) manual.* Suffolk, England: Thames Valley Test Company.

Saxton, J., McGonigle-Gibson, K., Swihart, A., Miller, M., & Boller, F. (1990). Assessment of the severely impaired patient: Description and validity of a new neuropsychological test battery. *Psychological Assessment, 2,* 298–303.

Sherer, M., & Adams, R. L. (1993). Cross-validation of Reitan and Wolfson's Neuropsychological Deficit Scales. *Archives of Clinical Neuropsychology, 8,* 429–435.

Sheslow, D., & Adams, W. (1990). *Wide Range Assessment of Memory and Learning.* Wilmington, DE: Jastak Associates.

Spiegal, R., Brunner, C., Ermini-Fünfschilling, D., Monsch, A., Notter, M., Puxty, J., & Tremmel, L. (1991). A new behavioral assessment scale for geriatric out- and in-patients: The NOSGER (Nurses' Observation Scale for Geriatric Patients). *Journal of the American Geriatrics Society, 39,* 339–347.

Stern, R. A., Arruda, J. E., Hooper, C. R., Wolfner, G. D., & Morey, C. E. (1997). Visual Analogue Mood Scales to measure internal mood state in neurologically impaired patients: Description and initial validity evidence. *Aphasiology, 11,* 59–74.

Sweet, J. (in press). Neuropsychological assessment in rehabilitation, neurology, and psychiatry. In R. Rozensky, J. Sweet, & S. Tovian (Eds.), *Psychological assessment in medical settings.* New York: Plenum Press.

Sweet, J., Moberg, P., & Westergaard, C. (1996). Five year follow-up-survey of practices and beliefs of clinical neuropsychologists. *The Clinical Neuropsychologist, 10,* 202–221.

Wechsler, D. (1987). *Wechsler Memory Scale—Revised.* San Antonio, TX: The Psychological Corporation.

Wechsler, D., & Stone, C. (1945). The Wechsler Memory Scale. *Journal of Psychology, 19,* 87–95.

Weintraub, S., & Mesulam, M. M. (1988). Visual hemispatial inattention: Stimulus parameters and exploratory strategies. *Journal of Neurology, Neurosurgery, and Psychiatry, 51,* 1481–1488.

Werner, H. (1937). Process and achievement: A basic problem of education and developmental psychology. *Harvard Education Review, 7,* 353–368.

White, R. F. (Ed.). (1992). *Clinical syndromes in neuropsychology.* Amsterdam: Elsevier.

White, R. F., Diamond, R., Krengel, M., Lindem, K., & Feldman, R. G. (1996). Validation of the NES in patients with neurological disorders. *Neurotoxicology and Teratology, 18,* 441–448.

Wolfson, D., & Reitan, R. M. (1995). Cross-validation of the General Neuropsychological Deficit Scale (GNDS), *Archives of Clinical Neuropsychology, 10,* 125–131.

2

Developments in the Psychometric Foundations of Neuropsychological Assessment

ELBERT W. RUSSELL

The last decade for neuropsychology has been a fruitful period for developing a new psychometric methodology. The major development in methodology has also initiated a significant theoretical advance. The methodological development has been the creation of computerized scoring programs. The construction of these programs utilized new methods to norm large test batteries. These methods, in turn, required the perfection of a methodology theory related to groups or batteries of tests. The theory may be called a test set theory. While there have been many developments in regard to individual tests, this chapter will concentrate on those aspects of neuropsychology that are related to this development of computerized assessment batteries.

THEORY DEVELOPMENT

At present, neuropsychologists are only partially aware of the scoring programs and many do not realize that the new methods used in cognitive measurement require a major conceptual change in methodology. Many basic concepts need to be rethought. While new, these methods will not supplement older methods of test development but will extend the traditional concepts to batteries of tests. In order to create the computerized scoring systems, the authors were forced to deal with the ways in which a group of tests are integrated so as to create an integrated battery. The new concepts related to integrated batteries include coordinated norming, consistent scaling, and correction for age, gender, and education.

ELBERT W. RUSSELL • Veterans Administration Medical Center, Miami, Florida 33143

The Central Difference between Approaches

Since at least the 1940s, there has been an ongoing controversy in neuropsychology concerning the general methods or approaches to assessment. Originally the opposition was between qualitative and quantitative methods (Goldstein & Scheerer, 1941). The critique of the quantitative method then was roughly the same as the present critique by the process approach (Milberg, Hebben, & Kaplan, 1986; Kaplan, 1988). Other methodological divisions include the opposition between the fixed battery and the flexible battery, the division between the process and the psychometric approaches, and even the division between the neurological (medical) and the psychological models. These approaches are not exclusive of the other methods, so it was common to use a mixture of flexible and psychometric methods. Nevertheless, the different methods had many ramifications relating to the way assessment was carried out.

Recently it became apparent that most of the distinctions can be attributed to a single basic difference in method. The basic underlying division was between what is called the hypothesis-testing method and the pattern analysis method. This difference appears to be fundamental and most of the other differences in method are derived from this distinction. For instance, the essential differences between the flexible and the fixed battery are derived from the different requirements imposed by the pattern and the hypothesis-testing approaches.

In their pure form, each method requires different testing and interpretation procedures. The ramifications produce most of the differences in theory and method. Most neuropsychologists are not aware that this difference is so crucial, since they mix the methods. The recent methodology developments in neuropsychology, other than test construction, are related to the pattern analysis method. Consequently, it becomes necessary to understand the difference in these methods before the extent and impact of the developments can be appreciated.

Hypothesis-Testing Method

Although the name "hypothesis testing" is of recent origin, the name applies to the traditional method of assessment in psychology. In this method the psychologist selects and utilizes tests in order to answer a question. In hypothesis testing, the question is framed as a hypothesis instead of a question (Russell, 1994). The hypothesis-testing method attempts to answer assessment questions in a serial fashion. A test or group of tests is used to answer a question or to test a hypothesis. In this method, the examiner begins with a question, usually related to the question in the consultation. If the question is "Does this patient have brain damage," the hypotheses would be "This patient has brain damage—disprove it." Previously in psychology, the psychologist would simply attempt to determine whether the patient had brain damage; in any case, the method of assessment is the same.

With hypothesis testing, if a person is thought to have a particular condition, then a test that is designed to determine whether the patient had that condition would be selected. The score that the patient obtains or the way in which he or she obtained it, would answer the question. For example, when the question is whether a person has brain damage, if the score on a test for brain damage is in the impaired range or the patient answered in a way that indicated impairment, then this would be evidence that the patient has brain damage and the hypothesis would be accepted. Or if the question is whether a person could read at a certain level, then a test of reading would be selected.

Tests are selected to answer a question. Thus, the hypothesis-testing method is basically a one-question–one-test approach. The examiner might use additional tests to support the first test. Thus, in the pure form of the method a group of tests is used only to obtain redundancy. Since most tests are designed to answer a particular question or to measure a specific condition, the method works well in most situations. It works well enough to be the principal methodological foundation for psychological assessment.

After obtaining an answer to the initial question, the examiner usually does not end the examination. Rather, he or she continues to investigate other questions. There is a methodological problem at this point, since the answering of one hypothesis does not in itself suggest another question (Russell, 1994). In the hypothesis-testing procedure, the tests the examiner uses to obtain the next question are not derived from the answer to the previous hypothesis. The derivation of new questions is not part of the pure hypothesis-testing method. The previous answer establishes constraints, but gives no clue as to which of many directions an examiner may proceed. If the patient has brain damage, the examiner may investigate the location, the pathology, the functions to be stressed in rehabilitation, and so forth. However, it is the situation and the neurological and psychological knowledge that the neuropsychologist brings to the case that determine the sequence of questions. The method is generally that of informal algorithms (Bauer, 1994; Russell, 1994).

In any case, further questions will require new tests to answer the new questions. This procedure of asking a series of questions may be called multistage, serial hypotheses, or ongoing hypothesis testing. The process continues until all of the relevant questions are answered. The length of the battery increases with each additional question. The reason that such neuropsychological batteries are lengthy is that there are a number of questions to be answered. In practice the method may become more complicated in that the examiner may need to compare tests and so administer two or more nonredundant tests. However, this procedure is the beginning of pattern analysis.

There is an alternate method that many neuropsychologists who advocate hypothesis testing recommend, which is not a pure hypothesis-testing method. This method advocates using a fixed or relatively fixed "core" (Bauer, 1994) or "basic battery" (Lezak, 1995, pp. 121–123). The neuropsychologist is looking for relatively impaired test scores to provide an indication as to the condition of the patient, which will then provide hypotheses to test. This method is a rudimentary form of pattern analysis.

The Flexible Battery. The hypothesis-testing process works best with a flexible battery. The flexible battery that is produced by the pure hypothesis-testing approach is unintegrated. The various tests are selected according to their relation to a series of questions and not according to their relation to each other. Thus, this method employs a group of tests that have no intrinsic relation to each other.

Lezak's (1995) designation of fixed batteries as "ready-made batteries" (pp. 123–125) is quite appropriate for neuropsychologists who are using the hypothesis-testing method. However, the rationale for a fixed battery is derived from the pattern analysis method and not the hypothesis-testing method. In this regard, Lezak's critique completely fails to understand the reasons for and method of using a fixed battery.

The Research Method of Hypothesis Testing. The clinical assessment hypothesis-testing concept is not the same type of hypothesis testing that is a well-developed research method. The basic method is well known in psychology. The research method uses groups of subjects (except in a few specifically designed individual case studies). The minimal number of groups is two: an experimental and a control group. The subjects are randomly assigned to the two groups or the subjects are matched on relevant variables. An experimental condition is applied to the experimental group and not the control group. A significant difference disconfirms the negative or null hypothesis. Tests of significance or power tests are utilized to determine whether the research study supports the hypothesis. Of course, in most cases the experimental process is much more complex. Which elements of the research method are part of the clinical assessment method called hypothesis testing?

In research one proceeds, using data gathered from many persons, to test a hypothesis, which is derived from a theory. This is a complex process in which the aim is to support a theory, so the process proceeds from the subjects to the theory. In assessment one reverses the direction and proceeds from a theory to an individual case. The hypothesis is that according to a certain theory this case should exhibit certain test results. (In the question mode certain test results, as determined by the relevant theory, will answer the question.) If the tests results are as hypothesized, then the patient's condition is considered to be that which the theory maintains. This process is almost the opposite of the hypothesis-testing process in research studies. Psychologists using the term "hypothesis testing" in assessment should keep these distinctions in mind.

Pattern Analysis

The pattern analysis method compares tests with each other in order to discover a pattern that reveals information about a condition. The pattern analysis method is primarily concerned with the relationships between tests rather than the scores or level of functioning on particular tests (or the manner that the subject used to obtain the score). The relationships between tests is derived from the relative level of scores on two or more tests. Knowledge of the relationship has been derived from research findings or clinical lore.

Contributions by Reitan. Probably, Reitan's most important contribution to neuropsychology will be his development of the pattern analysis method. While still in Halstead's laboratory, he apparently realized that different types of brain damage affected the various tests in Halstead's battery differently, so that he could determine the type of brain condition by observing test differences. Halstead may have had some conception of this patterning, since he was looking for factors composed of groups of tests. Later, Reitan added tests and changed the scoring of several of the Halstead tests in order to create more scores reflecting the effects of different types of brain damage. Thus, Reitan perfected the method of pattern analysis on an inferential level. He realized that it was necessary to establish a fixed battery in order to observe patterns. If one keeps changing tests, patterns between tests cannot be observed, since no stable basis exists.

Comparisons. The basis for the pattern analysis method is to examine interrelationships by comparing tests to each other. It is the comparisons and not the individual test scores that are crucial. Comparisons demonstrate dissociations between test scores (Russell, 1994). The research method of double dissociation is well known in neuropsychology (Teuber, 1955). In pattern analysis assessment the method is extended and applied to the test scores in a battery as a multiple dissociation (Russell, 1994). In the inferential manner the test battery scores are examined to see what patterns are present. It is these patterns that answer the questions asked of the neuropsychologist. When the tests in the battery are well selected according to coverage (Russell, 1994), the battery presents a model of the functioning of the whole brain (Russell & Starkey, 1993). When certain comparisons, which may involve many tests, are isolated and verified through research, they may be formalized. This is accomplished through creating indexes, formulas, or other formal means (Russell & Polakoff, 1993; Russell & Russell, 1993). The advantage of these formal methods is that they can be validated mathematically. The impressionistic findings that are the usual outcome of neuropsychological research are difficult to cross validate. The method and value of pattern analysis has been discussed in several places (Bauer, 1994; Russell, 1984, 1986, 1994).

Concept of a "Set" of Tests

The theoretical basis for pattern analysis is the concept of a test set or set of tests. A fixed battery that meets certain requirements constitutes a set. The definition of a set is related to that of a group of tests. The group and the set of tests constitute two kinds of batteries.

Definition

A group battery, or simply a battery, is defined as any collection of more than one test. This would include a randomly assembled collection as well as a set. A set is here defined as: (1) a group of tests, (2) which is integrated, that is, completely organized according to at least one specified principle, and (3) which has a common or standard metric relationship between tests. Thus, a fixed battery may be either a group or a set battery. The flexible battery is invariably a group battery.

Integration. The principle of organization is a way of selecting and ordering the group of tests. There are various ways in which tests can be organized according to a specified principle. Basically, integration requires establishing a specific principle in order to organize the relationships between the tests within a battery. Tests are selected according to the principle so that each test takes a specific place in the battery. For instance, when the principle is coverage by area, each test must represent a different area of the brain and all of the major areas of the brain must be represented. The tests are not redundant except when redundancy is a principle. These relationships between tests are determined and fixed by the nature of the object that the tests are representing. In the case of coverage, the location of functions in the brain determines the selection of tests. Under ordinary circumstances, the selected tests cannot be changed without destroying the integration. There may be many principles of organization other than coverage.

The most common principles are those of coverage by function and area (Russell, 1994, 1986; Russell & Starkey, 1993). The principle of coverage by function requires that all of the known functions of the brain be included in the battery by means of representative tests. The principle of coverage by area requires that all areas of the brain be included by representative tests.

The organizing principle may apply to only certain capacities such as the assessment of language or memory. In regard to aphasia, the Boston Aphasia Examination (Goodglass & Kaplan, 1983a) is still the model of how set batteries should be designed. Its coverage of both function and area was based on the most accepted theory of aphasia and it used a consistent metric. In regard to memory, two batteries are outstanding: the Wechsler Memory Scale—Revised (Wechsler, 1987) and the Memory Assessment Scale (Williams, 1991).

A particular pathology may be the basis of selection such as epilepsy. There are other principles, which cannot be discussed here, used to design and integrate batteries such as redundancy, efficiency, and rehabilitation needs (Russell, 1994; Russell & Starkey, 1993).

Standard Metric Relationship. The standard metric relationship requires (1) coordinated norms and (2) a common metric. This ensures equivalent test scores. There are a number of methods to establish equivalency (Russell, 1994). Pattern analysis is almost never concerned with the mere pass or failure of a test. Rather, the relationships between tests are established by the relative level of scores of the various tests. Thus, equivalent scores are essential (Russell, 1994; Russell & Starkey, 1993, pp. 49–50). Coordinated norms mean that all of the tests are normed on the same sample or that a statistical "bridge" is used to ensure their equivalence. Such coordinated norms are necessary to overcome the problem of differences in samples (Russell, 1994; Russell & Starkey, 1993). There must be an equivalency between scores for them to be accurately compared.

A common metric simply means that all of the tests use the same form of scales. It is difficult to compare scores when the battery uses a mixture of Wechsler scores, T-scores, and raw scores, especially when there is a mixture of impairment and attainment scales. The standardization of the scores requires the utilization of the same scaling procedure for all tests in the battery.

In the set battery, the combination of a fixed integrated battery and an equivalent metric creates a consistent background against which the differences between test results are due to differences within and between people, not differences between test norms. Accurate comparisons between test scores can be observed. As such, the interrelationships within the battery reflect the interrelationships between functions in the brain.

A number of batteries of tests that are in standard use can be considered to be sets by this definition. The Weschler Adult Intelligence Scale—Revised (WAIS-R) is a set as are almost all of the Wechsler tests. The principle used to organize the Wechsler intelligence tests is not very adequate. It was apparently only the selection of the most accurate tests of intelligence for both verbal and nonverbal ability. The psychometric requirements have been better met than any other tests. If the Minnesota Multiphasic Personality Inventory—2 (MMPI-2) is conceived of in terms of scales rather than the data pool, it is also a set battery. There are many other batteries, especially in regard to children's testing, that meet the criteria for a set.

Aspects of a Set Battery. The only way to test the whole person is with a set battery. A flexible battery that is developed during pure hypothesis testing does not attempt to examine the whole person. Rather, it is designed to answer a series of specific questions (Russell, 1984). If a person, even an expert, is putting together a battery under the pressure of test administration, it is unlikely that all of the known functions of the patient will be sampled; that is, unless the examiner has a preestablished group of tests in mind that have such coverage. Of course, in this case the examiner is using a fixed battery, if only informally. Even if other tests are added, one cannot cover the whole person without having a conception of a battery that covers the whole person, and that is a fixed battery. Most neuropsychologists using a fixed battery feel quite free to add or even drop some tests when the situation requires. This does not change the nature of the battery, since the tests were selected and normed as a fixed battery.

The fixed battery has been severely criticized (Lezak, 1995, pp. 123–125) as being a battery that indicates the examiner has a general lack of knowledge about how to conduct neuropsychological testing and that the examiner using a fixed battery is "naive" or "inexperienced." Such comments demonstrate an abysmal ignorance of the nature of the pattern analysis method. By contrast, the competent use of a set battery to perform pattern analysis requires more expertise than the use of a flexible battery in hypothesis testing. In addition to utilizing the same neurological and assessment knowledge that a hypothesis-testing method utilizes, pattern analysis requires more extensive knowledge of psychometrics and particularly knowledge of how tests interact with each other. Consequently, the expertise required for the competent pattern analysis use of a fixed battery is greater than that required for hypothesis testing.

Absolute Scales

There is another development that has recently appeared in a few tests that is important for the future development of test batteries. This is the appearance of absolute scales. An absolute scale is one that covers the entire range of a function, from zero (theoretically) to the full adult range. Zero is often unattainable in psychological scores; so the bottom of a scale is the lowest score for which a reliable score can be obtained. In practice such tests have an extended range from a below-average IQ of a young child to a superior adult IQ. In many areas, such as memory or tapping speed, a zero is obtainable.

Another attribute of absolute scales is that they are not age or education corrected. The WAIS-R requires the examiner to take two steps before obtaining an IQ. In the first step the raw scores are transformed into absolute scales. These are summed and then these sums are compared to norms to obtain the IQ scores. Thus, for the WAIS there are already absolute subtest scores, although not absolute ability index scores.

There is no advantage to the neuropsychologist to have different batteries for children and adults. In testing there is an awkward time period around age 17 when the adult and children's tests do not fuse very well. The reasons for this break are apparently more historical than structural. They are related to Wechsler's development of the adult test before he developed the children's version. At present, the Stanford Binet reaches adulthood and the top of the Weschler Intelligence Scale for Children—3rd edition (WISC-III) (Wechsler, 1991) test range greatly overlaps the adult versions. By extending the WISC tests by about a third at the most, an absolute scale could be developed.

There are many advantages to absolute scales. In numerous situations people want to know how well a person can perform a function regardless of their age. For instance, few people would want to determine the competency of commercial airline pilots using age comparison norms. We want to know how well the pilot can fly the airplane and not how well he can fly it in comparison to people 55 years of age. Soon, psychological testing may be used to determine retirement rather than age, in which case absolute norms will be necessary.

There are other situations in which absolute norms are desirable. People with significant brain damage or dementia often will score below the bottom of the scales on many tests used to assess brain damage. In the area of neuropsychology there is an awkward position between the standard brain damage batteries and the dementia batteries. Since the level of functioning varies greatly around the juncture between moderate brain damage and dementia, it would be of great help to extend the standard brain damage tests into the dementia range by producing absolute scales. In fact, since brain impairment often reduces the performance of adults to a point below the average range of adult abilities, all neuropsychology tests should be full-range absolute scales.

The major disadvantage of such absolute scales is that they would be longer than the usual scales. The statistical means for reducing the time to administer the absolute scores have been developed. The most common method is to establish a basal and a ceiling. However, there are methods beyond the basal and ceiling scoring [see manuals for Peabody Picture Vocabulary Test (PPVT)] (Dunn & Dunn, 1981) and Wide Range Achievement Test (WRAT) (Jastak, Jastak & Wilkinson, 1984). Choca, Laatsch, Garside, and Arnemann (1994) introduced another method for shortening a long test: the Adaptive Category Test (ACAT). It is an adaptive or interactive program, which means that the program contains a set of rules that determine when sufficient information has been gathered by a subtest to predict an accurate score for the subtest. The score sheet gives the predicted scores for each of the original subtests in the original category test. From a methodological point of view, this general method could be used with absolute scales for other tests.

Neuropsychological set batteries would be much improved in their ability to measure functions if they were designed to measure functions extending from the normal adult range to that of young children or severely impaired patients. This would enable the neuropsychologist to model a person's cognitive abilities when there are great differences. My prediction is that this will become the standard method of testing within the next 20 years.

It would be helpful to almost every psychologist if the children's batteries could be fused with the adult tests. Some tests such as the WRAT and the PPVT have already accomplished this fusion. It would be fairly simple to unite the children and adult Wechsler tests. Companies could, at least, design the tests so that the child and adult test items were the same at the point of overlap.

Innovations

There are several recent innovations in neuropsychological computerized testing that appear to be outstanding and so deserve mention. The Choca Computer Category Test (Choca et al., 1994) scoring is related to the Halstead–Russell Neuropsychological Evaluation System (HRNES) scoring program (Russell,

1993). This program will be discussed and does introduce some novel methods that warrant explanation. As with the other scoring programs, this program provides the ability to use alternate, usually abbreviated, methods. The Category Test is apparently longer than is necessary. Consequently, a number of abbreviated forms have been developed. Of these the existing research appears to slightly favor the abbreviation by Russell, which is the Revised Category Test (RCAT) (Russell & Barron, 1989; Russell & Levy, 1987; Taylor, Hunt and Glaser, 1990). It appears to be the shortest form that adequately represents the original Category Test. Choca's (Choca et al., 1994) program is the only computer program that administers and scores the RCAT. In addition, Choca's program permits the use of the ACAT. Since the score sheet gives the predicted scores for each of the subtests in the original Category Test, while rearranging the order of the subtests, these scores can be entered into the HRNES program in place of either the full Category or the RCAT scores. The research evidence from two samples indicates that the ACAT correlates with the full Category Test at .96 and .95 (Choca et al., 1994). This is as accurate as the RCAT, with a correlation of .97 (Russell & Levy, 1987) and it would be faster for patients whose performance on the Category Test is quite good. The ACAT, however, retains the Category memory section, which introduces some contamination into the Category Test Scores.

The WISC-III (Wechsler, 1991) introduces two important innovations. First, for the first time since the Wechsler–Bellevue, a new subtest has been added to the Wechsler tests. This is a perceptual speed test, Symbol Search. The new subtest clarifies and defines the functions measured by the Digit Symbol and Digit Span tests. Digit Symbol is evidently a fairly pure measure of perceptual speed, though a new subtest is probably purer. Digit Span then becomes the core of a fourth factor traditionally called a distraction factor. Nevertheless, this factor appears to be a short-term memory factor. Thus, the WISC-III now contains four separate factors.

The second innovation is the coordination of the Wechsler Individual Achievement Test (WIAT) (Wechsler, 1992) with the WISC-III. This produces what is evidently the best method of determining academic learning disabilities. From a theoretical point of view, this combination is utilizing the concept of coordination (Russell, 1994) to expand the WISC-III into a set battery that covers more functions than the original Wechsler tests.

Creating the coordinated battery and adding the new perceptual speed test to the WISC-III may presage a new direction for intelligence tests, that of attempting to systematically cover all cognitive functions. The creation of an equivalent combination of Wechsler tests for adults would be quite beneficial for neuropsychology.

COMPUTER DEVELOPMENTS: COMPARISON OF NDS, CNEHRB, AND HRNES

Of all the major methodological developments in neuropsychological assessment during the last decade, the application of computer processing is evidently the most important. Aside from the development of new tests, it is the only area in neuropsychology in which a major advance has occurred. The recent advances have occurred primarily in the areas of administration and scoring.

Administration and Interpretation

Both computerized administration and scoring are more closely related to the psychometric approach than to the process approach, although Kaplan and her students have utilized computer scoring quite effectively in such tests as the California Verbal Learning Test (CVLT) (Delis, Kramer, Kaplan, & Ober, 1987) and the MicroCog battery (Powell et al., 1993). Nevertheless, when they have utilized computer scoring, they have transformed the test or battery into a fixed test or even a set battery. Thus, computerization can be seen as a logical ramification of set battery theory and the pattern analysis method.

Most neuropsychologists are apparently unaware of the number of programs that are administered by computer. The major programs in this area have been thoroughly reviewed previously (Kane & Kay, 1992). My own opinion is that computer administration is the direction in which neuropsychological testing will proceed. Computers not only permit more efficient administration than by technicians, but their speed permits the simultaneous scoring of many parameters that are not possible using examiner scoring methods.

Although initially there was some seminal work accomplished in neuropsychology in regard to computer interpretation, this work has not progressed to any great extent in almost 20 years (Russell, 1995). Due to a great deal of resistance within the field of neuropsychology, computerized interpretation has not been developed. Since this form of computerization has recently been thoroughly examined in another paper (Russell, 1995), it will not be discussed here.

Computer Scoring Programs

General computerized scoring programs are so new that they have not been evaluated to any extent, much less compared. In the following section, the scoring programs based on the Halstead–Reitan Battery (HRB) will be examined and compared in some detail. Since these programs are both set batteries and computer scoring programs, they will be examined from both perspectives.

The amount of time and effort required of an examiner to use normative tables for batteries as extensive as these batteries, with corrections for age, education, and gender, is almost prohibitive. When examiner scoring was used for one of these programs (Russell & Starkey, 1993) in the developmental stage, it required at least 2 hours for a person who was familiar with the program to complete the task. In the computerized form it now requires about 15 to 20 minutes to score all 60 measures. In the future, computerization will permit the development of even more complex programs that require extensive scoring in neuropsychology, since they make such programs practical.

Although the computerized scoring of batteries was originally largely designed simply to provide faster and more accurate scoring, the creation of these systems of scoring somewhat inadvertently produced sets of tests. As such, it created a major advance in neuropsychology. While sets of tests had been in existence, at least since the creation of the Wechsler–Bellevue Intelligence Scale, no coherent theory related to sets had been devised. As such, the innovation of these set batteries initiated the formulation of the theory related to sets of tests.

Apparently, the first at least partially computerized scoring for a battery of tests was the Luria–Nebraska Neuropsychological Battery (LNNB) (Golden, Hammeke, & Purisch, 1980). It was based on Christensen's interpretation of Luria's method of testing. The coverage appeared to favor verbal abilities (Russell, 1980), but so did Luria's system. In creating a scoring system, Golden used coordinated norms and a common metric. Thus, the scoring system constituted a set, which was later computerized. Since I am not particularly familiar with this method of assessment, I will not attempt to deal with it in this chapter.

General Description of HRB Programs

Three published computerized scoring programs have been devised based on the HRB. These are the Neuropsychological Deficit Scale (NDS) (Reitan, 1991), the Comprehensive Norms for an Extended Halstead Reitan Battery (CNEHRB) (Heaton, Grant, & Matthews, 1991), and the Halstead–Russell Neuropsychological Evaluation System (HRNES) (Russell, 1993). A general examination of these three computer scoring programs finds many aspects in common. All three programs are IBM-compatible programs; the NDS and CNEHRB are DOS programs, while the HRNES is a Windows program. All three use the HRB and WAIS or WAIS-R as the core of the battery. The CNEHRB and HRNES add other tests to provide measures for what appear to be deficiencies in the original HRB.

The concept basic to these programs is that by properly transforming raw scores into scale scores, the scores can be made equivalent. Thus, the scores can be numerically directly compared. In addition, the HRNES and CNEHRB have age, education, and gender corrections. The corrections attempt to equalize the scores across age, gender, and intellectual ability levels. The correction for intellectual ability attempts to equate the scores to the patient's premorbid level. The single-best indicator of premorbid ability is education (Vanderploeg, 1994).

For all programs the scores can be printed and stored. In addition, the programs allow one to observe the test results without printing them. Both the HRNES and CNEHRB have a method for transporting the scores into a data file using a text format for research purposes.

From the start, the HRNES was designed to be more than a scoring system for the HRB. It was designed to extend not just the battery but the method pioneered by Reitan in order to create a new complete system of assessment. The system was designed for pattern analysis (Russell & Starkey, 1993, Chapter 5).

Battery Composition

NDS. The Neuropsychological Deficit Scale was first published by Reitan in 1987. In this program Reitan captures much of his thinking that is used to determine the existence of brain damage and the lateralization of damage. Basically, Reitan's computer program (1991) consists of several indices derived from the same data. The General Neuropsychological Deficit Scale (GNDS) is a new index to take the place of the Halstead Index. The Left Neuropsychological Deficit Scale (LNDS) and Right Neuropsychological Deficit Scale (RNDS) are lateralization scales. Together they lateralize brain damage.

The NDS is strictly a classical HRB program. It utilizes all of the HRB tests and some of the WAIS scores. Only the HRB tests are utilized and they all need to be entered for the program to work. Although not advised by Reitan, if necessary the examiner can substitute an estimated "missing data" number for a missing score. For this purpose, the mean raw score for the test should usually be used.

The norms that are used were evidently derived from Reitan's experience and they generally correspond to norms derived from other studies in the younger age range. While the scores are transformed into a scale having five steps, the program is not designed to produce scale scores to be used in interpretation analysis. Most of Reitan's analyses are performed with raw scores. The program can be considered an informal set in that the scales are based on extensive experience which gives them a rough equivalence.

CNEHRB. The Comprehensive Norms for an Extended Halstead–Reitan Battery (Heaton, Grant, & Matthews, 1991) was published in 1991. Originally it was intended to be an extensive set of norms for the HRB and some additional tests. Later, a computer scoring program was constructed to calculate scores from these norms. The CNEHRB norms and program utilize the HRB as the core group of tests, but add nine tests to this core in order to better cover functions and brain areas.

The CNEHRB constitutes a set. The selection of tests was based on the principle of coverage of all of the brain's functions and areas. A large proportion of the tests in this battery, including the WAIS but not the WAIS-R, were derived from coordinated norming. The scale scores use the *T*-score metric. The scores are corrected for age, education, and gender. Any selection of tests can be scored separately.

At this point, the CNEHRB has been reviewed by Fuerst (1993) and recently by Fastenau and Adams (1996). The review by Fuerst (1993) pointed out some problems with the computer portion of the program. However, it did not review the underling norming procedure used by the program. One of the main criticisms, that the program was copy protected, has been rectified. The critique discussed many minor weaknesses in the program but any special program will have problems. The review barely addressed the major question, that of the then existing alternatives. At the time the program was published, there were no alternatives except hand scoring for people who used the HRB but did not use Reitan's traditional method. Although the author discussed the difficulty of using the CNEHRB norms without the program, he did not emphasize the tremendous advantage there is in using a computer program.

There are two computer alternatives today, the NDS and the HRNES. Even though the computer program for the CNEHRB is not as well designed as the more recently published HRNES program, the CNEHRB program is still a very acceptable alternative.

The review by Fastenau and Adams (1996) dealt with the norming procedures without discussing the computer program aspect of the CNEHRB. They point out some of the problems that are also discussed in this chapter, such as the use of the WAIS and not the WAIS-R for their original norms. Their major criticisms concern what they consider to be excessive conversions, inappropriate use of multiple regression, and unnecessarily subdividing the normative data into too many divisions, i.e., age, sex and education. They even suggest that the authors redo the entire set of norms using their statistical methods.

Heaton, Matthews, Grant, and Avitable (1996) answer these objections quite well. Their primary and legitimate defense was that the criticisms of Fastenau and Adams were based on statistical concepts that are theoretical speculations (1996). This paper considers that the statistical methods used for norming the CNEHRB are adequate and well accepted.

In defense of their method, Heaton et al. (1996) present the first study which demonstrates that age and education corrections do increase the accuracy of the AIR index of brain damage above that derived from using uncorrected data. The improvement in percent of correct assessment for both brain damaged and normal subjects was quite large for subjects at the extremes of both the age and education ranges. For instance, above age 60 the raw score correctly identified only 39% of the normals while the corrected scores identified 94% of the subjects. This demonstration that age and education corrections will improve the accuracy of a test battery indicates that such corrections do improve the accuracy of the HRNES as well as the CNEHRB.

Finally, Heaton et al. (1996) state that, while there may be some faults with their norms, no other set of norms is as extensive or as well designed. Neither Fastenau and Adams (1996) nor Heaton et al. (1996) discussed the HRNES. This present writing compares the HRNES and CNEHRB to determine their accuracies. Certainly, there are no other sets of norms that are as adequate as the norms used in these two programs.

HRNES. The Halstead–Russell Neuropsychological Evaluation System (Russell, 1993) is also an extended HRB. However, most of the added tests are different from those used in the CNEHRB, but they are generally popular tests. The HRNES was derived from a previous version of this battery, the Halstead, Rennick, Russell Battery (HRRB) (Russell, Starkey, Fernandez, & Starkey, 1988).

The HRNES uses an original method to obtain coordinated norming, which basically predicts the scale scores from a set of index tests (Russell, 1987). The raw scores, which are corrected for age, education, and gender, are transformed into what are titled *C*-scores. *C*-scores use 100 for the mean and 10 for each standard deviation. While the norms are derived from a set battery, any selection of tests can be scored for a particular patient. The manual thoroughly discusses the derivation of the scores, including the norming population. It also provides extensive information concerning the parameters of the tests that are included and discusses the theory on which the battery is based.

Both the CNEHRB and HRNES add tests to the HRB core to make an extended battery. The particular tests that were added to each battery are discussed in detail elsewhere (Heaton et al., 1991; Russell, 1993, 1994).

Both programs use either the WAIS or WAIS-R. However, the WAIS-R that is used by the CNEHRB is derived from the original Psychological Corporation norms and not from the CNEHRB norming sample. Thus, while having excellent norms, the WAIS-R scores are not directly related to the CNEHRB sample.

In regard to the HRNES, about one third of the Wechsler test data was originally derived from WAIS tests (Russell, 1993, p. 54). The scores for the WAIS tests were converted to the WAIS-R equivalents by subtracting the difference between subtest and IQ means from the WAIS scores. This is as accurate as using *T*-scores (Russell, 1992). The HRNES computer program allows the examiner to use WAIS scores in addition to the WAIS-R scores by transforming them from the WAIS-R to the WAIS equivalent. This is accomplished by adding the difference between the subtests or IQs to the WAIS-R scores. This is the same method in reverse that was used in norming (Russell, 1993, pp. 17, 54–55). The WAIS-R Comprehension subtest is scored by the program, although its norms are not as extensive as the other subtests. It was not used in examining brain-damaged subjects during the last years of data collection. Unfortunately, the manual was not clear about this situation.

The HRNES has been reviewed four times at this point. The reviews are so recent that they cannot be discussed to any extent in this chapter. The review by Lezak (1995) was highly critical, but it was almost entirely incorrect in its statements. This chapter corrects the errors that were made.

The other three reviews were favorable (Lynch, 1995; Mahurin, 1995; Retzlaff, 1995). Lynch reviews all three programs briefly. The HRNES is recommended for clinicians who do not want the traditional HRB battery, but all three are approved. The reviews by Mahurin and Retzlaff are too recently published to be examined in this chapter.

Input

In all three programs, raw scores are entered and the scores are transformed into scale scores. In the HRNES the data can be entered using a mouse. Data entry time is relatively fast for the three programs, in the range of 15 to 30 minutes, depending on the number of tests scored. All three greatly increase efficiency and accuracy. The WAIS-R or WAIS may be scored through their own computer programs and then the scale scores can be used in the various neuropsychology programs. (The HRNES uses age-corrected scale scores.)

Data entry is straightforward, although the CNEHRB and NDS require a fairly considerable amount of small computations for indices and some tests. For instance, they require calculating the Category Test score and changing minutes and seconds into minutes for the Tactual Performance Test (TPT). In the CNEHRB, the number of blocks that are correctly placed for the TPT time must be prorated into time. The average impairment rating must also be calculated. These calculations may require a small hand calculator. The HRNES performs all calculations for the examiner except a few that require only elementary counting.

The scoring of individual tests and even administration of tests may vary among the programs. The NDS, of course, strictly uses Reitan's methods of administration and scoring. For the most part, the CNEHRB uses Reitan's methods. The HRNES is a development from Rennick's methods (Russell & Starkey, 1993, p. 51; Russell, Neuringer, & Goldstein, 1970) rather than directly those of Reitan. In addition, when research demonstrated a method for creating a more efficient method such as the RCAT (Russell & Levy, 1987), the new methods were utilized in the battery. Consequently, the examiner must read the administration instructions in the manual carefully before using this system.

Output

All of the programs permit the scores to be printed and stored. The output raw scores and scale scores can also be displayed on the screen. This allows one to look at the test results without printing them. (The HRNES does this through the commands "Print" and then "Text File.") The CNEHRB program scrolls the entire results section to the bottom unless it is stopped by pressing the space bar or break button. It is difficult to "catch" these scores, so this is a drawback to visually observing the results on the screen.

The printed results are fairly extensive for these programs. The CNEHRB prints the summary results in a condensed form so that all of the results are printed on a few pages. This enables the neuropsychologist to easily append the results to a written report. The HRNES and CNEHRB both provide profiles of the test results so that the results can be observed graphically. In addition, the HRNES provides two indices of brain damage and a lateralization index.

The HRNES printout has three sections: a score section, a graph section, and an input section. The first, or score section, prints the raw score, a corrected raw score (corrected for age, gender, and education), and the scale score for each test. (In some cases, such as the Digit Span and the Corsi Board, the raw score is not the inputted score but the traditional score such as the number of digits one can remember for the Digit Span.) The graph section presents the test scores so that one may visualize the amount of impairment for each test. This section is organized strictly by function rather than by interest, e.g., all executive functions are placed together. In some cases, a test that involves more than one functional area may be repeated. Since this area is by functions, it can serve as a guide to neuropsychologists when writing their report, in that many reports are organized by function.

Special Features

Research Data. Both the HRNES and the CNEHRB have a method for exporting the scores into a data file using a text format. As such, the data derived from testing does not need to be reentered into a statistical program by hand, but can be exported directly into a research program's statistical data files. Thus, the programs can be used to gather data for research purposes. This can greatly reduce the tedious entry work of research.

Score Averaging. The HRNES has a scoring feature that allows one to compare tests. This is a computational procedure that allows one to mathematically compare the scale scores of any single score or group of tests to another single score or group. A formula is computed by the program that corrects for the difference in standard deviations so that the comparison is mathematically exact. If the examiner wished to compare immediate memory tests to long-term memory tests, they could be selected and the combined scores of each group would be calculated. This provides a mathematical method of looking at patterns. The WISC-III (Wechsler, 1991) already uses such a formula to compare the WISC-III subtests with the WIAT subtests (Wechsler, 1992).

Correction for Premorbid IQ. One other feature that the HRNES program contains is a method for entering an IQ to replace the education level. The computer program allows a psychologist to enter a Full Scale IQ (FSIQ) in the client menu. This takes precedence over the education correction. For instance, a business man has only a high school education; but other information, including the WAIS-R, which he previously had taken, showed that he had a FSIQ of 120. The FSIQ of 120 can be entered into the program and it will take precedence over the education level in determining the correction.

The results of formulas estimating premorbid IQ can also be used to correct the HRNES scores. These formulas take into consideration items in addition to education. An IQ estimate from any of various formulas for premorbid IQ can be entered as the person's IQ/education level. This method will correct all HRNES scores, not just the person's IQ. Consequently, the correction of other battery tests need not be an intuitive estimate. For instance, if a formula gives a WAIS-R premorbid FSIQ of 110 for an individual, this can be entered and the computer program will compare the person with a high school education against college-educated norms instead of high school norms.

Coverage

For a general neuropsychology battery, the most important aspect is coverage. There should be adequate coverage of both locations and functions. That is, as much as possible, there should be tests for all of the areas of the brain and all major types of functions. All three computer programs recognize the need for coverage and have dealt with this need in various ways. This requirement has been covered previously (Russell, 1994), so it will not be discussed to any great length here.

NDS. The NDS uses only HRB scores and some of the WAIS tests (Reitan, 1991). Reitan believes that these tests are sufficient for a complete neuropsychological examination. Since the tests have been thoroughly discussed elsewhere (Reitan, 1991; Reitan & Wolfson, 1985), they need not be examined here. It should be pointed out that Reitan and Wolfson have developed computer programs for scoring the Reitan Adolescent and Children's batteries (Reitan, 1992; Reitan & Wolfson, 1986b). No other neuropsychology HRB programs have been created for these age groups.

CNEHRB. Both the CNEHRB and the HRNES batteries recognize that the traditional HRB, even with the inclusion of the WAIS or WAIS-R, had rather large holes in regard to both functions and areas. Both programs added tests to the original HRB. The CNEHRB contains a test, Digit Vigilance, that is specifically designed to measure attention. It also uses the Wisconsin Card Sort and the Thurstone Word Fluency Test as frontal tests. The Seashore Tonal Memory along with the Digit Span tests serve as immediate memory tests. Digit Span is evidently a left-hemisphere verbal test, whereas the tonal memory test seems to be a right-hemisphere test (Heaton et al., 1991). The Boston Naming Test is also used but in its experimental version.

HRNES. The HRNES has adopted several well-known tests such as the Boston Naming Test (Goodglass & Kaplan, 1983b), WRAT-R, Reading (Wilkinson, 1993) and the Peabody Picture Vocabulary Test—Revised (Dunn & Dunn, 1981). The HRNES uses two fluency tests—the H-Words (Russell & Starkey,

1993; Russell et al., 1970) and Design Fluency (Russell & Starkey, 1993)—as left and right frontal tests. Some other tests were designed for the battery based on well-known tests. The Miami Selective Learning Test is an extended version of the Buschke Memory test (Buschke, 1973) and the Analogies test is based on the general analogies method. The Gestalt Identification test is a completely new test (Russell & Starkey, 1993). It is a test of the occipital area of the brain. It has both a verbal and a visual form, so it should be able to cover the lesions that occur in either the right or left occipital areas of the brain (Russell, Hendrickson, & VanEaton, 1988). Clinical experience indicates that it measures a fairly crystallized ability. As such, it is not highly sensitive to brain damage in general, but it is sensitive to focal lesions in the occipital lobe.

Also, the test may be useful in assessing certain forms of dyslexia. The word section appears to be related to problems with dyslexia. The words are simple, and mild to moderate dyslexics can read them with no trouble. Many dyslexics do not recognize the partial forms of the "words" as rapidly as do normal readers, even though their recognition of the "objects" is normal.

Both the HRNES and CNEHRB batteries contain enough memory tests to constitute a memory battery in themselves (Russell, 1994). In fact the coverage of forms of memory is somewhat greater than the coverage by the Wechsler Memory Scale—Revised (WMS-R). The HRNES provides separate scoring for Digits Forward and Backward, since Digits Forward is considered to be a purer measure of immediate memory than either Digits Backward or Digit Span. The WMS-R has no equivalent of the TPT Memory and Location included in the HRNES.

In addition to traditional uses, the tests have been found to be helpful in the identification of malingering, since patients often do not think of them as memory tests. Malingerers often do well on these tests while completely failing other memory tests. The HRNES makes some changes in administration and scoring primarily in order to increase efficiency in this long battery. The changes do not appear to affect interpretation.

Scales

Derivation. While both the CNEHRB and HRNES have age, education, and gender corrections and scale scores, they differ in method of derivation, method of correction, and the type of scales. The CNEHRB normalized the raw score data for each test using a mean of 10 and a standard deviation of 3. The intervals are the same as the WAIS-R subtest scales. This procedure both equated the scales and converted them to attainment scales. The scales were then corrected for age, education, and sex using multiple regression. Since the authors, on the basis of an unpublished study, thought that there was little variation between the ages of 20 and 35, the correction was set to be the same as 34 for these ages. The regression analysis produced formulas used to correct the scores for age, education, and gender, while converting the scale scores to *T*-scores.

The HRNES accomplished the same objectives of producing scale scores and age, gender, and education corrections but in a different manner. The scale score conversions were based on the raw score data and the corrections were made to the raw scores. The scaling method is called reference scale norming (Russell, 1987; Russell & Starkey, 1993, pp. 33–34). The method for creating the scale scores was complicated. Essentially, the scores for each test were predicted from an index similar to the Average Impairment Score (AIS) scales. Since brain-damaged subjects scores were not normally distributed (Russell, 1987), this method corrected without producing a normal distribution of scores. Second, when new tests were added to the battery, their scale scores were statistically converted, using this reference scale norming, so that they were coordinated with the rest of the battery.

The correction method did not use reference scale norming but was entirely based on the normal sample. The brain-damaged subjects were not used to produce the age, gender, and education corrections. In regard to age, liner regression was used to predict the midpoint in every age decade for each measure, i.e., the scores for age 55 are the same from 50 to 59. The predicted scores were entered into the computer programs.

The method for creating education corrections was different from that of the CNEHRB. It was based on the average WAIS-R FSIQ for each of several education levels. Rather than using education directly derived from a linear regression formula, the average FSIQ was obtained for each of four education levels: below high school (<12 years of education), high school (12 years), college degree (16 years), and graduate school (20 years). An unpublished study, completed by the author, found that the changes in IQ occurred in steps at each graduation level. IQ tends to be related more to degrees obtained than to number of years. That is, there was little difference among subjects who did not graduate high school regardless of the highest grade obtained. Subjects who did not obtain a college degree were not statistically different from those who only passed high school. This was also true of college graduates with less than an advanced degree.

Consequently, the HRNES uses only four levels of correction: less than a high school graduate (10 years), high school graduate (12 years), college graduate (16 years), and an advanced graduate degree (20 years). The correction is accomplished by using a linear regression prediction of the HRNES test scores equivalent to the mean WAIS-R FSIQ level for each of the four education levels. The person with 12 years of education has a correction on all HRNES scores equivalent to a WAIS-R FSIQ of 101, which is the mean FSIQ for subjects with a high school degree.

The correction for gender was restricted to two measures: the Grip Strength and Tapping Speed. Our findings and other research (Dodrill, 1979; Heaton et al., 1986) had indicated that only these tests were significantly different for the two sexes.

Fineness of Scales. The CNEHRB emphasizes (manual, p. 21) that one of the advantages of the computer program is that the computer scoring is somewhat more precise than looking up scale scores in the CNEHRB tables. However, overall this is not exactly correct. The fineness of a scale, i.e., the number of points between each major interval in the final form of the scales, is determined by the least fine scaling at any point in the conversion process. That is, if the test raw score contains only 1 point per standard deviation, any scale derived from those raw scores will have only 1 point per standard deviation. On the other hand, if a raw score scale has 15 points per standard deviation and the scale score has only 3 points, the final scale score will have only 3 points. The least fine step in a scaling process determines the fineness of the completed scale scores.

In regard to the CNEHRB, the determining point is generally the scale score normalization conversion that has 3 points per standard deviation. The computer program will not provide any finer scoring. The final T scores will have 3.66 points between standard deviations, which round to either 3 or 4 points. An example from the CNEHRB will illustrate this point. At age 45 with 12 years of education, the Category T score of 52 represents raw scores that range from 28 to 35 or 8 raw score points. The number of raw score points that each scale score represents can be obtained by examining the CNEHRB manual (Heaton et al., 1991, Appendix C, p. 46). The interval covered by each scale score is also the number of raw scores that each T score will cover. Although the T score corrections are somewhat finer and different from those derived from the manual, since a regression formula is used to derive them, the computer program will not provide any finer scoring than that found in Appendix C. The correction process simply shifts this range up or down the T score range, depending on the subjects age, education, and gender. While the increased fineness is technically true for the normative tables, it does not increase the fineness of the scales. The grossness of the scales for both the CNEHRB and the HRNES is so great that this difference is essentially meaningless.

The HRNES conversion to scale scores has 4 points per standard deviation, so that its scales are a little, though generally not significantly, finer than the CNEHRB. The correction process for the HRNES is accomplished by changing the raw score to a corrected raw score. This process has no effect on the fineness of the C scales.

The fineness of the correction for both the age and education levels is less for the HRNES. The age intervals are 10 years each and the education is limited to four levels. In regard to age, the grossness of the scales means that lack of exactness is due more to the size of the scale interval than to the age interval. In regard to education, four levels is probably as exact as the relationship between IQ and education level will allow.

For example, Table 7 provides the range of scores that are related to the cutting point for impairment. It gives the raw score range for the HRNES and the raw score and T-score range for the CNEHRB. Since the correction for the HRNES is made on the raw scores, it does not affect the C score intervals. For instance, at this level (Table 7) the HRNES raw score range for the Category Test is 5 points, from 61 to 66. The equivalent CNEHRB range is 9 raw score points, from 74 to

83. A score anywhere in this range will give a T score of 36. The T-score range is 4 points, so the next lower T score will be 33. The regression equation will shift the whole range for the T scores, but the interval between T scores, when rounded, will remain either a 3 or 4. These interval differences will produce changes in the scale scores that may be called a rounding effect. The differences between the CNEHRB T-score intervals and the HRNES C-score intervals are generally not significant, but they do produce many relatively minor variations in the tables that occur later in this chapter.

Distribution. The distributions of neuropsychological raw scores have been found to be skewed (Dodrill, 1988; Russell, 1987). This even applies to scores obtained from a normal sample (Dodrill, 1988). Consequently, the shape of the distribution in neuropsychology needs to be taken into consideration. The HRNES norming procedure (Russell, 1987; Russell & Starkey, 1993) creates scale scores with equal intervals. For the CNEHRB, the normalization procedure transforms the raw scores into a normal distribution. The extent of the skewness can be obtained from Heaton et al. (1991, Appendix C, pp. 46–47), by counting the number of raw score points between each scale score interval. For example, with Trails B, the scale score interval of 18 contains two seconds; the interval of 10 has 8 seconds, while the scale score of 3 has 40 seconds. Thus, the raw scores were strongly skewed toward the lower scores. Almost all of the raw scores are skewed. The normal distributions for T scores (Heaton et al., 1991, p. 18), both normal and brain damaged, were obtained through the normalization procedure and not from the raw data.

The Computer Program Norms

Perhaps the two most important aspects of a battery are the derivation of the sample and equivalency between subtests. Evaluations that are oriented toward hypothesis testing emphasize the derivation, which should be an unbiased sample of the relevant normal population. Equivalency is of little concern, since the aim of hypothesis testing is to determine the existence of impairments for individual tests. Pattern analysis, which is dependent on comparisons, is more concerned with a constant standard for all tests in the battery than with accurate representation of normality. The assessment of impairment can be determined by research that sets cutting scores rather than using arbitrary points on the standard distribution.

There is a problem concerning the derivation of a sample, which is that samples of a theoretically normal population are never exact representatives of the normal population. The ability of any study to obtain a completely unbiased sample of the normal population is almost impossible. Probably, the most adequately normed tests for adults were the WAIS and WAIS-R. Yet, when the WAIS was renormed as the WAIS-R, there was almost an 8-point difference between the FSIQs of the two tests. But supposedly represented the "normal" population. The difference could not be due to the entire population's IQ increasing 8 points in 26 years. Obviously the difference was due to better norming of the WAIS-R.

Thus, every normal sample is biased to some degree. When there are independently normed tests in the battery, there is an unknown variation between tests due to these biases. Lezak's (1995, pp. 154–157) book recognizes this problem but states that ". . . this is usually not a serious hardship . . ." (p. 157). In other words, variation in norms is not terribly important. Nevertheless, a large portion of her criticisms of tests and specifically of the HRNES battery (pp. 714–715) is a critique of the norms.

The HRB norms have varied substantially from study to study (Fromm-Auch & Yeudall, 1983). For the computerized programs the question is: How accurate are the norms of the three batteries? This can be determined by: (1) examining the norming procedure; (2) comparing these norms with norms previously obtained for the HRB; and (3) comparing these norms with the best normed test, the WAIS-R.

Norming Procedure

NDS. The usual norming criteria do not apply to the NDS (Reitan, 1991), since the norm cutting points were derived from Reitan's experience. The only question is: How closely do his norms agree with other procedures? This will be examined later. The cutting point used to separate the normal subjects from brain-damaged subjects was apparently derived statistically. This is the General Neuropsychological Deficit Scale (GNDS) index that Reitan is using to replace the Halstead Index. One needs the program to compute the GNDS, but it may be even more accurate than the Halstead Index (Russell, 1995).

CNEHRB and HRNES. The CNEHRB and HRNES should be examined together, since these are the two extended HRB batteries. The sample for the CNEHRB is composed differently from that of the HRNES. The CNEHRB norming process was based on the normal distribution, while the HRNES derives scale scores through predicting them from an index composed of both controls and brain-damaged subjects (Russell, 1987; Russell & Starkey, 1993). The CNEHRB manual devotes considerable space to demonstrating the normality of the sample. In addition, the CNEHRB devotes considerable space to what is called a validation process. This is in reality a reliability measure and not a validation measure. The sample is randomly split into two parts, which are then compared. They are found to be very highly correlated. Almost any large sample that is split will be highly correlated. Other tables demonstrate that the sample T scores have a normal distribution. However, this does not demonstrate that the raw scores or the means for the sample tests are the same as the means of the population of the United States which the CNEHRB is supposed to represent.

The HRNES used a different method for determining scale scores (Russell, 1987; Russell & Starkey, 1993) in which the scale scores were derived from both the control and brain-damaged groups. The brain-damaged group, as with all brain-damaged groups (Dodrill, 1988; Russell, 1987), was skewed so the criteria of a normal distribution do not apply. The central question is whether the sample is representative of the national population as a whole.

Representativeness of the Sample. For a study of its size, the description of the CNEHRB subject sample in the manual was quite inadequate (Heaton et al., 1991). Many of the standard questions were not discussed. Table 1, in this chapter, provides the basic subject statistics for the two batteries.

Many authors criticize norming samples for being negative neurological or medical samples. A medical sample is composed of subjects who were given a neurological examination but were found to have no neurological problems. The CNEHRB avoids statements concerning the negative neurological composition of their sample, so that the reader does not know what percentage of the sample were negative neurological subjects. It only states that the subjects completed a structured interview, which probably consisted of a questionnaire that is similar to the one that the NDS and HRNES used.

The HRNES sample was composed of patients who had negative neurologicals. Thus, technically, the sample represents a cross-section of veterans who were suspected of having a neurological problem but were found to be normal. As such, this represents exactly the population to which a neuropsychological examination usually applies.

Another important aspect of collecting neuropsychological normative data is the criteria used to select the subjects. The criteria used help evaluate whether the sample is representative of the population. The HRNES manual (Russell & Starkey, 1993, pp. 27–32) fully states these criteria which were: (1) all subjects tested in the author's laboratory from 1968 to 1989; (2) they had a definite neurological diagnosis of pathology or a negative neurological examination; and (3) they were administered the entire core battery. (There were relatively few missing data.) These criteria excluded almost half of the patients tested during this time who completed the full core battery. The selection criterion and the method of obtaining the sample in the various centers are not provided for the CNEHRB.

Sample Size and Collection Sites. The adequacy of the representation of a sample to the normal population is less dependent on the size of the sample than on how typical it is. For instance, a sample of 500 subjects gathered from 12 locations may not be representative of the country as a whole if the locations are all college campuses. Although the sample could be large and conform to all the requirements of a normal curve, it would not represent the normal population.

The regional composition of the CNEHRB sample is not clear. While the text lists 11 sites by name, in which some part of the sample was gathered, it does not state how many subjects came from each location. A large proportion of this CNEHRB sample is the same as that reported in a previous study (Heaton et al.,

1986, p. 6), which used only three sites. Unlike the norming study, in the previous study the authors (Heaton et al., 1986) carefully provided the number of subjects from each site. There were 553 subjects in the original Heaton et al. (1986) study, while the CNEHRB norming sample had only 483 subjects. Subjects less than 19 years old were eliminated from the norming sample. Probably the eliminated subjects are about the number that would account for the difference between the Heaton et al. (1986) original sample and the CNEHRB sample. In addition, all of the examiners from all of the sites were trained by technicians or supervised by senior staff members at one of the three collection sites in the Heaton study (Heaton et al., 1986, p. 6). Thus, it is evident that the number of subjects who came from any site other than the three Heaton et al. (1986) sites must have been so few as to be of no normative significance.

Consequently, one may assume that, in spite of the listing of 11 sites, all or most all of the subjects for this study were derived from only three centers and the characteristics of the sample would reflect the three centers. The sites were medical schools in the northern or western part of the United States where the intellectual ability of students would be somewhat greater than for the United States as a whole. Thus, the probability is that the subjects in this sample, at each level of education, had a somewhat higher intellectual ability for the CNEHRB sample than the national average. The average education level for the CNEHRB sample was 13.6 years, while the WAIS FSIQ was 113.8. Thus, the norms do not constitute a truly representative sample of the nation.

While the HRNES sample was derived from only two centers, these were VA Medical Centers, which provided service to the military personnel of the country. Since most military personnel were originally obtained by draft, they would represent a cross-section of the country. Although Miami is only one location, it is highly cosmopolitan and the veterans come from all parts of the country. Except for psychiatric patients, the patients at a VA Medical Center are equivalent to those of a general hospital. By the time most VA patients entered the VA Medical Centers for this study, war injuries had healed or stabilized or the patient had died, so combat injuries constitute a very small portion of the physical problems that VA patients exhibit. The mean WAIS-R FSIQ for the normal comparison group was 102 and their educational level was 12.7. Consequently, while not completely typical, there is no reason to believe that the HRNES sample is any less representative of the general population than that of the CNEHRB. The decision as to the representativeness of the samples must rely on comparisons to the other well-normed samples such as the WAIS and WAIS-R.

Apparently, parts of the total CNEHRB extended battery were not given at all of the locations. Consequently, a somewhat different battery was given in different locations. The data for neither the Boston Naming Test (Heaton et al., 1991, p. 5) nor the WAIS-R (Heaton supplement) were gathered as part of the study. Consequently, they are not coordinated with the rest of the data, and thus cannot be considered part of the data set. They may be used for clinical assessment, with caution.

For the HRNES, during the period of data collection, the tests composing the extended battery were gradually added to the battery after they had been tested in clinical use. The coordination of the additional tests was achieved through use of the index norming method. The scores for the new tests were predicted using linear regression from the index composed of core HRB tests that had been used throughout the period of collection.

Sample Statistics

Examining the sample statistics demonstrates some significant differences between the samples. These statistics are provided in Table 1.

Age. The mean age of the HRNES sample, 44.6, is somewhat older than that of the CNEHRB, 41.8, or approximately 45 and 42. The difference represents the different settings in which the data were collected. The HRNES data evidently represent the age of neurological patients at a general hospital, while that of the CNEHRB represent patients at university hospitals.

Gender and Race. Neither study had an adequate sample of women, although the proportion of women in the CNEHRB was larger. Since the HRNES sample was obtained from the VA system, only 12% of the normal sample was women. Comparison of the differences between genders with other studies

TABLE 1. Statistical Data for the Subject Samples Used in the HRNES and CNEHRB

	Computer batteries	
Data	HRNES	CNEHRB
N Normal	200	378 (486)[a]
N Brain damaged	576	392
Mean age	44.6 (13.3)	41.8 (16.7)
Mean education	12.7 (2.9)	13.6 (3.5)
Percent females	12	34.4
Percent nonwhite	12	No information
Mean FSIQ WAIS	NA	113.8 (12.3)
FSIQ WAIS-R	102 (12.5)	NA
FSIQ WAIS-R Alternate[b]	NA	99.6 (15.2)
Number of locations	2	11 (3)[c]
N per location	Manual p. 27	No information
Negative neurologicals	Yes	No information
Years to collect	21	15

[a]Base sample plus validation sample.
[b]The WAIS-R subjects were not part of the original sample.
[c]Evidently, almost all of the subjects were recruited from three sites.

(Heaton et al., 1986) found the small VA sample to be representative. The HRNES had 12% nonwhites, which is about the same ratio as that in the nation. There is no information concerning the racial makeup of the CNEHRB. Considering the locations where data were gathered, the number of nonwhites may have been low.

Education and Intelligence. The education and IQ levels of the CNEHRB are higher than that of the HRNES. The mean education level of the CNEHRB was 13.6 as opposed to 12.7 for the HRNES normal sample. In addition, the mean WAIS-R FSIQ for the HRNES was 102 as opposed to an equivalent of 106 for the CNEHRB (since the original sample of the CNEHRB used the WAIS comparisons that required transforming the WAIS scores into WAIS-R scores by adding 7 to the VIQ and 8 to the FSIQ and PIQ). This means that the subjects that were used to norm the CNEHRB were 5 IQ points above the normal subjects used to norm the HRNES. Since the age and education corrections used by these programs were based on their respective samples, one would expect that the norms for the CNEHRB would be higher than for the HRNES. Since the CNEHRB general IQ is higher than average, all of the scores in the battery may be somewhat higher than the average for the general population in the United States. Those of the HRNES more closely reflect the national norm. Nevertheless, both batteries had acceptable norming and can be considered adequate for neuropsychological assessment.

Comparison to Other Normed Samples

In addition to the method of derivation, other types of evidence are needed to determine the accuracy of the norms such as the comparison with other norms. In effect, the accumulating evidence from a comparison with other norms produces a type of construct validity for the norms. Since the function of norms is to represent a population accurately, a poorly normed set that more accurately corresponds to sets of norms that are known to be representative is preferable to a presumably well-derived set that deviates from other sets of norms. Such evidence may be provided by comparing a new set of norms with either a measure whose norming is exceptionally well done or to a group of norms derived from previous studies of the same population.

While the HRNES norms have previously been compared to other established norms (Russell & Starkey, 1993, pp. 32–33), they have not been compared to the CNEHRB and NDS norms. Table 2 (raw norms) compares the HRNES, the CNEHRB, and the NDS norms to the norms derived by Dodrill (1988), Fromm-Auch and Yeudall (1983), and Pauker (1977, 1981). The norms appear to be the most complete sets available, although they are by no means the only sets of norms (see Fromm-Auch & Yeudall, 1983). Since only the three computerized norming tables have extensive scale scores, a comparison with other studies must rely on mean raw scores. These are provided in Table 2 for two ages, 30 and 75. Age 30 represents the approximate mean for Dodrill's and Fromm-Auch and Yeudall's

TABLE 2. Comparison among Norming Studies by Dodrill, Fromm-Ache, and Yeudall (FA & Y), Pauker, HRNES; CNEHRB; and NDS

Tests	Normative studies, age 30						Normative studies, age 75			
	Dodrill[a]	FA & Y[b]	Pauker[c]	HRNES[d]	CNEHRB[e]	NDS[f]	Pauker[c]	HRNES	CNEHRB	NDS[g]
WAIS-R FSIQ[h]	100	111	104	101	106[g]	NA	104	102	110[g]	NA
Category	35.7	30	43	37	31	35	71	71	67	35
Trails A	25	24	—	26	25	33	—	50	48	33
Trails B	66	53	—	68	58	75	—	121w	120	75
Speech	5	4	5	5	4	8	9	9	7	8
Rhythm	3 (27)	2	3	4 (26)	3 (27)	4 (26)	5	5 (25)	5 (25)	4 (26)
Aphasia	2	—	—	4	4	—	—	4	5	—
Cross	2	—	—	2	2	—	—	2	3	—
Percp Dis	4	—	—	4	3	—	—	10	4	—
TPT Tot	13.6	9.4	14.7	13.9	11.1	12.1	24.75	24.2	23.4	12.1
TPT Dom	—	4.5	—	6.1	4.6	—	—	8.7	8.6	—
TPT Non	—	3.1	—	4.4	3.8	—	—	9.9	9.1	—
TPT Both	—	1.8	—	2.6	2	—	—	6.4	5.6	—
TPT Mem.	8	8	7	8	8	7	4.3	6	6	7
TPT Loc.	5	6	4	5	5	6	1	2	1	6
Tapp. Dom	52	51	42	49	52	52	33	39	48	52
Tapp. Non	—	46	—	44	47	47	—	34	45	47
Grip Dom	—	52	—	47	51	—	—	38	43	—
Grip Non	—	50	—	43	47	—	—	34	40	—
Peg Dom	—	64	—	66	61	—	—	88	86	—
Peg Non	—	69	—	71	65	—	—	95	92	—

[a]Mean age was 27.8.

[b]Mean age was 28. Authors did not specify IQ by age.

[c]Derived from T conversion tables (Pauker, 1988), age 29, FSIQ 108.

[d]Scores interpolated to equal age 30.

[e]Scores are in most cases the midpoint for the interval corresponding to a T score of 50.

[f]Scores are the midpoint for category 1 (Reitan, 1991, p. 79).

[g]WAIS score transformed to equal WAIS-R.

[h]Mean raw scores for males with a high school level education at approximately age 30 and 75.

studies, which had a limited number of subjects in the upper age range. Due to the limited data in the upper age range, the two studies were not included in the 75-year-old section. Although included in both age ranges, the NDS scores do not change, since they are not corrected for age. The table presents the basic scores used in the HRB and the WAIS-R FSIQ.

The Samples. Of these norms, Pauker's were the earliest to be derived. Based on the description of the data collection process, they should represent one of the most adequately derived set of norms to be assembled. The results were often lower than the norms that were traditional in the field, so they have been largely ignored. In addition, they were never completed, in that the *N* for some of the age–education cells in the original study was too low. However, Pauker (1988) employed a process using overlapping cells, which is similar to the process of smoothing a curve to create a full table of norms (Pauker, 1981). The data used in Table 2 of this chapter were obtained from these tables.

Dodrill's (1988) norms were probably the best norms that have been produced for a limited age range. However, the mean age was 27.77, and there was no attempt to separate subjects by age. The subjects were patients with negative neurological histories who were carefully selected. However, the aspect of this study that ensured its greater accuracy was that Dodrill's data conformed to the WAIS-R FSIQ of 100 and had a normal distribution, apparently due to some selection of data.

The study by Fromm-Auch and Yeudall (1983) has been used widely. However, it appears to represent scores that are too high. Their mean WAIS FSIQ is 119.1, which when converted to the WAIS-R is still 111. In addition, the subjects are young with a mean age of 25.4. Thus, their norms would be expected to represent a population with considerably better than average ability. Consequently, they should not be used for most assessments.

For the HRNES and CNEHRB, the raw scores were obtained by attempting to present the most exact score equivalent to a *T* score of 50 (*C* score of 100) for each age. The occasional large range of raw scores for each *T*-score interval means that any chosen raw score may vary from the scores presented in the table by a number of digits, while remaining within the range. In regard to the CNEHRB, since the raw scores were apparently skewed, the normalization procedure produced intervals with varying numbers of raw scores.

Results. An examination of Table 2 demonstrates that the various norms are surprisingly similar, considering differences in norming locations and situations. To some extent the sets of norms are interchangeable. However, there are differences, and in a few places this difference is important. Individual measures within the batteries performed somewhat differently from one set to another.

In regard to the different sets of norms, the NDS is roughly equivalent to the other sets at age 30. It should provide approximately similar results to the other norms at that age. However, there is no age correction for these norms. When dealing with moderate to severe brain damage, the effect of damage is so strong that such correction may not be necessary. However, when the damage is mild, which it often is in forensic cases, the variation in ability produced by age may create a false assessment. At the 75-year level there is a great discrepancy between the NDS norms and the other sets. With the NDS norms a normal 75-year-old person could easily score in the brain-damaged range on almost all tests and the index.

Pauker's norms are lower than the other sets especially at the 30-year level. By contrast, the Fromm-Auch and Yeudall (1983) norms are the highest. Dodrill's norms fall between these extremes and constitute the model for norms at this age. The HRNES norms fall close enough to Dodrill's norms to be equivalent on most scores. The CNEHRB is somewhat higher than the HRNES, but the difference is not great at this age level. Not surprisingly, the results of the various sets tend to parallel the IQ level, with perhaps the exception of Pauker's norms, which are lower than one might expect for the FSIQ level.

At the age of 75, the HRNES, CNEHRB, and the Pauker norms are similar. The CNEHRB norms are higher than the HRNES norms for the WAIS-R equivalent, Category Test, Speech Perception, Perceptual disorders, and Tapping and Grip Tests, but the rest of the tests are within a few points of each other. Even these differences are not great except perhaps for the WAIS-R equivalent and Tapping.

Examination of the individual tests demonstrated several interesting effects. The greatest discrepancy appears to be the Tapping scores. This is especially true for the 75-year age. The HRNES scores are almost 10 points below the CNEHRB, and Pauker's norms are lower still. All three studies administered the test in approximately the same way, so that the method of administration does not appear to be a decisive factor. The CNEHRB norms are somewhat higher for all tests, but this is not as great as the Tapping difference. The one factor that appears to explain this difference is motivation. The HRNES scores were given as part of the clinical examination, so there was no incentive to "push" one's performance. The subjects for the CNEHRB were largely control subjects who may have wanted to demonstrate their ability. Tests such as Rhythm, which appear to be less affected by motivation, had more equal scores.

Another interesting finding was the effect of age on the TPT time for both the HRNES and the CNEHRB. At 75 years, the nondominant hand takes longer than the dominant hand. The ratio between hands changes with age, so that the traditional ratio between hands only holds for lower ages. Since this is true for both the HRNES and the CNEHRB, it is undoubtedly a genuine effect. The effect is probably due to reduced memory at the older age. In fact, this reduced memory can be observed in the low TPT Location scores at this age.

WAIS-R Comparison

In regard to comparing the program norms to a well-normed test, probably the WAIS and especially the WAIS-R are the most adequately normed cognitive ability measures in existence. Since either the WAIS or WAIS-R was included in all three computer scoring programs, they will be used to help determine the adequacy of the norming for the programs. The value of comparing the WAIS and WAIS-R to the program norm lies in the fact that the WAIS and/or the WAIS-R were normed with the rest of the battery, so that they represent the accuracy of the entire battery. The HRNES utilizes the WAIS-R age-corrected scores without additional correction, except for education level. However, the WAIS-R was given at the same time as the other scores, so its scores do represent the same sample as the rest of the HRNES.

The CNEHRB corrected the scale scores and IQs from the WAIS in the same manner as it did for the rest of the battery. The CNEHRB variations found for the WAIS variations due to age represent the same corrections that were applied to all of the tests in the CNEHRB. Thus, the WAIS findings apply to the entire CNEHRB battery.

NDS. For the NDS, there was no attempt to compare the scale score ranges either to an accepted normal distribution or to the WAIS in Table 3. In the NDS manual (Reitan, 1991, p. 79), the range numbers 0 and 1, which are considered to be within the normal range, have WAIS Verbal and Performance IQ scores of 90+ and 82–89, respectively. Both the CNEHRB and the HRNES set the brain-damaged range at well above 90 for the WAIS at all ages (see Table 3).

As an example, since the WAIS VIQ is 7 points higher than the WAIS-R, the CNEHRB VIQ is 98. By contrast, the cutting point for Reitan's norms is 81 and below. Thus, it is much lower, and thus more difficult to obtain a score in the brain-damaged range. Since other scores are less conservative, this WAIS cutting point appears to reflect Reitan's concept that the WAIS is less affected by brain damage than HRB tests, rather than being a statistical finding.

CNEHRB and HRNES. The WAIS-R comparisons of the CNEHRB and the HRNES are provided in Table 3.[1] The WAIS-R was chosen on the base score rather than the WAIS, since it is used more often today. However, the norming for the CNEHRB was accomplished entirely with the WAIS. The WAIS-R norms that are provided were derived from the norms used by the Psychological Corporation for the norming of the WAIS-R and they are completely unrelated to the norming process of the CNEHRB (Heaton, 1992).

Table 3 compares various IQ scores for the two batteries at three age levels. The education was held constant at the high school level, since this is the average

---

[1]It is relatively easy to check the findings reported in this chapter by running the raw scores on the three programs. Since any scale score represents a range of raw scores, the obtained score may be somewhat different than the score presented in the tables. This is due to a rounding effect. Generally, the central score in a range is presented. However, when the *T* score was not equivalent to the central score, another more representative score may have been selected.

TABLE 3. WAIS and WAIS-R IQ Comparisons for CNEHRB and HRNES at Various Age Levels

	WAIS & WAIS		HRNES		CNEHRB		
Scale	WAIS-R score	WAIS equiv.	C-score	T-score equiv.	T score[a]	Difference	WAIS-R T score[b]
Age 25, education 12							
VIQ	100	107	102	52.00	50	−2.00	50.00
PIQ	100	108	102	52.00	50	−2.00	51.00
FSIQ	100	108	102	52.00	51	−1.00	51.00
VIQ	88	95	92	42.00	36	−6.00	41.00
PIQ	90	98	95	45.00	39	−6.00	43.00
FSIQ	90	98	95	45.00	39	−6.00	42.00
Age 45, education 12							
VIQ	100	107	102	52.00	48	−4.00	47.00
PIQ	100	108	102	52.00	48	−4.00	49.00
FSIQ	100	108	102	52.00	49	−3.00	47.00
VIQ	92	99	95	45.00	39	−6.00	43.00
PIQ	90	98	95	45.00	37	−8.00	43.00
FSIQ	90	98	95	45.00	36	−9.00	41.00
Age 74, education 12							
VIQ	100	107	102	52.00	43	−9.00	42.00
PIQ	100	108	102	52.00	42	−10.00	46.00
FSIQ	100	108	102	52.00	42	−10.00	42.00
VIQ	97	104	100	50.00	38	−12.00	42.00
PIQ	97	105	100	50.00	38	−12.00	42.00
FSIQ	97	105	100	50.00	38	−12.00	42.00

[a]WAIS-R scores were converted into WAIS equivalents before entering them into the CNEHRB program.
[b]WAIS-R scores converted to T scores by the CNEHRB program.

in our society. Two IQ levels were obtained for each age level. They are the equivalent to a WAIS-R score of 100 and the level in which either the HRNES or the CNEHRB reached the impaired level, below a T score of 40. The latter score provides a measure of the accuracy of the tests to assess brain damage. Age 45 was selected as the age near the sample mean for these batteries. Age 74 is the highest age that the WAIS-R norms extend. Age 25 was somewhat arbitrarily selected to represent the young subjects.

Since the CNEHRB uses the WAIS, an equivalent WAIS score related to the WAIS-R score of 100 is found in column 3. The equivalent C scores and T scores are provided for the HRNES. The CNEHRB T scores, column 6, are those derived from the WAIS score, column 3, that are equivalent to the WAIS-R scores in the second column. The difference between the HRNES and CNEHRB T scores are given in column 7. Finally, the T scores derived by the CNEHRB computer program from the Psychological Corporation WAIS-R norms are presented in column 8.

In discussing the IQ scores, it should be kept in mind that the IQs themselves are age-corrected scores. The HRNES simply uses the IQs without correction for age, while the CNEHRB normalizes the IQ and then corrects for age. The mean HRNES scores are compatible with the WAIS and WAIS-R for each age level. They run a little above the average, with a C score of 102. In regard to the CNEHRB, since the program corrects the IQs, which are already corrected for age, the changing T scores represent a change in the data base for the CNEHRB. Three effects are observable. First, for the mean the CNEHRB WAIS scores are close to the average at the 25-year age level, since the T score is 52. This means that for the rest of the tests in the CNEHRB there is probably a close correspondence to the national population mean at the younger age level.

Second, the difference between the tests increases as the age increases. This is observed for the CNEHRB at age 74 in that the T scores are near 40 for the WAIS IQs of 107 or 108.

Third, the CNEHRB scores become impaired more rapidly with the reduction of IQ than do the HRNES scores. That is, the difference between the two tests is greater for IQ scores below the mean than at the mean. This effect also increases with age, so that on the CNEHRB by age 74, a WAIS FSIQ score of 105 indicates the existence of brain damage. The equivalent T score is 38, which is below 40. They are higher than the national norm as indicated by the WAIS. Thus, they will indicate brain damage too easily not only for the WAIS but for the entire set of measures. The intervals for the CNEHRB T scores are between 3 and 4 points, so part of this difference could be due to a rounding artifact. In summary, the findings indicate that the CNEHRB norms are apparently a little too high in the older age ranges and that this difference becomes greater with the lower scores.

From the WAIS-R comparisons and from the comparisons with other norms, it is evident that the HRNES is at least as accurate as the CNEHRB. In addition, at the older age ranges the CNEHRB appears to be somewhat too high compared to the general population of the United States. At the older age ranges, the CNEHRB will tend to give people T scores that are too low, so that people may be designated as impaired when they are not. Thus, in regard to impairment the HRNES appears to be more conservative than the CNEHRB, especially in the older age ranges.

Other Support for the HRNES Norms

There are some other studies that support the HRNES norms that were not included in these norming studies. It is such studies that will eventually determine the adequacy of the two norming systems. They furnish a type of construct validity for the battery. Probably the strongest support for the HRNES comes from the HRNES Wechsler Memory Scale (WMS) norms. The first norming of the WMS (Russell, 1975) was evidently too high (Crosson, Hughes, Roth, & Monkowski,

1984; Haaland, Linn, Hunt, & Goodwin, 1983). When the WMS was renormed (Russell, 1988), it agreed quite closely with Crosson and co-workers' (1984) estimate of what the norms should be. The renormed data were obtained as part of the norming of the entire HRNES, so it indicates that the other HRNES test norms are probably accurate.

Another study that supported the HRNES norms was completed by Kay, Morris, and Starbuck (1993). Using airline pilots, both the CNEHRB and HRNES age- and education-corrected norm scores were generally equivalent to those obtained by the pilots in the same age and education categories.

In regard to the Boston Naming Test, whose norms are correlated with the rest of the HRNES, when an older age sample with less than average education was examined (Lichtenberg, Ross, & Christensen, 1994), the scores were comparable or somewhat lower than those derived from the equivalent HRNES age- and educated-corrected norms (Russell & Starkey, 1993). The education level for the sample was 11.1 years. The most comparable group to the HRNES age 75 with <12 years education was the group of white subjects with an age from 70 to 74 years. This group had a Boston Naming Test score of 48.9, while the HRNES score was 52.

Comparison of HRNES and CNEHRB Scale Scores

Comparison of HRNES and CNEHRB must be related to scale scores. In these batteries a correction has been made for age, education, and gender, so that each one of these dimensions should be examined.

Age Scale Scores

The largest effect on test scores is produced by age. Most of the tests used in the HRNES and CNEHRB are affected by age. These effects are examined in Table 4, which provides a *T*-score comparison of the HRNES and CNEHRB at three age levels that span the adult ages. The levels are 25, 45, and 75. The tests that the HRNES and the CNEHRB have in common are provided and include almost all of the HRB tests.

The scores compare the HRNES and CNEHRB at each age level by obtaining the *T* scores for each battery from the same raw scores. The raw scores are the HRNES raw scores at each age level that are equivalent to a *C* score of 100. However, in order to compare scores, the *C* scores are transformed into *T* scores by subtracting 50. The *C* scores and their equivalent *T* scores are not provided for the HRNES, since they are all 100 for *C* scores or 50 for *T* scores. The Cross Drawing (Spatial Relations) is the only exception. It had so few scores at this level that it was 102. The CNEHRB *T* score is the *T*-score equivalent to the HRNES raw score. It is obtained by placing the HRNES raw score in the CNEHRB computer

TABLE 4. Differences between HRNES, CNEHRB T Scores at 3 Age Levels for Males with a High School Level Education

| | AGE | | | | | | | | |
| | 25 | | | 45 | | | 75 | | |
Test	HRNES Raw[a]	CNHRB T score	Diff[b] T score	HRNES Raw[a]	CNHRB T score	Diff[b] T score	HRNES Raw[a]	CNHRB T score	Diff[b] T score
Category	34	48	-2.00	49	44	-6.00	71	52	2.00
Trails A	24	52	2.00	34	44	-6.00	50	43	-7.00
Trails B	62	49	-1.00	86	45	-5.00	121	49	-1.00
Speech	5	48	-2.00	7	43	-7.00	9	45	-5.00
Rhythm	3 er	50	0.00	4 er	49	-1.00	5 er	52	2.00
Aphasia	3	54	4.00	4	50	0.00	4	52	2.00
Cross	2	57	5.00	2	58	6.00	2	60	8.00
Percp Dis	4	45	-5.00	6	43	-7.00	10	39	-11.00
TPT Tot	11.8	47	-3.00	17.3	44	-6.00	25	49	-1.00
TPT Dom	5.8	43	-7.00	7	43	-7.00	8.7	50	0.00
TPT Non	3.8	47	-3.00	6.2	43	-7.00	9.9	49	-1.00
TPT Mem	8	49	-1.00	7	43	-7.00	6	47	-3.00
TPT Loc	5	49	-1.00	4	50	0.00	2	57	7.00
Tapp Dom	48	40	-10.00	45	39	-11.00	39	38	-12.00
Tapp Non	43	40	-10.00	40	38	-12.00	34	35	-15.00
Grip Dom	50	44	-6.00	45	41	-9.00	38	43	-7.00
Grip Non	46	44	-6.00	41	42	-8.00	34	45	-5.00
Peg Dom	70	43	-7.00	75	40	-10.00	90	46	-4.00
Peg Non	74	42	-8.00	80	44	-6.00	100	46	-4.00

[a]The raw score is equivalent to a HRNES C score of 100 for each age. A HRNES C score of 100 is equivalent to a T score of 50.
[b]This is the difference between the CNEHRB T score and the HRNES T score.

program for a male with a high school education at the required age level. Finally, a difference is obtained between the CNEHRB T score and the HRNES equivalent T score. The last column for each age holds this difference. A minus means that the CNEHRB T score was less than the HRNES T score.

Results. The results of this procedure, as indicated in Table 4, show some patterns. The overall pattern is that the C and T scores, as indicated by the HRNES equivalent T scores, are fairly close at the 25- and 75-year levels but somewhat farther apart at the 45-year level. Since both the HRNES and the CNEHRB use linear regression to obtain the scores, this curvilinear finding needs to be explained. The CNEHRB scores plateau from 20 to 34, while the HRNES norms do not. The age correction regression lines of the HRNES and CNEHRB T scores converge at the older age levels. The difference at age 45 is close to the greatest difference between the two sets of norms.

The C and T scores represent raw score ranges of several scores. On the few tests that were examined, the ranges were similar. For instance, the HRNES Category test for an equivalent T score of 50 has a raw score range of 48 to 53. The equivalent range for the CNEHRB with a T score of 44 is 48 to 59. Thus, the differences between the CNEHRB T scores and the HRNES equivalent T scores represent a real but a small difference in norming. Nevertheless, the variability between tests appears to be greater than any general effect.

Individual Tests. This comparison denotes some differences among individual tests. The greatest differences occur among the motor tests, particularly Tapping. At the 45-year level, the T score for the CNEHRB is 11 points lower on the dominant hand and 12 points lower for the nondominant hand for the CNEHRB Tapping. This difference was seen in the raw scores as well. The CNEHRB subjects tapped faster than the HRNES subjects at each age level. Unlike some of the other measures, this discrepancy increased with age.

This difference is not found for the Rhythm or Aphasia tests, which are roughly the same for both batteries at all ages. The difference in scores for the Cross Drawing (Spatial Relations) is undoubtedly an artifact of the large raw score intervals at the normal level. The size of the difference for Trails A at age 75 is apparently partly artifactual due to a rounding effect. A raw score of 49, 1 point below the score given in the table, would produce a CNEHRB T score of 48 with a difference of only -2 from the HRNES equivalent T score.

The large difference in regard to TPT Location is also artifactual due to large raw score intervals. However, it is interesting that at the age of 75 a score of 2 is normal for the HRNES and 1 for the CNEHRB. These scores are considerably below the traditional cutting point for brain damage, which was 5. This supports Pauker's (1977) original finding that around 70 the mean localization score was 2.

Education

The second type of correction that the HRNES and CNEHRB make is for education. Education provides a method to estimate premorbid ability levels. The CNEHRB program uses a linear correction for years of education, so the correction is based directly on the subject's years of education. The HRNES education correction is not direct but is based on the average WAIS-R FSIQ for each of four education levels (below high school, high school, college, and advanced degrees).

Table 5 presents the difference in T score or T-score equivalents between the HRNES and CNEHRB produced by the education correction. The differences were found by using the HRNES raw scores that were equivalent to a C score of 100 (or a T score of 50) at each educational level. The raw scores were entered into the CNEHRB program to obtain the equivalent T score. However, each of the education levels also contained the general difference that existed for the high school level, which was found at age 45. In order to obtain a pure measure of the difference that education alone produced, the scores from the high school level were subtracted

TABLE 5. Differences between HRNES and CNEHRB T Scores at Age 45, for Males at the High School Level and Three Education Levels with the High School Level Scores Removed and the Difference between Males and Females at the High School Level

| | Male education level differences | | | | Female difference |
| | *T* score minus HS scores | | | *T* scores | |
Test	<HS	BA	Grad.	HS	HS
Category	1.00	−3.00	−2.00	−6.00	0.00
Trails A	0.00	−4.00	−7.00	−6.00	0.00
Trails B	0.00	−2.00	−7.00	−5.00	−2.00
Speech	2.00	−1.00	−5.00	−7.00	0.00
Rhythm	2.00	2.00	−3.00	−1.00	0.00
Aphasia	3.00	−1.00	0.00	0.00	−3.00
Cross	1.00	−3.00	−6.00	6.00	0.00
Percp Dis	2.00	−2.00	−3.00	−7.00	−4.00
TPT Tot	−1.00	−2.00	−1.00	−6.00	0.00
TPT Dom	−2.00	3.00	5.00	−7.00	−5.00
TPT Non	0.00	1.00	−1.00	−7.00	−3.00
TPT Both	0.00	−2.00	−1.00	−6.00	0.00
TPT Memory	4.00	4.00	12.00	−7.00	0.00
TPT Loc	−4.00	−5.00	−2.00	0.00	0.00
Tapp Dom	1.00	−2.00	−4.00	−11.00	6.00
Tapp Non	1.00	−1.00	−3.00	−12.00	5.00
Grip Dom	0.00	−3.00	−3.00	−9.00	11.00
Grip Non	0.00	0.00	0.00	−8.00	10.00
Pegboard D	2.00	0.00	5.00	−8.00	−6.00
Pegboard N	−2.00	3.00	3.00	−6.00	−4.00

from each education level other than that of high school. This pure education difference is the difference between each education level and the high school level. Thus, the scores in columns 2, 3, and 4 indicate the pure effect of education levels with the general effect at the high school level removed. The high school scores would be zero throughout, so these were not presented. The high school level scores in this table, which were presented in column 5, represent the actual difference between the CNEHRB and the HRNES at the high school level for subjects who are 45 years old. A minus means that the CNEHRB T score was lower than the HRNES T-score equivalent. The actual T-score difference between the CNEHRB and the HRNES at each educational level for age 45 may be obtained by adding the high school score (column 5) to each of the other education level scores.

The results derived from this table demonstrate that the general differences between the CNEHRB and HRNES at age 45 are variable with no noticeable trend. Individual measures show trends, but these vary from test to test. Much of the difference between scores is due to the rounding effect. However, it is expected that the CNEHRB will be inaccurate below 8 years of education or above 20 years, since the events that caused an individual to obtain education in these ranges are generally not related to ability.

The TPT dominant hand has a somewhat constant effect in that the scores increase in the positive direction. However, those of the nondominant hand decrease. These effects cancel each other so that the TPT total score shows almost no effect. The reason for this occurrence is not clear. In the case of the motor tests, Tapping and Grip Strength, the trend is for the difference to increase. The faster speed for CNEHRB Tapping is even greater with people who have a higher education. The most probable explanation for this trend is still motivation.

Gender

The effect of gender is also examined in Table 5, and is accomplished by comparing the CNEHRB and HRNES scores for females at the high school, age 45 level. The difference in Table 5, column 6, is the relative difference that gender produces between the CNEHRB and the HRNES. The difference is obtained by subtracting the female difference between the two programs from the male difference at the high school level, presented in column 5. For instance, on Trails B, females tend to score 2 T scores less than do males, so their total T scores on the CNEHRB will be 7 T scores below the HRNES equivalent T scores. The males will be 5 points less. A difference of 2 points could represent a rounding effect.

As has been found in almost all studies, the only significant difference between men and women for the HRB tests is in regard to the motor tests. For both the CNEHRB and the HRNES, the male scores are better than the female scores on Tapping and Grip Strength. The positive difference in Table 5, column 6, for the females means that their T scores are more similar to the males on the HRNES than the CNEHRB.

By contrast, the Pegboard difference is in the opposite direction. In this instance, the reason is fairly clear. The HRNES does not correct the Pegboard for gender. Previous literature (Heaton et al., 1986) had not indicated the presence of this difference, so it was not considered in norming. This appears to have been a mistake, especially since this is one motor activity where females do better than males. Using the CNEHRB norms at age 45 with a high school education, the females can complete the dominant hand Pegboard in about 65 seconds, while it takes the males 85 seconds. The difference in regard to the nondominant hand is about the same. Where relevant, this difference should be taken into consideration in interpretation.

Standard Deviation

All of the calculations given in the previous tables were based on the mean for each measure. To make a thorough comparison, the effect of the scale intervals needs to be examined. Here the scores related to standard deviations are investigated. Table 6 compares the scores of the HRNES and the CNEHRB at the mean and at each of two standard deviations below the mean. In order to make the comparison, the raw score for the HRNES are used as a gauge against which the CNEHRB scores are compared. The raw scores equivalent to the mean and first two standard deviations were used. For the HRNES, these are C scores of 100, 90, and 80. The equivalent T scores would be 50, 40, and 30.

The HRNES raw scores, which were obtained from these intervals, were entered into the CNEHRB computer program and the CNEHRB T scores were derived (Table 6). Next, the difference between these T scores was obtained by subtracting the HRNES equivalent T score from the CNEHRB T score, so a minus indicates that the CNEHRB is less than the HRNES.

An inspection of the results presented in Table 6 indicates that the CNEHRB scores for the Trail Making and Tapping tests are less than the HRNES at the mean, and the differences become greater as one proceeds away from the mean. The other tests vary; some, such as Location, even become more impaired for the CNEHRB. Minor variations may be due to rounding adjustments. With the exception of Trail Making and the Tapping tests, the difference between the two computer programs is negligible. It is surprising, considering the great difference in the method of determining scale scores, that there are not greater differences.

At least part of the difference in regard to the Trail Making Test B is that its distribution was not linear when brain-damaged subjects were plotted for the HRNES. In order to take this effect into account, the regression line for the HRNES Trails B scale scores was reset by hand.

Cutting Scores for Brain Damage

The major question in regard to tests of brain damage is the difference between the two programs in designating impairment scores. The impairment score

TABLE 6. Comparison of CNEHRB T Scores and T Score Differences Equivalent to HRNES Raw Scores for the Mean and 2 SD T Scores for Age 45 Years and Education 12

| | Raw and T score for 3 SD intervals | | | | | | | | |
| | HRNES $T = 50$ | | | HRNES $T = 40$ | | | HRNES $T = 30$ | | |
Test	HRNES Raw	CNHRB T	Diff[a] T	HRNES Raw	CNHRB T	Diff[a] T	HRNES Raw	CNEHRB T	Diff[a] T
Category	49	44	-6	73	40	0	98	27	-3
Trails A	34	44	-6	69	27	-13	104	15	-15
Trails B	86	45	-5	189	28	-12	339	15	-15
Speech	7	43	-7	15	33	-7	24	29	-1
Rhythm	4 (24)	49	-1	7 (23)	40	0	10 (20)	34	4
Aphasia	4	50	0	11	37	-3	18	29	-1
Cross	2	58	8	4	34	-6	5	23	-7
Percep	6	43	-7	24	30	-10	43	24	-6
TPT Tot	17.3	44	-6	32.3	32	-8	46.7	28	-2
TPT Dom	7	43	-7	11.9	36	-4	17	32	2
TPT Non	6.2	43	-7	11.8	31	-9	16.3	27	-3
TPT Both	3.9	44	-6	8.6	32	-8	13.4	28	-2
TPT Mem	7	43	-7	6	36	-4	4	29	-1
TPT Loc	4	50	0	3	46	6	1	35	5
Tapp Dom	45	39	-11	35	27	-13	26	15	-15
Tapp Non	40	38	-12	31	22	-18	22	10	-20
Grip Dom	45	41	-9	39	36	-4	32	31	1
Grip Non	41	42	-8	35	37	-3	29	32	2
Peg Dom	75	40	-10	118	26	-14	161	17	-13
Peg Non	80	44	-6	124	22	-18	168	22	-8

[a] This is the difference between the CNEHRB T score and the HRNES equivalent T score given above.

generally determine whether a patient is considered to be brain damaged. Although the two programs have somewhat different sets of T scores for the same raw score, each program uses a different cutting point to designate the existence of impairment. The HRNES uses one-half standard deviation below the mean or a C score equal to 95 and below (equivalent to a T score of 45). In contrast, the CNEHRB uses scores less than a full standard deviation or a T score below 40. The critical scores and the range of scores related to the critical scores are provided in Table 7.

Table 7 provides the critical male raw score and range of scores that separate the normal from the impaired scores for both the HRNES and the CNEHRB at age 45 with a high school (12 years) education level. It also provides critical raw scores for age 75 with a high school education and critical raw scores for the graduate level (20 years) of education at age 45. These age and education levels represent extremes of the corrections made by the programs and indicate the difference in impairment scores for age and education. The critical or cutting score is the first score that is equal to the impaired range. For impairment scales, such as the Category Test, it is the lowest impaired raw score and for attainment scores it is the highest impaired raw scores. These scores are accompanied by a plus or minus. The plus indicates that the score is impaired as well as all higher scores and the minus indicates the score is impaired as well as lesser scores. The critical T score is also provided for the CNEHRB. It is not provided for the HRNES, since it is in all cases, except for the Cross Drawing, a C score of 95, which is equivalent to a T score of 45.

In order to define more exactly the critical scores, the ranges of raw scores, all of which are equivalent to the critical T score, are provided. That is, every score within the specified range if placed into the program will give the critical T score. For age 45 and the high school level, the range of raw scores is given for both programs. For the CNEHRB, the range of T scores is given for the highest T score below 40 and also the range of the T scores that apply to the highest T score below 40.

The last 4 columns present the effect of age and education on the impairment cutting point. Age 75 demonstrates the effect of the older age levels on the cutting points, while the graduate degree education level (20 years) illustrates the effect of education or IQ level. The range is not given since it would be approximately the same as the ranges for the high school, age 45 level.

In regard to the results, examination of the table at the high school, age 45 level demonstrates that the differences found in the other tables are not repeated here. The scores that were higher for the CNEHRB in the other tables are not necessarily higher with these cutting points. For instance, it takes a higher score for Categories on the CNEHRB to indicate impairment than on the HRNES. The Trails B test is about the same, while Trails A has a lower score for the CNEHRB to indicate impairment. Overall, the two programs indicate impairment at about the same level using the different cutting points. Apparently, setting the cutting point differently for the two batteries canceled much of their differences. The Tapping speed norms are still higher for the CNEHRB.

TABLE 7. Comparison of the Impairment Cutting Scores Used by the HRNES and the CNEHRB[a] for Ages 45 and 75 and Education Levels of 12 (High School) and 20 (Graduate Degree)

| | Males, high school, age 45 | | | | | | Age 75, ed 12 | | Age 45, Ed 20 | |
| | HRNES[b] | | CNEHRB, T score <40 | | | | HRNES | CNEHRB | HRNES | CNEHRB |
Test	Raw	Range	Raw[c]	Range	T	Range	Raw[b]	Raw[c]	Raw[b]	Raw[c]
Category	61+	61–66	74+	74–83	36	38–34	83+	108+	43+	36+
Trails A	51+	51–59	42+	42–49	36	38–34	67+	61+	43+	32+
Trails B	117+	117–150	111+	111–130	36	38–34	152+	237+	90+	67+
Speech	11+	11–12	10+	10–12	36	38–34	13+	13+	8+	6+
Rhythm	5 (25)+	5 (25)	8 (22)+	8–9 (21)	37	39–35	6 (24)+	10 (20)+	3 (27)+	6 (24)+
Aphasia	7+	7–8	9+	9–12	37	39–35	7+	9+	4+	5+
Cross	4+	4	3+	3–4	34	43–26	4+	4+	4+	4+
Percep Dis	14+	14–18	10+	10–13	37	39–35	18+	10+	12+	7+
TPT Tot	24.6+	24.6–28.5	23.1+	23.1–28.4	36	38–34	32.7+	60+	18.0+	19.2+
TPT Dom	9.3+	9.3–10	9.4+	9.4–12.9	36	38–34	11.0+	17.5+	6.9+	9.4+
TPT Non	9.1+	9.1–10	6.7+	6.7–8.6	39	41–37	13.0+	27.0+	6.6+	5.4+
TPT Both	6.2+	6.2–7.3	5.4+	5.4–6.8	36	38–34	8.7+	16.0+	4.6+	4.0+
TPT Memory	6–	6	6–	6	36	38–34	5–	3–	8–	6–
TPT Location	3–	3	1–	1	35	39–32	1–	0–	4–	4–
Tapping Dom	40–	40–37	46–	46–43	39	40–36	35–	41–	42–	49–
Tapping Non	35–	35–34	41–	41–38	38	40–36	30–	39–	37–	44–
Grip Dom	42–	42	39–	39–34	36	38–33	35–	34–	42–	46–
Grip Non	38–	38	37–	37–30	37	39–35	31–	26–	38–	37–
Pegboard Dom	97+	97–107	83+	83–89	35	37–33	111+	120+	80+	71+
Pegboard Non	102+	102–112	81+	81–86	39	42–35	118+	123+	81+	81+

[a] Impairment is indicated by a HRNES T scores = < 45 and a CNEHRB T scores <40.
[b] All raw scores for the HRNES in this table are equivalent to a T score of 45, except the Cross Drawing (Spatial Relations), which is 50.
[c] This is the least impaired CNEHRB raw score that is in the range, which has a T score of <40.

The differences at age 75 are variable, but the HRNES generally requires a higher score to indicate impairment. For instance, a HRNES score of 83 indicates impairment for the Category test, while the CNEHRB requires a score of 108. Thus, it is more difficult to obtain a score indicating impairment at age 75 for the HRNES. The large difference between the HRNES and the CNEHRB for the TPT Time tests at age 75 is an artifact due to the different methods that the HRNES and the CNEHRB use to prorate the unplaced blocks.

A high level of education, indicated by the 20 year level, reverses this tendency. Here, in general, the CNEHRB requires a higher score than the HRNES to indicate impairment. However, in both instances of greater age or education the test scores are variable, and one needs to examine individual test scores to determine which program provides a lower impairment score. Two exceptions are the Tapping Test and the Pegboard Test. In both cases a lower score indicates brain damage for the HRNES than the CNEHRB. (The Pegboard uses an impairment scale, so a lower score has a higher raw score.)

Increasing Accuracy

The accuracy of most tests or indices for the existence of brain damage is based on a single cutting point. This produces an all-or-nothing scale. In the actual situation, brain damage impairment does not act this way. Rather, the normal group and the brain-damaged group each has a distribution that overlaps. The cutting point for separating the brain-damaged subjects from the normal subjects is usually set at the point of overlap. As such, it does not reflect the distribution of cases. A more exact and realistic method would be to provide a scale showing the chance that a person would be brain damaged at each scale score point. Such a scale for the HRNES average impairment score (AIS) is provided in Table 8. This table was derived from the norming data used for the HRNES, so it may be applied to the HRNES scores.

TABLE 8. Percent of Subjects that Are Brain Damaged for Each AIS Scale Score[a]

Measures	AIS scale scores									
	105	102.5	100	97.5	95	92.5	90	87.5	85	82.5
% Normal	10.1	35.5	25.5	10.5	7	7	1.4	2	1	0
% BD[b]	0.0	2.1	9.7	10.6	10.2	12.5	7.5	8.7	8.7	30
Sum Norm	100	89.9	54.4	28.9	18.4	11.4	4.4	3	1	0
Sum BD	0	2.1	11.8	22.4	32.6	45.1	52.6	61.3	70	100
Total[c]	0	2.2	17.8	43.6	63.9	79.8	92.2	95.3	98.5	100

[a]Raw scores were converted to percent of normal or percent of brain-damaged subjects.
[b]BD, brain damaged subjects.
[c]Total accumulative percent of both groups that are brain damaged for each interval.

The original data for the control and brain-damaged groups were converted into percent scores representing the percent of the entire group to which the score belonged (Guilford, 1965, pp. 34–36). This was done to equate the groups and eliminate the base rate effect. This produced the percent normal and the percent brain damaged in the table. Then, the accumulative percent for each group was obtained as the sum of normals and the sum of brain-damaged subjects. The brain-damaged group had a positive accumulation. However, the normal group had a negative accumulation, representing the number of normal subjects remaining at each level as one proceeded into the brain-damaged range. The total is the accumulative percent of both groups that are brain damaged for each interval. The total was obtained with this formula: Sum BD/(Sum BD + Sum Norm) × 100. Since this is the accumulative percent of brain-damaged subjects at each interval, it is the chance, in percentage, that a subject with a particular AIS score has brain damage.

Examination of the table indicates that a person with a AIS score of 95 has only little more than a 50% chance of being brain damaged, even though the person's score is in the brain-damaged range. In contrast, if the AIS score is 102 and above, the person has only a 2% chance of being brain damaged. If the score is 82, the chance is almost 80%. At a score of 90, the chance is over 90% that the person has brain damage.

It should be noted that these HRNES AIS data were obtained without age and education corrections. However, they represent a group with a mean approximate age of 45 and a high school education. Since the HRNES correction procedure transforms the raw scores at each age or education level to be equivalent to the age of 45 with a high school education, this table should be relatively accurate for all ages and education levels.

The subjects used to construct this table were medical patients who had no incentive to do poorly, in that neither compensation nor forensic judgment would be affected by the test outcomes. As such, it is probable that few if any functional conditions, such as hysteria or malingering, were included. When such functional cases are examined, neither these nor any cognitive test results will accurately portray the level of a patient's functioning. Thus, it is crucial to determine the possible functional condition or psychopathology of a patient before neuropsychological test results can be trusted.

CONCLUSION

The examination of the three published computerized scoring systems has uncovered some definite findings. First, it is evident that all three systems are valid in their own manner. The NDS is the most authentic representation of the traditional HRB procedure. The HRB procedure relies on inference to a great degree and on the accumulated knowledge of Reitan and other adherents. The NDS permits a measure of the existence of brain damage, the GNDS. At least at lower age ranges the GNDS is as accurate and may be more accurate than any existing index. In addition, the NDS permits a measure of lateralization, using the RNDS and LNDS. These also appear to be as valid as any other method. The scoring procedure does not interfere with a further analysis based on test scores using methods advocated by Reitan and Wolfson (1985, 1986a). The NDS appears to be accurate for ages below 40, but it becomes progressively less accurate at higher age levels. Those using the NDS must take this into consideration in the interpretation.

In regard to the HRNES and CNEHRB, it is clear that both are valid and either can form the basis of a neuropsychological examination that is considerably more advantageous than examiner scoring. The derivation of both the HRNES and CNEHRB norms are more representative of the entire general population at all age ranges than any other set of norms. Each of the other alternative norms that have been developed over the years has certain rather severe problems. Although both are valid, the HRNES and CNEHRB each reflect a slightly different population sample. The CNEHRB norms are more related to a normal or slightly above normal, highly functioning population, while the HRNES norms are more typical of patients who appear for neurological evaluations and are found to be normal.

While better than any other scales used with neurological assessment, neither the *C* scores nor the *T* scores are as finely graded as would be desirable for many measures. Often this produced a variability in this study that made comparisons somewhat inexact. The comparison between the two programs were made less precise and thus more inaccurate by this problem. Consequently, it is thought that both systems need finer scale scores, probably at least 5 points per standard deviation.

Major Effects

The comparison of the CNEHRB and HRNES related to age found that the norms for the CNEHRB are somewhat higher than the HRNES at the middle-age range, around 45, but become more alike at the older age range. In regard to the WAIS, the norms are high enough so that a person with a FSIQ of 105 is in the brain-damaged range at age 74. This might have indicated that the norms were too high for other tests, since all the tests were normed on the same population. Nevertheless, on investigation the overall pattern for the *C* and *T* scores for the other tests in the HRNES and CNEHRB batteries did not find such a great discrepancy. As indicated by the HRNES equivalent *T* scores, the scale scores for the HRNES and CNEHRB are fairly close at the 25- and 75-year levels but somewhat further apart at the 45-year level. There were some differences between the CNEHRB and HRNES scale scores at 75. Except for Trails A, Perceptual Disorders, Tapping, and Grip, the differences were not significant and could be accounted for by rounding effects.

The effect of education on tests between the CNEHRB and HRNES was variable with no noticeable trend. The exception was Tapping speed, which was greater for people who have a higher education than for those who do not. The effect of gender was only found for motor tests. As expected, males were faster and stronger than females on the Tapping and Grip Strength tests. However, female T scores are more similar to the males on the HRNES than the CNEHRB. In contrast to the other motor tests, females were faster on the Pegboard for the CNEHRB. The norming procedure for the HRNES does not correct for a gender difference on the Pegboard.

The difference between the HRNES and the CNEHRB produced by scaling as observed at the first and second standard deviation below the mean was variable but surprisingly small. The only difference was that the Trail Making and Tapping test T scores, which are lower for the CNEHRB scores than the HRNES at the mean, become greater as one proceeds away from the mean.

The major question concerning these programs was their relative sensitivity to brain damage as indicated by the designation of impairment. In this regard the impairment score differences were often not the same as those found for T scores and raw scores. The two programs have different cutting points to designate the existence of brain damage impairment. The HRNES uses a one-half standard deviation below the mean or a C score of ≤ 95 (equivalent to a T score of 45), while the CNEHRB uses below a full standard deviation or a T score below 40. Apparently, setting the cutting point differently for the two batteries canceled out much of their differences for the critical impairment scores at the high school and age 45 level. In many cases the HRNES actually indicates the existence of brain damage impairment at a more stringent, i.e., less impaired raw score level, than the CNEHRB. At age 75, the HRNES generally requires a higher score to indicate impairment, while at a higher level of education the CNEHRB requires a more stringent score. However, the individual test scores are quite variable. The two exceptions are the Tapping Test and the Pegboard Test, both of which require lower scale scores on the HRNES to indicate impairment.

Minor Findings

There were some minor findings that were unrelated to the differences between the programs. The traditional ratio of speed between the dominant and nondominant hands for the TPT was found to be strongly age related. While the traditional ratio held for the younger ages, the older people, approximately 60 and above, actually took less time to complete the board with their dominant hand. Second, from the CNEHRB norms it was apparent that women completed the Grooved Pegboard more quickly than men, although they do not do as well on gross motor tasks.

Summary

Overall, the similarities between the two programs were greater than the differences. Some of the differences in norms were canceled by the use of different cutting scores for impairment. The differences that were found were variable, with the exception of those related to the Tapping tests and to a lesser extent the other motor tests. Here, the CNEHRB had faster normal Tapping speeds. As a result, it had lower T scores throughout the analysis. This may be due to a higher achievement motivation for the CNEHRB subjects that was related to the data gathering settings.

The overall general conclusion is that all of these programs are well qualified for their purposes. The NDS is suitable for people using the strict Reitan approach. For neuropsychologists using an extended HRB approach, both the HRNES and CNEHRB are sound. They have somewhat different norms, though they are surprisingly similar when the individual test variability is considered. Both are far better than any other alternative set of norms.

Considering the increased efficiency and accuracy of the programs, every neuropsychologist who uses many of the HRB tests should utilize at least one of the programs. Because of their greater validity compared to alternatives, they will undoubtedly become a requirement for forensic cases.

THE FUTURE OF NEUROPSYCHOLOGY ASSESSMENT

What do the findings concerning computerized scoring portend for the future? Some occurrences are clear. Since no other types of batteries have been validated (Russell, 1995), these scoring systems are demonstrably more accurate and valid than other batteries in neuropsychology, except possibly the LNNB. Tests have been added to the basic HRB, which indicates that it will probably continue to be changed. Other set batteries will eventually be developed and validated. The computerized batteries may not resemble the HRB as it is presently constructed. However, just as the Wechsler intelligence tests displaced heterogeneous collections of cognitive ability tests, such computerized sets of tests will displace ad hoc batteries.

Farther into the future it is evident that computerized administration of tests will displace most of the examiner testing except for the new tests that have not been computerized. The computer-administered batteries will also score the tests, using absolute scales along with age, gender, and premorbid corrections. Finally, basic computer interpretive systems will sketch the outline of a case. Already the HRNES and NDS contain several interpretative aspects such as indices of brain damage and lateralization indices. In addition, the HRNES contains a method of comparing tests. These interpretive features will serve to form a skeleton around which a full report may be created.

The advantages of such a system in which a computer administers, scores, and makes basic interpretations are clear. The first is efficiency. Several patients can be tested at once and technicians can be used to run most stages of the assessment process. More measures can be administered and scored in the same amount of time than can the traditional examiner administration and scoring methods. Second, it is obvious that such a system will be more accurate than examiner scoring. Third, such a method will aid research in that data can be collected with much less effort. Finally, such a system will have more reliability and demonstrated validity than other methods. Computer systems including the interpretive elements are completely reliable in that the program does not vary from one testing to another. The validity of such programs can be determined and errors corrected. Once incorporated into the system, the validity will remain constant across examinations, while the validity of ad hoc batteries varies with each person and each administration.

It will take time for this methodology to become accepted and put into practice. Perhaps as Kuhn (1980, pp. 150–151) contends the present generation of neuropsychologists will need to retire before the new paradigm can be fully accepted. Nevertheless, such computerization does offer a new paradigm for assessment to the future generations of neuropsychologists.

REFERENCES

Bauer, R. M. (1994). The flexible battery approach to neuropsychological assessment. In R. D. Vanderploeg (Ed.), *A guide to neuropsychological practice* (pp. 259–290). Hillsdale, NJ: Erlbaum.

Buschke, H. (1973). Selective reminding for analysis of memory and learning. *Journal of Verbal Learning Behavior, 12,* 543–550.

Choca, J., Laatsch, L., Garside, D., & Arnemann, C. (1994). *CAT: The computer Category Test.* Manual. Toronto: Multi-Health Systems.

Crosson, B., Hughes, C. W., Roth, D. L., & Monkowski, P. G. (1984). Review of Russell's norms for the Logical Memory and Visual Reproduction subtests of the Wechsler Memory Scale. *Journal of Consulting and Clinical Psychology, 52,* 635–641.

Delis, D. C., Kramer, J. H., Kaplan, E., & Ober, B. (1987). *CVLT: California Verbal Learning Test— Research Edition.* New York: Psychological Corporation.

Dodrill, C. B. (1979). Sex differences on the Halstead–Reitan Neuropsychological Battery and on other neuropsychological measures. *Journal of Clinical Psychology, 35,* 236–241.

Dodrill, C. B. (1988). *What constitutes normal performance in clinical neuropsychology?* Paper presented at the 97th Annual Convention of the American Psychological Association, Atlanta, Georgia.

Dunn, L. M., & Dunn L. M. (1981). *PPVT, Peabody, Picture Vocabulary Test—Revised, Manual.* Circle Pines, MN: American Guidance Service.

Fastenau, P. S., & Adams, K. M. (1996). Heaton, Grant, and Matthew's Comprehensive Norms: An Overzealous attempt. *Journal of Clinical and Experimental Neuropsychology, 18,* 444–448.

Fromm-Auch, D., & Yeudall, L. T. (1983). Normative data for the Halstead–Reitan neuropsychological tests. *Journal of Clinical Neuropsychology, 5,* 221–238.

Fuerst, D. R. (1993). A review of the Halstead–Reitan Neuropsychological Battery norms program. *The Clinical Neuropsychologist, 7,* 96–103.

Golden, C. J., Hammeke, T. A., & Purisch, A. D. (1980). *Manual for the Luria–Nebraska Neuropsychological Battery.* Los Angeles: Western Psychological Services.

Goldstein, K., & Scheerer, M. (1941). Abstract and concrete behavior. An experimental study with special tests. *Psychological Monographs, 53* (2, Serial No. 239).

Goodglass, H., & Kaplan, E. (1983a). *The Assessment of aphasia and related disorders* (rev. ed.). Philadelphia: Lea & Febiger.

Goodglass H., & Kaplan, E. (1983b). *Boston Naming Test—Booklet.* Philadelphia: Lea & Febiger.

Guilford J. P. (1965). *Fundamental statistics in psychology and education* (4th ed.). New York: McGraw-Hill.

Haaland, K. Y., Linn, R. T., Hunt, W. C., & Goodwin, J. S. (1983). A normative study of Russell's variant of the Wechsler Memory Scale in a healthy elderly population. *Journal of Consulting and Clinical Psychology, 51,* 878–881.

Heaton, R. K. (1992). *Comprehensive norms for an expanded Halstead–Reitan Battery: A supplement for the Wechsler Adult Intelligence Scale-Revised.* Manual. Odessa, FL: Psychological Assessment Resources.

Heaton, R. K., Matthews, C. G., Grant, I. & Avitable, N. (1996). Demographic corrections with comprehensive norms: An overzealous attempt or a good start. *Journal of Clinical and Experimental Neuropsychology 18,* 121–141.

Heaton, R. K., Grant, I., & Matthews, C. G. (1986). Differences in neuropsychological test performance associated with age, education and sex. In I. Grant & K. M. Adams (Eds.), *Neuropsychological assessment of neuropsychiatric disorders* (pp. 100–120). New York: Oxford.

Heaton, R. K., Grant I., & Matthews, C. G. (1991). *Comprehensive norms for an expanded Halstead–Reitan Battery.* Norms manual and computer program. Odessa, FL: Psychological Assessment Resources.

Jastak, J. F., Jastak, S. R., & Wilkinson, G. S. (1984). *Wide Range Achievement Test, Revised (WRAT-R): Manual.* Wilmington, DE: Jastak Associates.

Kane, R. L., & Kay, G. G. (1992). Computerized assessment in neuropsychology: A review of tests and test batteries. *Neuropsychology Review, 3,* 1–117.

Kaplan, E. (1988). A process approach to neuropsychological assessment. In T. Boll & B. K. Brynt (Eds.), *Clinical neuropsychology and brain function: Research, measurement and practice.* Washington, DC: American Psychological Association.

Kay, G. G., Morris, S., & Starbuck, V. (1993, October). *Age and education based norms control for the effects of occupation on pilot test performance.* Paper presented at the Annual Meeting of the National Academy of Neuropsychology, Phoenix, AZ.

Kuhn, T. S. (1980). *The structure of scientific revolutions.* Chicago: University of Chicago Press.

Lezak, M. D. (1995). *Neuropsychological assessment* (3rd ed.). New York: Oxford.

Lichtenberg, P. A., Ross, T., & Christensen, B. (1994). Preliminary normative data on the Boston Naming Test for an older urban population. *The Clinical Neuropsychologist, 8,* 109–111.

Lynch, W. J. (1995). Microcomputer-assisted neuropsychological test analysis. *Journal of Head Trauma Rehabilitation, 10,* 97–100.

Mahurin, R. K. (1995). Halstead–Russell Neuropsychological Evaluation System (HRNES). In T. C. Conoley and James C. Impara (Eds.), *12th mental measurements yearbook* (pp. 448–451). Lincoln: University of Nebraska Press.

Milberg, W. P., Hebben, N., & Kaplan, E. (1986). The Boston process approach to neuropsychological assessment. In I. Grant & K. M. Adams (Eds.), *Neuropsychological assessment of neuropsychiatric disorders* (pp. 65–86). New York: Oxford.

Pauker, J. D. (1977). *Adult norms for the Halstead–Reitan Neuropsychological Test Battery: Preliminary data.* Paper presented at the Annual Meeting of the International Neuropsychological Society, Sante Fe, NM.

Pauker, J. D. (1981). *T-Score conversion tables for Halstead–Reitan Neuropsychological test Battery for adults.* Unpublished manuscript, Clarke Institute of Psychiatry and University of Toronto, Toronto, Canada.

Pauker, J. D. (1988). Constructing overlapping cell tables to maximize the clinical usefulness of normative test data: Rationale and an example from neuropsychology. *Journal of Clinical Psychology, 44,* 930–933.

Powell, D., Kaplan, E., Whitla, D., Wientraub, S., Catlin, R., & Funkenstein, H. (1993). *MicroCog: Assessment of cognitive functioning* [manual and computer program]. San Antonio: Psychological Corporation.

Reitan, R. M. (1987). *The Neuropsychological Deficit Scale for Adults: Computer program.* Tucson, AZ: Neuropsychology Press.

Reitan, R. M. (1991). *The Neuropsychological Deficit Scale for Adults Computer Program, Users Manual.* Tucson, AZ: Neuropsychology Press.

Reitan, R. M. (1992). *The Neuropsychological Deficit Scale for Older Children Computer program.* Tucson, AZ: Neuropsychology Press.

Reitan, R. M., & Wolfson, D. (1985). *The Halstead–Reitan Neuropsychological Test Battery: Theory and clinical interpretation.* Tucson, AZ: Neuropsychology Press.

Reitan, R. M., & Wolfson, D. (1986a). The Halstead–Reitan Neuropsychological Test Battery. In D. Wedding, A. M. Horton, & J. Webster (Eds.), *The neuropsychology handbook* (pp. 134–160). New York: Springer.

Reitan, R. M., & Wolfson, D. (1986b). *The Neuropsychological Deficit Scale for Younger Children: Computer program.* Tucson, AZ: Neuropsychology Press.

Retzlaff, P. (1995). Review of the Halstead–Russell Neuropsychological Evaluation System (HRNES). In J. C. Conoley and J. C. Impara (Eds.), *12th mental measurements yearbook* (pp. 451–453). Lincoln: University of Nebraska Press.

Russell, E. W. (1975). A multiple scoring method for the assessment of complex memory functions. *Journal of Consulting and Clinical Psychology, 43,* 800–809.

Russell, E. W. (1980). *Theoretical bases of the Luria–Nebraska and the Halstead–Reitan Battery.* Paper presented at the 88th Annual Convention of the American Psychological Association, Montreal, Canada.

Russell, E. W. (1984). Theory and developments of pattern analysis methods related to the Halstead–Reitan battery. In P. E. Logue & J. M. Shear (Eds.), *Clinical neuropsychology: A multidisciplinary approach* (pp. 50–98). Springfield, IL: Charles C. Thomas.

Russell, E. W. (1986). The psychometric foundation of clinical neuropsychology. In S. B. Filskov & T. J. Boll (Eds.), *Handbook of clinical neuropsychology* (vol. 2, pp. 45–80). New York: Wiley.

Russell, E. W. (1987). A reference scale method for constructing neuropsychological test batteries. *Journal of Clinical and Experimental Neuropsychology, 9,* 376–392.

Russell, E. W. (1988). Renorming Russell's version of the Wechsler Memory Scale. *Journal of Clinical and Experimental Neuropsychology, 10,* 235–249.

Russell, E. W. (1992). Comparison of two methods for converting the WAIS to the WAIS-R. *Journal of Clinical Psychology, 48,* 355–359.

Russell, E. W. (1993). *Halstead–Russell Neuropsychological Evaluation System, norms and conversion tables.* Unpublished data tables available from Elbert W. Russell, 6262 Sunset Dr., Suite PH 228, Miami, FL, 33143.

Russell, E. W. (1994). The cognitive–metric, fixed battery approach to neuropsychological assessment. In R. D. Vanderploeg (Ed.), *A guide to neuropsychological practice* (pp. 211–258). Hillsdale, NJ: Erlbaum.

Russell, E. W. (1995). The accuracy of automated and clinical detection of brain damage and lateralization in neuropsychology. *Neuropsychology Review, 5(1),* 1–68.

Russell, E. W., & Barron, J. H. (1989). A difference that is not a difference: Reply to Vanderploeg. *Journal of Consulting and Clinical Psychology, 55,* 317–318.

Russell, E. W., Hendrickson, M. E., & VanEaton, E. (1988). Verbal and figural Gestalt Completion Tests with lateralized occipital area brain damage. *Journal of Clinical Psychology, 44,* 217–225.

Russell, E. W., & Levy, M. (1987). A revision of the Halstead Category Test. *Journal of Consulting and Clinical Psychology, 55,* 898–901.

Russell, E. W., Neuringer, C., & Goldstein, G. (1970). *Assessment of brain damage: A neuropsychological approach.* New York: Wiley.

Russell, E. W., & Polakoff, D. (1993). Neuropsychological test patterns in men for Alzheimer's and multi-infarct dementia. *Archives of Clinical Neuropsychology, 8,* 327–343.

Russell, E. W., & Russell, S. L. K. (1993). Left temporal lobe brain damage pattern on the WAIS. Addendum. *Journal of Clinical Psychology, 49,* 241–244.

Russell, E. W., & Starkey, R. I. (1993). *Halstead–Russell Neuropsychological Evaluation System* [manual and computer program]. Los Angeles: Western Psychological Services.

Russell, E. W., Starkey, R. I., Fernandez, C. D., & Starkey, T. W. (1988). *Halstead, Rennick, Russell Battery* [manual and computer program]. Miami, FL: Scientific Psychology.

Taylor, D. J., Hunt, C., & Glaser, B. (1990). A cross validation of the Revised Category Test. *Psychological Assessment, 2,* 486–488.

Teuber, H. L. (1955). Physiological psychology. *Annual Review of Psychology, 6,* 267–296.

Vanderploeg, R. D. (1994). Estimating premorbid level of functioning. In R. D. Vanderploeg (Ed.), *Clinicians guide to neuropsychological assessment* (pp. 43–68). Hillsdale, NJ: Erlbaum.

Wechsler, D. (1987). *Wechsler Memory Scale—Revised, manual.* San Antonio, TX: Psychological Corporation.

Wechsler, D. (1991). *Wechsler Intelligence Scale for Children—Third Edition (WISC-III).* Manual. San Antonio, TX: Psychological Corporation.

Wechsler, D. (1992). *Wechsler Individual Achievement Test* (WIAT). Manual. San Antonio, TX: Psychological Corporation.

Wilkinson, G. S. (1993). *The Wide Range Achievement Test 3. Administration Manual.* Wilmington, DE: Jastak Associates.

Williams, J. M. (1991). *The Memory Assessment Scale* (test and manual). Odessa, FL: Psychological Assessment Resources.

3

The Clinical Utility of Standardized or Flexible Battery Approaches to Neuropsychological Assessment

GERALD GOLDSTEIN

Recently, Kane (1991) wrote an extensive review article on the matter of standard and flexible neuropsychological test batteries in which he described the two approaches to assessment, provided the historical backgrounds of both methods, and reviewed a number of tests commonly used in individualized or flexible assessments. In this chapter, I will be dealing with different but complementary matters. For the most part, the chapter will be devoted to a description of the two approaches and an examination of their theoretical foundations. It will be proposed that practice issues are of secondary significance, and that the question of whether one administers the same or different tests to every patient is a relatively trivial matter. It can be stipulated in advance that most practicing clinicians now use a combination of fixed and flexible assessment methods, and that fixed batteries, as strictly defined, are primarily used in research settings in which it is necessary to obtain a large database.

Lezak (1995) has pointed out that there is really no such thing as a fixed battery in a historical sense, since fixed batteries have changed dramatically over the years. With regard to the Halstead–Reitan Battery (Reitan & Wolfson, 1993), there is only a moderate resemblance to the battery initially described by Halstead (1947) in *Brain and Intelligence*. Similarly, the Luria–Nebraska battery (Golden, Purisch, & Hammeke, 1985) has changed over its briefer history, with the latest edition having alternate forms, a new intermediate memory scale, and a qualitative scoring system. The reverse point cannot be documented as clearly, but it is

GERALD GOLDSTEIN • Pittsburgh VA Health Care System, and University of Pittsburgh, Pittsburgh, Pennsylvania 15260 commonly understood that most advocates of flexible batteries do not give an entirely different set of tests to each patient. Rather, they generally give a usually brief series of the same tests, or "core battery" (Hamsher, 1990), to each patient for purposes of initial screening.

I propose that the essential differences between fixed and flexible battery approaches are not based on these practical matters, i.e., what one does, but on theoretical issues, i.e., what one believes. To begin, the fixed battery approach is relatively new to clinical science, while the flexible approach can probably be traced back to antiquity in the way in which physicians examined their patients. "Fixed batteries" only emerged recently in medicine with the advent of autoanalyzers and other computer-assisted laboratory procedures. More pertinent to clinical neuropsychology, the fixed approaches appear to have emerged from American psychometrics, while the flexible approach emerged from European behavioral neurology. The flexible approach is clearly rooted in a medical model, while that is not necessarily the case for the fixed battery approach. As we will try to show, it appears to be based largely in what we will characterize as a "laboratory model."

The view that the differences between the approaches are largely philosophical in nature is supported somewhat by the fact that there are no data that attest to the superiority or inferiority of one or the other approach as indicated by commonly accepted outcomes. These outcomes include accuracy of diagnosis relative to objective external criteria, success of rehabilitation outcome based on recommendations contained in the neuropsychological report, accuracy of prognosis, or prediction of behavior. There are really no data attesting to the superiority of fixed or flexible batteries with regard to these matters. Representatives of each side have presented anecdotes attesting to the superiority or inferiority of one method or the other, but they tend to counterbalance each other.

THEORETICAL FOUNDATIONS OF THE FIXED BATTERIES

What eventuated in the fixed battery approach to neuropsychological assessment most likely began in Ward Halstead's Chicago laboratory during the 1930s. Some of the conceptual roots can be traced back to earlier times, but I know of no predecessor to Halstead's project for neuropsychology. Basically, that project was the establishment of a laboratory to which patients could come to be evaluated with a series of standard procedures that could be administered in the same way and using the same instructions with all patients. The procedures themselves were to be derived from the corpus of experimental neuropsychology and were to consist of instruments with established validity and reliability. The laboratory was devoted to furthering the understanding of human brain–behavior relationships through study of a variety of abilities. Halstead had an elaborate theory of biological intelligence and its relationship to the frontal lobes, which is not currently widely accepted but has great relevance to the development of standard neuro-psychological test batteries.

This laboratory model was also taken up by Teuber (1959) and his group. Teuber called for bringing the "brass instruments" of the experimental laboratory into the clinic. We hasten to add that Teuber and his collaborators were not and are not advocates of the fixed battery approach to neuropsychological assessment. However, they were and remain advocates of the use of validated laboratory procedures administered under standard conditions. In any event, despite numerous theoretical differences, both Halstead and Teuber ran laboratories rather than clinics, and one can imagine the kinds of reinforcement given to junior investigators and technicians who deviated from established procedures.

The first component of the fixed battery approach therefore appears to be the use of objective procedures that can be administered in a standard fashion. An outgrowth of this practice has been the use of technicians in assessment and a departure from the traditional medical model in which patients are personally examined by their physicians. The use of laboratory procedures, however, does not make assessment fixed. It becomes fixed when all of the procedures are routinely administered to all patients. Advocates of the fixed approach argue that this practice assures that one evaluates areas that may be of importance, but that may be missed using an individualized approach assessing only initially apparent areas requiring evaluation. This consideration may be of importance, but there are other relevant matters involved. In the psychometric tradition, a battery, as such, is somewhat sacrosanct, and the component tests are not meant to be interpreted individually, but in relation to each other. Calculation of important global scores are also dependent on administration of the complete battery.

Another part of Halstead's project had to do with quantification, and he performed two major factor analyses on the then-current version of his set of tests. If one subscribes to factor analytic theory and accepts the view that individual tests load on separate factors each of which represent separate abilities, then there is little question that all of the tests have to be given in order to make interpretations from a factor analytical perspective. To do otherwise is a compromise. There are obviously numerous questions concerning whether or not the Halstead–Reitan Battery is actually a battery in this sense and whether this approach is pertinent to neuropsychology; but it would nevertheless appear that an interest in factor analysis and related procedures has provided some impetus to the fixed battery approach. Interestingly, attempts to replicate modern confirmatory factor analyses have been compromised by investigators using somewhat different tests in their batteries (Newby, Hallenbeck, & Embretson, 1983).

In summary, the use of fixed battery approaches is thought to be based in a preference for objective, standard procedures, capable of being administered and scored by technicians, and the application of multivariate statistical methods to the psychometric development and framing of the assessment procedure. A third matter has to do with clinician objectivity. Utilization of a flexible approach typically requires knowledge of the history prior to interpretation, while the fixed approach makes no such requirement. Using the fixed approach, one can know the history in advance or make an interpretation based only on the test materials obtained during the assessment. This "blind diagnosis" matter is controversial; but whether one should do it or not is not the issue at hand here. The issue is the belief, or lack of it, that test data are interpretable independently and not conditional on the context in which the testing took place. I would accept the view, though never really stated that way, that founders and advocates of the American psychometric tradition believe that test scores are powerful. Numbers have meaning based on the often extensive and careful efforts made during test construction. These numbers are not unlike those used by physicians when taking blood pressure or temperature. This view, with regard to neuropsychology, stands in sharp contrast to what will be described regarding the flexible approach, where, perhaps drawing the analogy too far, the physician must personally observe the nurse taking the temperature or blood pressure to see how it is done, or to do it her- or himself.

Certain misunderstandings have arisen concerning terminology often associated with fixed batteries. These batteries are often characterized by their advocates as "comprehensive," while their critics sometimes describe them as "screening procedures." Both terms have been misinterpreted. As we have pointed out elsewhere (Goldstein, 1986), if by screening one means "screening for brain damage" in the sense of simply detecting its presence or absence, that is incorrect. Any degree of familiarity with the fixed batteries should indicate that they do more than that, and that they deal with numerous assessment issues such as locus and type of lesion, severity of impairment, prognosis, rehabilitative implications, and related considerations. The term "screening" is more appropriately applied in the sense that these batteries provide an overview of a variety of aspects of brain function, such as language or spatial abilities, without going into extensive detail about any one of them.

The term "comprehensive" is sometimes used to assert that advocates of fixed batteries believe that their procedures assess all aspects of brain function in extensive detail. It appears that this alleged claim has created a straw-man argument, in that no reputable advocate of the fixed battery approach really holds that view. Actually, the term "comprehensive" has taken on the meaning of a standard set of procedures that works well in most situations and that provides a meaningful assessment of the various domains and modalities of brain function for most patients. That is not to say that fixed batteries cannot have weaknesses in particular areas. The absence of memory tests in the Halstead–Reitan Battery has been noted on several occasions in the literature (Goldstein, 1990; Jones & Butters, 1983), as has the absence of sensitive spatial–constructional tasks on the Luria–Nebraska battery (Shelly & Goldstein, 1983). These deficiencies, however, are correctable, and advocates of fixed batteries have made numerous efforts to supplement their procedures in light of these criticisms. It is also generally acknowledged that patients with highly specific syndromes may require a more extensive evaluation. Obviously, a fixed battery cannot provide the detailed evaluation of an aphasic patient, for example, that a full aphasia examination can provide. Thus, "comprehensive" is really not meant to imply assessment of all areas in all possible detail. It really means a set of procedures that clinicians can utilize in most situations to provide a competent, appropriate assessment that is responsive to the needs of the referring agent and the patient. The major domains and modalities of brain function are assessed with these procedures, but it is important to note that there is an underlying theoretical issue regarding acceptance of the view that neuropsychological assessment is, in essence, an evaluation of domains and modalities. That is, the fixed-battery advocates may accept a theoretical structure that differs from the domain–modality structure that was really developed within behavioral neurology. We will turn to this issue in the following.

Let us start with an example from the criticism that the Halstead–Reitan Battery is lacking in memory tests. We would note the implicit assumptions here that: (1) memory is a domain of cognitive function separable from other cognitive functions such as language and perceptual–motor skill, and (2) the Halstead–Reitan Battery does not assess memory in ways that are different from the conventional memory tests. Thus, the theoretical response to the criticism is that memory is involved in essentially all cognitive abilities. You need memory to do the Category Test, the Tactual Performance Test, the Rhythm Test, and so on. The point is that memory may not operate in the brain in isolation, but is always involved in some aspect of problem solving, motor execution, or language comprehension or production. This view may have been stated, perhaps unclearly, by Halstead in his "Central Integrative Field (C) factor." As I understand it, by C Halstead meant something we might call memory, but he described it in terms of a background process representing the past against which new stimuli can be tested and integrated. The theory appears to resemble Piaget's concept of assimilation and accommodation (Piaget & Inhelder, 1973). Thus, the Category Test assesses memory because the subject must match the current stimulus with experience with other items.

The argument is raised that this approach to assessment cannot identify patients who "only" have memory disorders and are otherwise normal. Typically, patients with amnesic disorders associated with Korsakoff's syndrome or some patients with closed-head injury are mentioned to illustrate this point. The argument can be answered empirically, since numerous studies have shown that when patients with amnesic disorders are given complex tests of abstraction and problem-solving ability, they do not do well on them. Thus, the existence of a "pure syndrome" may sometimes be the product of an inadequate examination. The extensive controversy surrounding the so-called "Gerstmann syndrome" also lends credence to this view (Benton, 1961). Many of those involved in rehabilitation of head-injured patients now indicate that their patients' problems are not as much with memory itself as they are with "executive function," in this application connoting the capacity to use memory productively in organizing the problem solving.

To generalize from this example, we would indicate that brain function can be viewed in ways different from domains and modalities. If some alternative model is used, then it may be inappropriate to criticize a test procedure because it does not assess "language" or "memory" as long as that procedure provides a plausible alternative model of how the brain works. As I understand the original Halstead model, the brain works in an adaptive manner to deal with changes in the environment through evaluating new events against a central integrative field, an ability to absorb similarities and form abstractions, a capacity to suppress affective demands (perhaps something like attention), and various perceptual and motor skills that direct behavior. In many ways it is a different way of thinking about brain function from the domains and modalities or modularity-based views of behavioral neurology.

While the term "battery" is commonly used in psychometrics, it is difficult to find a concise definition. The most appropriate definition found in a standard dictionary is "An array or grouping of like things to be used together." While most psychometricians would probably agree with that definition, they would not say dogmatically that for a procedure to be used as a battery all of the parts must be administered. That assumption appears to be implicitly made, however, because the quantitative analysis of scores generally assumes complete data. Perhaps the most apparent example is based on the Wechsler intelligence scales. It is not appropriate to report actual IQ values unless all of the subtests are administered. One can "predict" or "estimate" IQs, but it is not appropriate to report values based on incomplete data as actual IQ values.

It is proposed on the basis of these considerations that advocates of fixed batteries in neuropsychology believe in an approach oriented toward quantification, multivariate analysis of data, and a number of psychometric procedures that may include factor analysis, cluster analysis, multidimensional scaling, computation of various combinatorial scores such as summary scores, indices, and composite scores based on administration of more than one test. To such individuals, the term "flexible" is readily translatable to the term "missing data." Missing data probably constitute the major nuisance to the application of multivariate statistical analysis.

Furthermore, advocates of fixed batteries typically do not subscribe to modularity or other specific localization models of brain function. Their modus operandi in neuropsychological interpretation is not directed to what has been described as the "pathognomonic signs" level of interpretation described by Reitan and Wolfson. That is, the goal is not that of identifying some specific identifiable syndrome, but rather that of assessing various dimensional aspects of brain function. It is, in many respects, a dimensional rather than a categorical approach. In that regard, it resembles multivariate battery approaches to such areas as intelligence, aptitude, or personality. Without necessarily accepting the numerous mathematical assumptions that underlie factor analysis, there is nevertheless a belief that crucial aspects of brain function can be evaluated best by examining the interrelationships among various functions, abilities, and skills. Such relationships are best elicited by a battery in which these relationships have been studied and are well understood on the basis of quantitative methods such as factor analysis or clinical experience with the battery. Indeed, it has been said that a good clinician may function by doing an intuitive factor analysis in her or his head. Acceptance of these considerations would suggest that the term "fixed battery" is a redundancy, since a battery is an instrument that necessarily contains a finite number of procedures. On the other hand, the term "flexible battery" is an oxymoron, because one cannot vary the number of tests used and assert that one is using a "battery."

THEORETICAL FOUNDATIONS OF THE FLEXIBLE BATTERIES

The use of flexible batteries is often associated with the process approach to neuropsychological assessment. While this association is inescapable, I will try to separate the two in the following manner. The process approach, named after Werner's (1937) "Process and Achievement" paper, stresses observation of the individual during testing in order to determine how a particular end result is achieved, since the same end result or test score may be achieved by numerous means. Many instruments, observational methods, and scoring systems have been developed within the theoretical framework of the process approach. These matters will not be discussed here. Rather, the discussion will be limited to the issue of fixed versus flexible batteries as described above, stipulating that advocates of the process approach generally do not use fixed, standard batteries.

Although what are now described as flexible batteries have been used since the beginning of psychological assessment, it probably became an advocacy issue following the development of the fixed battery approach to neuropsychological assessment that was largely accomplished by Ralph Reitan and numerous collaborators. I think that I am being historically correct in saying that advocacy of the flexible battery approach was in reaction to the Reitan group's work, and later to the approach taken by Golden and collaborators centering around the Luria–Nebraska Neuropsychological Battery (Adams, 1980; Spiers, 1981). This reaction included a number of points. It was suggested that it is not possible to do an adequate neuropsychological assessment of all domains of function in sufficient detail within the framework of a single procedure. Even if one could, time would be wasted in dealing with irrelevant matters, while one might possibly miss or not pay sufficient attention to crucial areas of concern. We should look at what is relevant in detail and not become involved with matters that are not pertinent to the patient in question. Thus, a flexible assessment might be more pertinent, but briefer, than a fixed assessment. In keeping with contemporary concerns, it may be more cost-effective.

One way of designing a flexible assessment is through the referral question. That is, the tests used are selected to be optimally responsive to the questions asked by the referring agent. This procedure is of particular value in settings in which referring agents are familiar with the basic scope of neuropsychological assessment and can frame their questions in detailed, appropriate, and answerable ways. Hamsher (1990) includes this criterion in addition to others in his description of the specialized or flexible approach. In what he calls the "individual-centered normative approach," assessment is characterized by a "core battery" plus a collection of specialized batteries appropriate to the referral question or the disease entity. The clinician has the opportunity to switch specialized batteries as information is obtained. Hamsher gives the example of an initial administration of a dementia battery, discovery of significant aphasic signs, and switching to an aphasia battery.

Most contemporary users of the flexible approach use the individual-centered normative approach rather than an informal, individualized bedside assessment or conversation with the patient. That is, they mainly use published, standardized tests that meet the appropriate psychometric requirements. The number of such tests is quite large by now, and we are thankful to the continuing encyclopedic work of Muriel Lezak for keeping track of this massive amount of material (Lezak, 1995) over a period of more than 20 years. Thus, the database for the flexible approach comes from the literature pertinent to the development of these tests, which in turn comes from the experimental neuropsychological research that provided the rationale for the particular test. For example, the original research with the Wisconsin Card Sorting Test came from the experimental work of Grant and Berg (1948), and later Milner (1963) and her group, and was followed by the psychometric work of Heaton (1980) that eventuated in the published, standardized version of the test that is now in common use. This practice-related database is in some contrast to what is used by the advocates of the fixed battery approach. These neuropsychologists depend heavily on the research done with the particular battery they use. The research involving other tests is often not relevant to their practice, because they do not use other tests. Thus, for example, clinicians who rely exclusively on use of the Halstead–Reitan Battery may only have an academic interest in the California Verbal Learning Test (Delis, Kramer, Kaplan, & Ober, 1987), because they do not use it in their practices. Correspondingly, users of the flexible approach may have little knowledge concerning interpretation of the Halstead–Reitan Battery, although they may make use of some of the individual tests. However, it should be noted that competent practice with either approach requires considerable knowledge of the experimental and basic neuropsychological literature.

Hamsher (1990) allies the flexible approach to the process of syndrome identification. As he says, "A very important role for clinical neuropsychology is to apply its scientific methodology for the study of behavior to the problem of diagnosing disorders of mental status, that is, *defining and identifying neurobehavioral syndromes*" [italics added] (p. 261). This matter is extremely crucial, because it reflects the more general controversy in health science between categorical and dimensional models. This very same debate is taking place in psychiatry, with strong sentiment for classifying at least the personality (Axis II) disorders on a dimensional basis. Within clinical neuropsychology, we are proposing the view that the flexible approach is strongly wedded to a categorical model, while the fixed battery approach is more strongly associated with a dimensional model. In neuropsychology, categories are not necessarily specific diagnoses, but may be syndromes reflecting a number of commonly co-occurring phenomena that have some structural or functional relationship with each other. The dimensions may be trait-like phenomena such as those referred to by Halstead and Reitan as adaptive abilities. As we suggested, these phenomena may be elicited with factor analysis, but that point is controversial and there are other ways of describing and measuring dimensional traits (e.g., various scaling procedures).

The flexible approach has the advantage of being more prepared to react rapidly to advances in clinical neuropsychology. That is, new tests can be adopted almost as soon as they are published. Thus, the Halstead–Reitan, and even the Luria–Nebraska batteries have been characterized as "old-fashioned" and their advocates have been criticized for being unresponsive to new developments in the field. However, the extent to which new developments are incorporated are dependent on the willingness of individual clinicians to give up some of the procedures with which they are familiar and to learn to use new tests. Nevertheless, while fixed batteries need not be old, it is more difficult to create a whole new battery than it is to develop a single new test.

One might suggest that the capacity of the flexible approach to incorporate new developments might allow for greater capability of keeping clinical practice more contemporary with developments in neuroscience and conceptual changes in clinical neuropsychology. For example, the growing concept of ecological validity of tests (Acker, 1990) and its realization through such instruments as the Rivermead Behavioural Memory Test (Wilson, Cockburn, Baddeley, & Hiorns, 1989) would appear to be more readily dealt with in the framework of a flexible assessment approach. Recent developments in basic memory research can be incorporated in a similar manner through new procedures like the California Verbal Learning Test (Delis et al., 1987). Advocates of the fixed battery approach might cite the ancient adage "If it ain't broke, don't fix it" in response to this point, particularly since the two most widely used fixed batteries have not changed in any fundamental way over many years.

Differing Brain Models

There is a basic issue regarding whether fixed and flexible approaches to assessment reflect differing conceptualizations of brain function. Do the two views have different models? That question would appear to be difficult to answer because if one considers just the two major fixed procedures, the Halstead–Reitan Battery is based on Halstead's model as modified by Reitan, while the Luria–Nebraska was based on Luria's theories. Elsewhere (Goldstein, 1986), we have indicated our belief that both batteries actually share the same scientific model and program, and that the theories of Halstead and Luria, while of obvious significance to neuroscience, did not direct the manner in which research with these batteries was conducted. That is particularly true for Luria, who had nothing personally to do with the research done with the Luria–Nebraska battery. If that is the case, then I would propose that the flexible approach is associated primarily with the concept of a modular brain (Moscovitch & Nachson, 1995), while the fixed approach is more consistent with the belief in a dimensional brain. Perhaps the best way to evaluate that view is through an examination of the role of syndromes in neuropsychological assessment.

Probably the most widely and thoroughly studied syndrome in neuropsychology is Korsakoff's syndrome or psychosis, and so we will use it as an introductory example (Butters & Cermak, 1980). Following the acute stage of the disorder, known as the Wernicke stage, the most prominent features are a severe anterograde amnesia, a retrograde amnesia for events occurring just prior to the onset of the illness, relatively well-preserved memory of early life, a frequent but not always present tendency to confabulate, relatively intact intellectual function, and personality changes in the direction of increased apathy, passivity, and lack of initiative. Identification of the syndrome utilizing neuropsychological tests is a reasonably straightforward matter, and clearly a specialized set of tests evaluating particular aspects of memory, learning, and general intelligence can readily identify the disorder. On the other hand, failure to administer appropriate tests of memory and new learning may result in failure to identify the syndrome. Indeed, in a classification study using discriminant function analysis, we found that the Halstead–Reitan Battery, which is short on memory tests, produced several false-negative errors for presence or absence of brain damage in patients with Korsakoff or Korsakoff-type amnesic disorders. On the other hand, the Luria–Nebraska battery, which has a memory scale, classified most of these same patients correctly (Goldstein & Shelly, 1984). We hasten to add that these findings were based purely on statistical analyses and not clinical judgment, which might have led to very different conclusions about these amnesic patients. However, just looking at the quantitative, psychometric structure of the Halstead–Reitan Battery, there appears to be some insensitivity to detection of this kind of specific syndrome. In the case of the Luria–Nebraska, there was more capability of identifying these patients as brain damaged, but our study did not deal with the matter of whether or not they could be accurately identified as having Korsakoff's syndrome.

There are several general points to be made from this example. First, in an investigation for the presence of a specific syndrome, a straightforward evaluation utilizing tests matched to the diagnostic criteria for Korsakoff's syndrome would appear to represent the most sensible way to proceed. Fixed batteries are typically not designed to identify specific neurobehavioral disorders, such as subtypes of aphasia or amnesia. However, since the specific syndromes are produced by brain damage, the fixed batteries should be able to detect the generalized consequences of brain dysfunction. Ideally, in a patient with a specific syndrome, a fixed battery should be able to detect the presence of brain damage and to provide a profile of relative strengths and weaknesses that may go beyond the criteria for the syndrome. For example, aphasic patients may be shown to have conceptual and perceptual–motor deficits that would not be made apparent using a specialized aphasia evaluation. Things become problematic, if not embarrassing, for the fixed batteries when the patient with a clear syndrome is not at least identified as brain damaged. That is probably the major reason for the recent expansion of the Halstead–Reitan Battery by some of its users and researchers (Heaton, Grant, & Matthews, 1991), and to some extent, of the Luria–Nebraska battery as well (Golden et al., 1985). Fixed batteries may be insensitive to highly specific disorders with little associated symptomatology unless the battery happens to contain tests that are sensitive to the particulars of those disorders.

The flexible approach varies in its flexibility, and may range from an informal bedside conversation to application of the individual-centered normative approach in which standardized, published tests are used and a core battery is generally included, but subsequent selection of tests is based on individual patient considerations. In the latter case, the clinician sometimes uses a core battery plus a number of specialized batteries, both of which amount to being fixed. The difference between this procedure and the fixed battery approach is essentially the use of multiple rather than single fixed batteries. Thus, the clinician may have available in addition to the core battery a "dementia" battery, a "learning-disability" battery, a "head-injury" battery, and so on. This procedure would appear to be particularly attractive, since it permits specialized assessment but still can accommodate testing by trained technicians. The model developed by the Benton laboratory in which well-standardized tests may be used in combination, but not in a uniform procedure, would appear to represent this approach. Thus, there is no "Benton Battery," but there is a series of quantified, valid, and reliable tests that can be used to address specific assessment areas (Benton, Hamsher, Varney, & Spreen, 1983; Benton, Sivan, Hamsher, Varney, & Spreen, 1994).

The more extreme flexible approach in which the clinician personally examines the patient and uses procedures, generally of an unstandardized type, based on previous patient responses and hypotheses formed during the examination no longer appears to have a prominent place in contemporary clinical neuropsychology. The "tests" themselves have been referred to, perhaps pejoratively, as "a bag of tricks," and major questions have been raised concerning the validity and reliability of this procedure as a whole. Even behavioral neurologists, who typically bear the brunt of this criticism, have begun to develop objective, quantitative tests. If these presumptions are correct, then the argument by advocates of fixed battery approaches that other approaches are subjective, idiosyncratic, and generally lacking in scientific rigor are perhaps less well-taken than they were in the past. While this historical process has not led to a reconciliation between advocates of fixed and flexible approaches, it has modified and clarified the pertinent issues.

Linear and Matrix Inference Models

I would like to develop the idea here that a major distinction between flexible and fixed battery advocates is that in making inferences, flexible battery advocates use a linear model, while fixed battery advocates use a matrix model. A linear inference model is used when an initial piece of information raises alternative hypotheses that are evaluated, following which alternative subhypotheses are formed, and the procedure is continued in an iterative manner until a conclusion is reached. It is based on syllogistic logical reasoning and may be characterized as a decision tree. The essence of identifying a syndrome would appear to be the sequential inclusion and exclusion of individual symptom possibilities. A matrix inference model is used when information is presented simultaneously, and an inference is made on a pattern detection basis. An anecdotal example of this process is watching Ralph Reitan make neuropsychological inferences in front of a group. Dr. Reitan always wanted all of the data presented on a 5 × 7 card. He would look at the card and immediately start interpreting. My guess is that he knew essentially instantaneously what the interpretation was by relating the test scores to each other, and extended time was only required to explain his inferences to others. My assumption is that he was making his interpretation by pattern recognition from the matrix of test scores.

Observing advocates of the flexible battery approach in action gives a different impression. Watching a colleague examine an aphasic patient once provided a totally different experience. First, the colleague, Dr. Harold Goodglass, not being an advocate of the fixed battery approach, wanted to see the patient himself rather than look at his test scores. After a brief initial conversation, Dr. Goodglass gave the patient a series of tasks to perform, during which it was apparent that he was ruling in and out various possibilities. The patient was asked to read and to write. Following writing, he was asked to see if he could read what he had written. On a reading task, he was asked to identify the words themselves and then asked to point to the appropriate word that would answer a question. It seemed that Dr. Goodglass was going through a logical, sequential series of steps to reach a diagnosis.

What are the appropriate quantitative foundations for linear and matrix models? Linear models are typically associated with univariate statistics, perhaps organized as a decision tree. Tests are considered one at a time, and scores based on combinations of test variables are rarely used. General summary scores, such as impairment indices, are also rarely used. Inference making is generally derived from examination of significant and nonsignificant findings, based either on comparisons between patients and controls or among patient groups. A body of experimental evidence is developed though this procedure, and characteristics of some syndrome are delimited. Subsequent clinical testing can then be used to determine whether or not these characteristics are observed. This process clearly describes the work done with Korsakoff patients. Therefore, we can now diagnose this disorder effectively through retracing the assessment steps taken by the investigators who did the original work. The model was clearly linear, sequentially ruling in and ruling out a number of alternatives. In its most elegant form, the linear model can produce double dissociations in which tasks of equal difficulty level are done at widely varying levels of performance in different diagnostic groups (Teuber, 1959). That is, task A may be done well by group 1 and poorly by group 2, while task B, which was shown to be of equal difficulty level in a general population, is done well by group 2 and poorly by group 1.

The matrix inference method makes use of performance profiles or patterns. A fixed battery is desirable because if the profile or pattern is to be detected, it is done best when all of its elements are present. Interpretations are made through simultaneous comparisons among multiple tests. Much, but not all, of the research providing the foundations for clinical interpretation involves administration of the complete battery to various patient groups. Thus, while much research has been done with the Halstead Category Test from the Halstead–Reitan Battery, that research may not be directly relevant to how one uses the Halstead Category Test in interpretation of the Halstead–Reitan Battery. The more pertinent studies were those that related performance on that test to other battery measures. Sophisticated interpretation cannot be made in the absence of a context of other test scores in which the Halstead Category Test appears.

This pattern recognition method was clearly enunciated in an important paper by Reitan (1964) in which he showed that clinical interpretation of Halstead–Reitan Battery data produced far more accurate classification of cases by type and locus of lesion than did application of univariate statistics. Reitan concluded that the information leading to accurate classification must be somewhere in the data, but the task of capturing the nature of that information has become a topic for extensive discussion and research. Indeed, the project of the Russell, Neuringer, and Goldstein (1970) neuropsychological keys was directly initiated by Reitan's comment. Ultimately, this activity led to attempts at computer-assisted interpretation, since if rules of interpretation could be objectified and the appropriate algorithms developed, then computers could be programmed not only to score but also to interpret neuropsychological test profiles (Adams, 1986).

The statistical basis for this pattern recognition approach is multivariate analysis. The first attempts at use of this branch of statistics were made by Halstead in the form of factor analyses of his battery of discriminating tests. Despite the controversial nature of factor analysis as a statistical tool, interest in it has persisted over the years, and contemporary investigators are now doing work with advanced methods, notably confirmatory factor analysis.

As we indicated above, factor analysis helps in describing the often complex pattern of interrelationships among tests and the dimensions of our test batteries. Aside from Halstead's four factors, other factor models have been proposed, including an effort to organize neuropsychological tests according to the factor-analysis-based concept of crystallized and fluid intelligence (Russell, 1980), and our own factor analytic studies in which we identified verbal, sensory–perceptual, problem-solving, and motor skill factors in the Halstead–Reitan Battery (Goldstein & Shelly, 1972). With the availability of confirmatory factor analysis, we can now test alternative hypotheses concerning factor structure.

Another widely used set of multivariate methods is multiple regression techniques. Discriminant function analysis has been one of the more widely used techniques, with more recent use of a related technique called logistic regression analysis. The issue here is accuracy of classification, utilizing multivariate combinations of test variables. There were several early studies using discriminant analysis done with the Halstead–Reitan Battery and a smaller number of tests selected from it demonstrating highly accurate classification rates (Wheeler, 1963; Wheeler, Burke, & Reitan, 1963). Some years ago, we showed that this method was superior to univariate methods with regard to accurate separation of cases into right-hemisphere and left-hemisphere lesion groups (Goldstein & Shelly, 1973). The original validation studies for the Luria–Nebraska Battery utilized discriminant analyses (Golden, Purisch, & Hammeke, 1978; Purisch, Golden, & Hammeke, 1978).

Cluster analysis, another related technique, is also used in classification, but it works on the basis of different mathematics and strategies. The major point is that in cluster analysis, subgroups are not previously identified, but arise from the analysis. The method is particularly applicable in situations in which there is a large heterogeneous database and there is some interest in identifying clusters of subjects that are similar among themselves within that database. It is of particular value in individual differences or subtyping research (Goldstein, 1994).

The current use of various multivariate analysis techniques is now widespread in neuropsychology, and their application is not restricted to fixed batteries. Having said that, however, it is important to note that it is necessary to have a large number of subjects, all of whom received the same procedures, to use these kinds of analyses. Subjects with only one piece of missing data have to be dropped from the analysis, with replacement by an estimated score usually viewed as an unsatisfactory practice.

Returning to clinical practice, it is easy to understand why advocates of the fixed battery approach might wonder why advocates of an at least unduly flexible approach would not want to take advantage of the important advances in neuropsychological interpretation contributed by multivariate research. The capability of conceptualizing one's test material dimensionally on the basis of factor analyses, or of making correct classifications on the basis of well-established prediction equations, or of appropriately identifying a subtype of a disorder based on findings coming from cluster analysis research would surely be desirable. The response to this challenge would appear to lie in one's evaluation of the success multivariate analysis has had with regard to accuracy and precision of prediction. We have not heard the last of this matter.

Clinical Applications and Implications

The considerations we have been raising clearly have relevance to the way in which one establishes a practice. In this section, I will elaborate on the proposal that the adoption of either a fixed, flexible, or mixed approach should relate to the nature of that practice. Such a decision requires consideration of practical, financial, professional, scientific, and clinical matters. Each of the aspects will be briefly considered.

Practical/Financial

There are many settings in which it is not possible for patient time or funding reasons to administer a fixed procedure as lengthy as the Halstead–Reitan Battery. Use of the Luria–Nebraska battery is an alternative here, but that solution might not be appropriate for scientific or clinical reasons. Many clinicians in this situation use targeted, brief batteries that are specifically responsive to the referral question. Many efforts have been made to develop short forms of the more popular tests in an attempt to deal with this situation. Computerized assessment may ultimately provide a better solution to this difficult problem area for neuropsychologists. As an editorial comment, I would add that neuropsychological assessment research has not done a very satisfactory job of abbreviating its procedures in a way that does not sacrifice quality and adequate thoroughness.

Professional

Choice of practice style often relates strongly to the nature of one's interaction with members of other professions. Sometimes, referring physicians want only brief, rapidly delivered reports that do not contain a great deal of detail but are responsive to specific questions. Others prefer longer, more detailed reports based on a full and comprehensive evaluation. Use of an extensive fixed battery generally fares better in the latter situation. Professional setting and activities are also relevant. In forensic work, for example, testing is generally quite thorough and lengthy with resources usually made available to accomplish such evaluations. While many forensic neuropsychologists do not advocate fixed batteries, it is my impression that many, if not most, of them incorporate major components if not complete fixed batteries into their lengthy testing. Furthermore, if not technically administering one of the standard fixed batteries, forensic neuropsychologists tend to accomplish the intent of such procedures through assessment of a wide range of abilities rather than through a narrowly focused evaluation for a specific syndrome. That is because they are generally asked to testify about broad functional adaptive abilities in addition to the particular details of some specific syndrome.

Scientific

If the clinician is functioning as a scientist–practitioner and is using patient data in research protocols, the use of at least a core fixed battery may be a necessity. One can use a flexible approach in clinical practice, but that practice may be accomplished independently from one's research. As we have detailed throughout this chapter, choice of practice style may be strongly based on one's scientific beliefs and theoretical framework. Issues such as localization theory, concern with identification of neurobehavioral syndromes rather than describing dimensions of behavior, and philosophy of science and scientific methodology all may become involved in determining the pattern of one's practice. It is worth repeating that the weight of scientific evidence does not favor either the fixed or flexible approach. However, there are some clinical matters worthy of consideration in making a decision concerning pattern of practice. We will turn to that topic in what follows.

Clinical

I would like to defend the view that the clinical utility of the fixed or flexible approach to assessment is related to the characteristics of the patient population in which one provides services. An entire volume has recently appeared that deals with the various roles of clinical psychologists in health settings to which the reader is referred for an extensive treatment of this significant matter (Sweet, Rozensky, & Tovian, 1991). The many issues raised there are quite pertinent to clinical neuropsychology. While clinical neuropsychology is a professional specialty, clinical neuropsychologists work in primary, secondary, and tertiary health care facilities, as well as in educational settings. More specifically, some are engaged in independent private practice and may become involved with patients at the primary care stage. Some work in general medical facilities, while others work in specialized acute neurology, neurosurgery, psychiatric, and rehabilitation settings. What one does in the way of assessment would appear to be highly influenced by the particular setting in which one works.

Primary Care. The neuropsychologist doing independent practice often receives referrals from neurologists and neurosurgeons and, when this is the case, can be viewed as functioning at the tertiary level, since the patient has already sought specialized care. However, the issues are somewhat different for the psychologist in a setting in which he or she has primary care responsibilities. Assuming that the psychologist is competent to do neuropsychological assessments, the issue would nevertheless revolve around screening. Extensive fixed or flexible batteries are rarely administered in primary care settings, and screening is all that is generally accomplished, often leading to a referral in positive cases. The issue of screening, however, may be more serious than simply determining whether or not to make a referral, because identification of significantly impaired performance could connote serious illness necessitating immediate care. Therefore, the underlying science at this level involves an understanding of the general principles of screening, as well as the specifics of neuropsychological screening research. That is, there should be some knowledge of the consequences of making false positives and negatives and the related distinction between sensitivity and specificity. There has been abundant research concerning the use of a variety of tests as screening for brain damage procedures. The empirical validity of such tests is an important issue. I would note here that the matter of screening is separate from the issue of single tests for brain damage and the well-established superiority of batteries. The issue is that all health care professionals should have some competency at primary care within their own areas of specialization and should ideally be capable of providing services in emergency rooms, rural clinics, or other primary care settings in which the use of specialized procedures may be completely unfeasible and/or inappropriate. Berg, Franzen, and Wedding (1987, 1994) have written a book containing extensive material on the content of neuropsychological screening. Clinicians in this "first-line" role should be particularly knowledgeable about mental status examinations and competent in their use. Some neuropsychologists have become competent through appropriate training in administering portions of the neurological examination, a skill that can be of significant value in an isolated, primary care setting.

General Medicine. Neuropsychologists in general medical settings, other than those that restrict their work to neurology, neurosurgery, or psychiatry services, have the task of assessing patients with a wide variety of illnesses, some of which may have consequences for brain function. Tarter, Edwards, and Van Thiel (1988) make the following comment about assessment of such patients:

> This evaluation could take one of two general forms: a standardized test battery such as the Halstead–Reitan Neuropsychological Test Battery or the Luria–Nebraska Battery, or alternatively, a specialized test battery can be composited that consists of standardized measures. Regardless of whichever assessment strategy is employed, the main objective is to obtain a profile of the person's cognitive capacities and limitations. (pp. 8–9)

It would appear that in medical settings, it is worthwhile to do more than screening, but since the presence or absence of brain damage has not yet been established in the majority of patients evaluated and the illness the patient has may not be associated with specific neuropsychological deficits, the most prudent form of assessment would appear to be a comprehensive battery. It may be one of the standard fixed batteries or a battery designed by the clinician, as long as it is sufficiently comprehensive to assess major cognitive functions. An individualized approach would not appear to be as appropriate unless the referral requests evaluation of a suspected specific neurobehavioral syndrome. Obviously, if a specific syndrome becomes apparent during the course of the general assessment, additional specialized testing would be indicated.

Psychiatry. The use of neuropsychological tests in psychiatric settings has a long and instructive history (Goldstein, 1985). Some neuropsychologists eschewed the application of neuropsychological tests to psychiatric patients, feeling that they were not appropriate procedures for such disorders. Without going into detail, it is my impression that historically, mostly clinical work with psychiatric patients has involved the use of fixed batteries. There is an abundance of research involving use of the Halstead–Reitan Battery with schizophrenic patients and a moderate amount with the Luria–Nebraska battery (Goldstein, 1991). I know of no body of research reporting on what is learned from administering a flexible battery to schizophrenic patients. However, extensive work has been done with individual tests, notably the Wisconsin Card Sorting Test, and information-processing tests of attention, such as reaction time tasks and various versions of the Continuous Performance Test procedure (Nuechterlein, 1991). Advice to the clinician working in a psychiatric setting with schizophrenic patients would depend on the purpose of the assessment. Without going into detail about the matter, it can be said that neuropsychological tests cannot diagnose schizophrenia. The performance of schizophrenic patients is exceedingly heterogeneous on our commonly used clinical tests (Goldstein, 1994). However, neuropsychological tests can be used to assess cognitive function in schizophrenic patients. For this purpose, the use of a fixed battery may be preferred, because so much research has been done with them and there is no single neurobehavioral syndrome that characterizes all of schizophrenia that might be elicited by a specialized or flexible assessment.

A different approach may be taken to other psychiatric disorders. Much is now known about neuropsychological aspects of depression, particularly with regard to memory (Watts, 1995). Specialized tests evaluating automatic and effortful processing in memory can be particularly helpful in the assessment of depressed patients. There are other psychiatric disorders that look more like specific neurobehavioral syndromes, notably attention deficit hyperactivity disorder (ADHD) and autism. Competent assessment of these cases requires specialized knowledge of the research literature regarding these disorders and their neuropsychological aspects. In all frankness, however, neither fixed nor flexible approaches have reached sophisticated levels in assessment of these disorders. In the case of ADHD, assessment generally involves detailed evaluation of attention itself, as well as executive abilities, but Barkley (1991) has made the following remark: "Children with ADHD do not have significant memory problems *nor do they have a particularly distinctive profile on standard neuropsychological test batteries*" [italics added] (p. 729). In the case of autism, we are only beginning to learn about the neurobehavioral aspects of this disorder through intensive study of high-functioning (IQ > 70 and verbal) cases (Minshew, Goldstein, Muenz, & Payton, 1992). At this point, it does not appear that the standard batteries capture the complex deficit pattern associated with autism, and the flexible approach is made difficult through limited understanding of the relevant areas to pursue.

Neurology and Neurosurgery. The matter of practice pattern is a controversial one for those working in an acute neurological or neurosurgical setting. Founders of both the fixed and flexible approaches worked in such settings, both groups claiming the superiority of their method. However, it can be assumed that once a patient is admitted to an acute neurology or neurosurgery service, the presence of brain damage is typically well established, and it is usually not necessary to engage in complex differential diagnostic procedures to determine whether the patient's symptoms reflect a structural brain disorder or to decide whether the condition is "functional" or "organic."

Whether to use a fixed or flexible battery in an acute setting would appear to be based on a number of considerations. As we have indicated, the identification of specific neuropsychological syndromes is generally straightforward and can be accomplished through administration of tests that assess the various criteria for that syndrome. Thus, if a patient's language suggests that he or she has Broca's aphasia, and one wishes to confirm that diagnosis, there are available numerous specialized tests that can be used to answer that question. With that aim in mind, there seems little point in administering a lengthy standard battery. In such cases, the application of a flexible "process approach" procedure can be quite helpful in eliciting more subtle but clinically relevant aspects of the patient's communication. This practice style is particularly relevant if that is the information the referring clinicians want; in this example, a detailed description and diagnosis of the patient's aphasia.

This pattern of practice would appear to be more desirable as level of specialization of the clinical service increases. That is, if one works only with stroke patients, head-injured patients, or aphasic patients, there would appear to be a need to utilize specialized procedures that provide detailed information. Information at this level of preciseness may be particularly important for diagnostic, management, and planning matters, and advocates of the flexible approach may be correct in stating that such detail cannot be provided by a standard, fixed evaluation.

There is nevertheless a role for standard batteries in acute settings, although it may not be as urgent for immediate treatment considerations as is the specialized examination. That role relates to the point that to the extent the specialized examination becomes increasingly focused, it increasingly fails to evaluate cognitive abilities that either may also be impaired or that provide compensatory strengths. Thus, giving the Halstead–Reitan Battery to the patient with Broca's aphasia may be quite worthwhile, if the severity of the aphasia does not proscribe its valid administration. It can reveal aspects of the patient's perceptual and motor skills, attention, problem-solving abilities, spatial skills, and related areas of function that the specialized aphasia examination cannot. Such information would have obvious value for prognosis and rehabilitation planning. It would appear that in an acute setting, the neuropsychologist should have the capability of doing both specialized and comprehensive assessments. In doing comprehensive assessments, there is always the choice of using a standard battery or using one's own collection of tests. As indicated above, the advantages of a standard battery are its psychometrics and the opportunity to make inferences based on the substantial research accomplished with the commonly used standard batteries.

Rehabilitation

Desirable practice patterns for neuropsychologists working in rehabilitation clinics and hospitals are also controversial. On the one hand, Bleiberg, Ciulla, and Katz (1991) come down foursquare for standard batteries:

> There are many reasons for using a formal neuropsychological test battery. The major test batteries have extensive normative and validation data and thus are useful for comparing a given patient with populations of various types and degrees of known pathology, as well as with "normal" populations. The major test batteries are also composed of multiple, overlapping tests that sample different areas of function, thus permitting the analysis of patterns of performance within an individual patient. Thus, the psychologist may identify intact as well as impaired areas of function, knowledge of both being necessary for the development of a rehabilitation plan. An analysis of patterns of performance also assists in an approximation of the patient's preinjury abilities, which has clinical as well as medicolegal utility. (p. 393)

Lezak (1987), while also emphasizing the need for a thorough neuropsychological assessment for rehabilitation planning, stresses the particular importance of evaluating the specific areas of executive function, capacity to take an abstract attitude, attention, and concentration. She recommends various observational procedures and specific tests to evaluate these areas, but does not recommend the use of any particular battery.

The Rusk Institute group does not advocate for a standard battery, but has used standard tests in its research such as the Wechsler Adult Intelligence Scale Block Design subtest and various cancellation tasks. In my opinion, the major contribution of this group in the area of assessment is that of linking cognitive testing with functional activities and defining for the psychologist the distinction between abilities as assessed with tests and functions as assessed by observation of the individual acting in a natural environment (Diller, 1987). The Rusk group has encouraged us to supplement our traditional cognitive tests with various forms of functional assessment, with the aim of determining whether the tests had ecological validity or capacity to predict function in everyday life (Acker, 1990). This work has been taken up by Barbara Wilson and her colleagues, who have developed tests specifically designed to be ecologically valid, and who have accomplished research correlating those tests with objective functional outcome measures (Wilson, 1987).

Based on these considerations, the neuropsychologist working in a rehabilitation setting may wish to utilize extensive testing, because of the complex nature of rehabilitation planning, but may also consider the tests used from the standpoint of their ecological validities. He or she may also wish to go beyond traditional testing through use of various forms of functional assessment and utilization of functional outcome measures.

Some Neuropathological Considerations

A consideration involved in selection of a fixed or flexible battery involves the disease process under study. It has become apparent in recent years that there are disease entities that are associated with multiple neuropsychological deficits with different deficits and deficit patterns appearing in different patients and at different stages of the disease. HIV infection is one of those disorders. Thus, a work group formed to make recommendations concerning assessment of patients with this disorder (Butters et al., 1990) suggest that a relatively comprehensive battery is required because of the diverse manifestations the disorder can take with regard to CNS impairment. Recently, Heaton et al. (1995) found that the number of tests used in earlier studies can be reduced, but there continues to be a need for comprehensive assessment. Studies of patients exposed to toxic substances such as organic solvents show a similar phenomenon (Morrow, Ryan, Hodgson, & Robin, 1990). While it is not uncommon for these individuals to have neuropsychological deficits, the deficits differ from individual to individual, and there is no prototypic pattern or syndrome. Multiple sclerosis is by definition a diffuse disorder in which there may be extensive variability in symptom pattern. The recent elegant studies of memory in multiple sclerosis patients (Rao, 1990) are of great significance, but do not imply that an adequate neuropsychological assessment can be restricted to memory. These individuals may have tactile, visual, conceptual, speech production, and perceptual–motor deficits, and these areas have to be evaluated in order to provide an adequate neuropsychological description of the patient with multiple sclerosis. While patients with these disorders do not necessarily require a fixed battery, they do require an extensive, reasonably comprehensive battery. A more focused specialized approach could lead to significant diagnostic error because of failure to evaluate areas that may be significantly impaired. The syndrome-seeking, linear approach does not appear to be optimal for these disorders. We see this situation as the converse of the case in which the patient has an isolated, specific syndrome that can be inadequately delineated by a fixed, comprehensive battery without subsequent specialized testing.

SUMMARY

The preference for fixed or flexible neuropsychological test batteries is not a matter of what one does, but one of a complex set of scientific and professional beliefs, probably based to a great extent on one's background, training, and experience. What one does is conditioned to some extent by situational factors and by practical and professional considerations. We have tried to show that the choice of approach involves not only the particular tests or the number of tests given, but is related to inference-making procedures and utilization of differing referential databases.

We have indicated that choice of approach is associated with concepts of brain function and with preference for categorical or dimensional classificatory systems. A particular interest in syndromes is associated with the flexible approach, while identifying patterns of adaptive abilities seems more compatible with the fixed battery approach. It was suggested that one approach may be more appropriate than the other in differing settings, and that assessment of specific disorders may be more adequately accomplished by one or the other approach, depending on the nature of the disorder.

ACKNOWLEDGMENT

Acknowledgment is made to the Department of Veterans Affairs for support of this work.

REFERENCES

Acker, M. B. (1990). A review of the ecological validity of neuropsychological tests. In D. E. Tupper & K. D. Cicerone (Eds.), *The neuropsychology of everyday life: Assessment and basic competencies* (pp. 19–55). Boston: Kluwer Academic Press.

Adams, K. M. (1980). In search of Luria's battery: A false start. *Journal of Consulting and Clinical Psychology, 48,* 511–516.

Adams, K. M. (1986). Concepts and methods in the design of automata for neuropsychological test interpretation. In S. B. Filskov & T. J. Boll (Eds.), *Handbook of clinical neuropsychology* (Vol. 2, pp. 561–576). New York: Wiley-Interscience.

Barkley, R. A. (1991). Attention deficit hyperactivity disorder. *Psychiatric Annals, 21,* 725–733.

Benton, A. L. (1961). The fiction of the Gerstmann syndrome. *Journal of Neurology, Neurosurgery, and Psychiatry, 24,* 176–181.

Benton, A. L., Hamsher, K. deS., Varney, N. R., & Spreen, O. (1983). *Contributions to neuropsychological assessment.* New York: Oxford University Press.

Benton, A. L., Sivan, A., Hamsher, K. deS., Varney, N. R., Spreen, O. (1994). *Contributions to neuropsychological assessment* (2nd ed.). New York: Oxford University Press.

Berg, R., Franzen, M., & Wedding, D. (1987). *Screening for brain impairment: A manual for mental health practice.* New York: Springer.

Berg, R., Franzen, M., & Wedding, D. (1994). *Screening for brain impairment: A manual for mental health practice* (rev. ed.). New York: Springer.

Bleiberg, J., Ciulla, R., & Katz, B. L. (1991). Psychological components of rehabilitation programs for brain-injured and spinal-cord-injured patients. In J. J. Sweet, R. H. Rozensky, & S. M. Tovian (Eds.), *Handbook of clinical psychology in medical settings* (pp. 375–400). New York: Plenum Press.

Butters, N., & Cermak, L. S. (1980). *Alcoholic Korsakoff's syndrome.* New York: Academic Press.

Butters, N., Grant, I., Haxby, J., Judd, L. L., Martin, A., McClelland, J., Pequegnat, W., Schacter, D., & Stover, E. (1990). Assessment of AIDS related cognitive changes: Recommendations of the

NIMH workshop on neuropsychological assessment approaches. *Journal of Clinical and Experimental Psychology, 12,* 963–978.

Delis, D. C., Kramer, J. H., Kaplan, E., & Ober, B. A. (1987). *California Verbal Learning Test: Manual.* San Antonio, TX: Psychological Corporation.

Diller, L. (1987). Neuropsychological rehabilitation. In M. J. Meier, A. L. Benton, & L. Diller (Eds.), *Neuropsychological rehabilitation* (pp. 3–17). Edinburgh, England: Churchill Livingstone.

Golden, C. J., Hammeke, T. A., & Purisch, A. D. (1978). Diagnostic validity of the Luria neuropsychological battery. *Journal of Consulting and Clinical Psychology, 46,* 1258–1265.

Golden, C. J., Purisch, A. D., & Hammeke, T. A. (1985). *Luria–Nebraska Neuropsychological Battery: Forms I and II.* Los Angeles: Western Psychological Services.

Goldstein, G. (1985). The neuropsychology of schizophrenia. In I. Grant & K. Adams (Eds.), *Neuropsychological assessment of psychiatric disorders: Clinical methods and empirical findings* (pp. 147–171). New York: Oxford University Press.

Goldstein, G. (1986). An overview of similarities and differences between the Halstead–Reitan and Luria–Nebraska neuropsychological batteries. In T. Incagnoli, G. Goldstein, & C. J. Golden (Eds.), *Clinical application of neuropsychological test batteries* (pp. 235–275). New York: Plenum Press.

Goldstein, G. (1990). Comprehensive neuropsychological assessment batteries. In G. Goldstein & M. Hersen (Eds.), *Handbook of psychological assessment* (2nd ed., pp. 197–227). New York: Pergamon.

Goldstein, G. (1991). Comprehensive neuropsychological test batteries and research in schizophrenia. In S. R. Steinhauer, J. H. Gruzelier, & J. Zubin (Eds.), *Handbook of Schizophrenia: Volume 5. Neuropsychology, psychophysiology and information processing* (pp. 525–551). Amsterdam: Elsevier.

Goldstein, G. (1994). Cognitive heterogeneity in psychopathology: The case of schizophrenia. In P. A. Vernon (Ed.), *The neuropsychology of individual differences* (pp. 209–233). San Diego: Academic Press.

Goldstein, G., & Shelly, C. H. (1972). Statistical and normative studies of the Halstead Neuropsychological Test Battery relevant to a neuropsychiatric hospital setting. *Perceptual and Motor Skills, 34,* 603–620.

Goldstein, G., & Shelly, C. H. (1973). Univariate vs. multivariate analysis in neuropsychological test assessment of lateralized brain damage. *Cortex, 9,* 204–216.

Goldstein, G., & Shelly, C. H. (1984). Discriminative validity of various intelligence and neuropsychological tests. *Journal of Consulting and Clinical Psychology, 52,* 383–389.

Grant, D. A., & Berg, E. A. (1948). A behavioral analysis of degree of reinforcement and ease of shifting to new responses in a Weigl-type card sorting problem. *Journal of Experimental Psychology, 38,* 404–411.

Halstead, W. C. (1947). *Brain and intelligence.* Chicago: University of Chicago Press.

Hamsher, K. deS. (1990). Specialized neuropsychological assessment methods. In G. Goldstein & M. Hersen (Eds.), *Handbook of psychological assessment* (2nd ed., pp. 256–279). New York: Pergamon.

Heaton, R. K. (1980). *A manual for the Wisconsin Card Sorting Test.* Odessa, FL: Psychological Assessment Resources.

Heaton, R. K., Grant, I., Butters, N., White, D. A., Kirson, D., Atkinson, J. H., McCutchan, J. A., Taylor, M. J., Kelly, M. D., Ellis, R. J., Wolfson, T., Velin, R., Marcotte, T. D., Hesselink, J. R., Jernigan, T. L., Chandler, J., Wallace, M., Abramson, I., and the HNRC Group. (1995). The HNRC 500—Neuropsychology of HIV infection at different disease stages. *Journal of the International Neuropsychological Society, 1,* 231–251.

Heaton, R. K., Grant, I., & Matthews, C. G. (1991). *Comprehensive norms for an expanded Halstead–Reitan Battery.* Odessa, FL: Psychological Assessment Resources.

Jones, B. P., & Butters, N. (1983). Neuropsychological assessment. In M. Hersen, A. S. Bellack, & A. E. Kazdin (Eds.), *The clinical psychology handbook* (pp. 377–396). New York: Pergamon.

Kane, R. L. (1991). Standardized and flexible batteries in neuropsychology: An assessment update. *Neuropsychology Review, 2,* 281–339.

Lezak, M. D. (1987). Assessment for rehabilitation planning. In M. J. Meier, A. L. Benton, & L. Diller (Eds.), *Neuropsychological rehabilitation* (pp. 41–58). Edinburgh, England: Churchill Livingston.

Lezak, M. D. (1995). *Neuropsychological assessment* (3rd ed.). New York: Oxford University Press.

Milner, B. (1963). Effects of different brain lesions on card sorting. *Archives of Neurology, 9,* 90–100.

Minshew, N. J., Goldstein, G., Muenz, L. R., & Payton, J. B. (1992). Neuropsychological functioning in non-mentally retarded autistic individuals. *Journal of Clinical and Experimental Neuropsychology, 14,* 749–761.

Morrow, L., Ryan, C., Hodgson, M., & Robin, N. (1990). Alterations in cognitive and psychological functioning following exposure to mixtures of organic solvents. *Journal of Occupational Medicine, 32,* 743–746.

Moscovitch, M., Nachson, I. (1995). Modularity and the brain: Introduction. *Journal of Clinical and Experimental Neuropsychology, 17,* 167–170.

Newby, R. F., Hallenbeck, C. E., & Embretson, S. (1983). Confirmatory factor analysis of four general neuropsychological models with a modified Halstead–Reitan battery. *Journal of Clinical Neuropsychology, 5,* 115–134.

Nuechterlein, K. H. (1991). Vigilance in schizophrenia and related disorders. In S. R. Steinhauer, J. H. Gruzelier, & J. Zubin (Eds.), *Handbook of Schizophrenia: Volume 5. Neuropsychology, psychophysiology and information processing* (pp. 397–433). Amsterdam: Elsevier.

Piaget, J., & Inhelder, B. (1973). *Memory and intelligence.* New York: Basic Books.

Purisch, A. D., Golden, C. J., & Hammeke, T. A. (1978). Discrimination of schizophrenic and brain-injured patients by a standardized version of Luria's neuropsychological tests. *Journal of Consulting and Clinical Psychology, 46,* 1266–1273.

Rao, S. M. (1990). Multiple sclerosis. In J. L. Cummings (Ed.), *Subcortical dementia* (pp. 164–180). New York: Oxford University Press.

Reitan, R. M. (1964). Psychological deficits resulting from cerebral lesions in man. In J. M. Warren & K. A. Akert (Eds.), *The frontal granular cortex and behavior* (pp. 295–312). New York: McGraw-Hill.

Reitan, R. M., & Wolfson, D. (1993). *The Halstead–Reitan Neuropsychological Test Battery: Theory and clinical interpretation* (2nd ed.). Tucson, AZ: Neuropsychology Press.

Russell, E. W. (1980). Fluid and crystallized intelligence: Effects of diffuse brain damage on the WAIS. *Perceptual and Motor Skills, 51,* 121–122.

Russell, E. W., Neuringer, C., & Goldstein, G. (1970). *Assessment of brain damage: A neuropsychological key approach.* New York: Wiley-Interscience.

Shelly, C. H., & Goldstein, G. (1983). Psychometric relations between the Luria–Nebraska and Halstead–Reitan Neuropsychological Test batteries in a neuropsychiatric setting. *Clinical Neuropsychology, 4,* 128–133.

Spiers, P. A. (1981). Have they come to praise Luria or to bury him: The Luria–Nebraska controversy. *Journal of Consulting and Clinical Psychology, 49,* 331–341.

Sweet, J. J., Rozensky, R. H., & Tovian, S. M. (1991). *Handbook of clinical psychology in medical settings.* New York: Plenum Press.

Tarter, R. E., Edwards, K. L., & Van Thiel, D. H. (1988). Perspective and rationale for neuropsychological assessment of medical disease. In R. E. Tarter, D. H. Van Thiel, & K. L. Edwards (Eds.), *Medical neuropsychology* (pp. 1–10). New York: Plenum Press.

Teuber, H.-L. (1959). Some alterations in behavior after cerebral lesions in man. In A. D. Bass (Ed.), *Evolution of nervous control from primitive organisms to man* (pp. 157–194). Washington, DC: American Association for Advancement of Science.

Watts, F. N. (1995). Depression and anxiety. In A. D. Baddeley, B. A. Wilson, & F. N. Watts (Eds.), *Handbook of memory disorders* (pp. 293–317). Chichester, Wiley.

Werner, H. (1937). Process and achievement: A basic problem of education and developmental psychology. *Harvard Educational Review, 7,* 353–368.

Wheeler, L. (1963). Predictions of brain-damage from an aphasia screening test: An application of discriminant functions and a comparison with a non-linear method of analysis. *Perceptual and Motor Skills, 17* (Suppl. 1), 63–80.

Wheeler, L., Burke, C. J., & Reitan, R. M. (1963). An application of discriminant functions to the problem of predicting brain-damage using behavioral variables. *Perceptual and Motor Skills, 16* (Suppl. 3), 417–440.

Wilson, B. A. (1987). *Rehabilitation of memory.* New York: Guilford Press.

Wilson, B. A., Cockburn, J., Baddeley, A. D., & Hiorns, R. (1989). The development and validation of a test battery for detecting and monitoring everyday memory problems. *Journal of Clinical and Experimental Neuropsychology, 11,* 855–870.

4

The Halstead–Reitan
Neuropsychological Battery

JAMES C. REED AND HOMER B. C. REED

HISTORICAL OVERVIEW

Two books published in 1947 were of interest to psychologists. The first book was Halstead's (1947) *Brain and Intelligence*. This book served as the development of what is now known as the Halstead–Reitan Battery of Neuropsychological Tests (HRB), which for the past nearly 50 years has had a major impact on the field of human clinical neuropsychology by (1) expanding knowledge on brain–behavior relations, and (2) validating studies that have influenced clinical practice. More research has been done with this battery of tests than any other single neuropsychological battery. In the 1930s and 1940s, Halstead's work was not universally accepted. Dr. Earl Walker, a neurosurgeon and colleague of Halstead at the University of Chicago, wrote, "since this battery was quite unique and a departure from most of the previous tests of brain functions, Dr. Halstead found some reluctance on the part of classical psychologists to accept his criteria" (Reed, 1984, p. 290). Dr. Paul Bucy, another neurosurgeon and also a colleague of Halstead, wrote

> Ward Halstead developed a method of assessing the patient's emotional and psychological situation which was relatively free of subjective evaluation by the examiner. The examination could be repeated in the same way over and over again and after considerable intervals. It was criticized by some as being too mechanical but I think this criticism was false. (Reed, 1984, p. 290)

JAMES C. REED • Wayland, Massachusetts 01778   HOMER B. C. REED • Neuropsychology Laboratory, New England Medical Center, Boston, Massachusetts 02111

Change is slow to occur; there are neuropsychologists still around who have some reluctance to accept the Halstead tests and there are those today who still criticize the HRB as being too mechanical. We think that criticism is false also.

The second book was written by Ernest Gardner (1947), *Fundamentals of Neurology*. It was widely used as a text in courses on physiological psychology and it helped many graduate students develop an appreciation and understanding of the central nervous system. In Chapter 18, Gardner wrote, "Lesions of association cortex in the major hemisphere may be followed by defects in the performance of purposeful acts (*apraxias*), whereas similar lesions in the minor hemisphere are not ordinarily followed by any symptoms" (Gardner, 1947, p. 277). Sometimes change does occur. It is now known and accepted that there is definite symptomatology resulting from lesions of the minor hemisphere. Construction apraxia, visuospatial defects, inability to copy simple geometrical figures, and some would say artistic abilities are recognized as right-hemisphere functions. Part of this knowledge and recognition stems from early studies done with the HRB (Reitan, 1955a, 1959, 1964; Reitan & Davison, 1974; Wheeler, 1964; Wheeler & Reitan, 1962, 1963; Wheeler, Burke, & Reitan, 1963). These represent a sample of many studies that contributed to an understanding of brain–behavior relationships and the validation of the HRB. The early studies were comprehensive. The discriminating power of each test in the battery was investigated, and for the aphasia examination the discriminating power of each item was studied. The tests and items were analyzed not only for sensitivity to the presence or absence of brain impairment but also to whether they were right-hemisphere indicators or left-hemisphere indicators. The Wheeler et al. (1963) study was the first use of the Mahalanobis Discriminant Function (1936) in psychological research. Reitan (1994) has written an extensive review of Halstead's contributions to neuropsychology and of the HRB and has presented a discussion of many of the early validating studies and their implications for rehabilitation.

Reitan (1988) outlined a model of brain–behavior relations, and he gave criteria that tests should meet in order to assess an individual's cognitive functioning with respect to the integrity of the brain. The neuropsychological battery should (1) evaluate the full range of neuropsychological functions dependent on the brain; (2) include tests that relate to the brain generally, as well as tests that tap specific areas of cortical function; (3) include tests in the neuropsychological battery that provide an equivalent representation of both cerebral hemispheres so that a balanced interpretation of the degree of deficit may be determined; and (4) be composed of tests where each test has been carefully validated for its sensitivity to cerebral damage.

One battery that meets these criteria is the HRB, and a brief description of the specific tests follows:

1. Category Test (CT): This test is a measure of nonverbal concept formation ability. It requires abstract reasoning and logical analysis skills and

the ability to benefit from knowledge of one's errors. It is the best single test in the battery to detect the presence or absence of brain damage (Reitan, 1995b). The score is the number of errors.

2. Tactual Performance Test (TPT): The test measures complex psycho-motor problem-solving skills, memory, and incidental learning. The test is sensitive to the presence or absence of brain dysfunction; it can be used to lateralize lesions to either cerebral hemisphere; and it has some capacity to localize on an anterior–posterior dimension. The subject is blindfolded and is required to insert ten blocks of different sizes and shapes into holes on a formboard, first with the preferred hand, next with the nonpreferred hand, and finally with both hands. After the task is completed, the subject is required to draw the shape of the board and the blocks and indicate their location on the board. Six scores are obtained (1) time in seconds for the preferred hand, (2) for the nonpreferred hand, (3) for both hands, (4) for total time, (5) for memory [number of blocks correctly drawn (TPTM)], and (6) for location [the number of blocks correctly located (TPTL)]. This last score is the second-best measure for detecting presence or absence of brain impairment (Reitan, 1995b).

3. Speech Sounds Perception Test (SSPT): This test is a measure of auditory discrimination. There are 60 items. Each item consists of four nonsense syllables. The subject hears one of the syllables for each item spoken over a tape and underlines that syllable on the test form.

4. Seashore Rhythm Test (SRT): There are 30 items in this test. The subject hears pairs of rhythms and the task is to mark S when the pairs are the same and D when different. The score is the number correct. Both SSPT and SRT traditionally have been regarded as measures of concentration and attention. The tests are sensitive to presence or absence of brain impairment. Their lateralization and localization status is a matter of continuing debate.

5. Index Finger Tapping Speed (IFT): This is a test of motor speed. The score is the average number of taps in five 10-second time periods, both for the preferred and nonpreferred hand. The test can be used to lateralize lesions to one of the two hemispheres.

The foregoing measures were part of the original Halstead Battery. Reitan and colleagues have added the following measures:

6. Trailmaking Test A and B (TMTA & B): On TMTA, numbers enclosed in circles are randomly arranged on a sheet of paper. The task is to draw a line connecting the circles in order starting at 1 and going to 26. On the TMTB, numbers and letters are randomly arranged. The task is to connect the circles by alternating between the numbers and letters (1 to A, A to 2, 2 to B, . . . to L to 13.) For both A and B, the time score is the number of seconds required to complete the tasks. Errors are recorded.

7. Grip Strength (GS): A dynamometer is used to obtain GS in the right and left hands. The score is the average in kilograms for two trials for each hand.
8. Reitan Aphasia Screening Test (AST): It samples receptive and expressive language and related language functions, e.g., naming, word and phrase repetition, articulation, reading, writing, arithmetic, spelling, and left–right disorientation, and it also provides measures of the ability to copy simple geometrical figures.
9. Sensory–Perceptual (SPE): The examination covers tactile finger recognition, fingertip number writing perception, and the ability to perceive visual, auditory, and tactile stimuli presented under conditions of single and double simultaneous stimulation.

Along with the HRB, it is customary to administer the appropriate Wechsler Intelligence Scale.

THE HRB AND NORMATIVE RESEARCH

The previous section gave a bird's-eye view of the early history of the tests along with a description of the battery. The purpose of this chapter is to describe the HRB as it exists today and to delineate its place in contemporary neuropsychology, both as a research instrument and as a tool for clinical practice. The battery still remains one of the most widely used neuropsychological test batteries in the United States and Canada and increasingly is being used abroad (Sheikh, Nagdy, Townes, & Kennedy, 1987; Preiss & Hynek, 1991). For the interested reader, there is a wealth of material that describes the clinical application of the battery (Reitan, 1984; Reitan & Wolfson, 1985, 1986a,b, 1988a,b, 1992a,b, 1993). In this chapter we will emphasize work that has appeared since Parson's (1986) thoughtful review. The recent research has been directed toward the sensitivity of individual tests, the development of normative data, and clinical and scientific applications in head injury, stroke, schizophrenia, aging, various disease conditions, and rehabilitation. In recent years the merits and demerits of the "fixed" versus the "process" approach have been reviewed, discussed, and rediscussed. In the course of this chapter we will examine each of the foregoing areas.

The HRB, Aging, and Normative Data

Variables that affect performance on the HRB, in addition to the integrity of the brain, are gender, education, and age, the latter more than the preceding two, but among the foregoing the relationships are complex and there are many interactions. Fitzhugh, Fitzhugh, and Reitan (1962) found that among patients hospitalized for chronic neurological disorders, younger patients scored better than older patients on tests that require problem solving, and the two groups were not significantly different on tests that were dependent on store information. Reed and

Reitan (1963) compared younger and older persons without evidence of brain damage, and their findings also indicated that younger persons were superior to older persons on tests that depend on abstract reasoning and immediate problem solving, but the older persons were slightly superior to the younger persons on tests said to be dependent on stored memory and experiential background.

Meyerink (1982), cited by Reitan and Wolfson (1986a), used the HRB and studied 125 subjects who were grouped into the age categories of 20–29 years, 30–39 years, 40–49 years, 50–59 years, and 60–70 years. Meyerink's subjects did not have evidence of cerebral disease and his results were similar to the previous findings. He found that tests of long-standing experiences and prior learning did not show change across the age groups; there was only limited change on tests of sensory input; complex motor functions showed substantial deterioration with age but not simple motor functions; language-processing ability decreased significantly with age; visual–spatial abilities appreciably deteriorated with advancing age, particularly in the age group 60–70 years; and finally, there was a pronounced curve of deterioration among abilities that involved abstraction, reasoning, and logical analysis. The group past 60 showed the largest decrement.

In general, as described in Reitan and Wolfson's (1986a) major review, the studies have shown that on problem-solving tests of the HRB there is a steady decline on these tests with age. The decline is minimal on tests that do not require problem-solving skills but instead measure stored information or well-rehearsed skills. Measures of vocabulary and general information from the Wechsler–Bellevue represent the tests most heavily dependent on stored information, whereas the CT, TPT, and TMTB represent the extreme of the problem-solving and cognitive speed/flexibility domain.

More recent research has also shown a relation between the HRB or portions thereof to age and education. In an extensive study, Heaton, Grant, and Matthews (1986) found that among normal controls, Wechsler Adult Intelligence Scale (WAIS) variables were more closely related to education than to age, whereas the opposite was true for HRB variables. For some tests there was also a gender relationship, e.g., finger tapping and dynamometer GS were influenced by gender (men being faster and stronger).

Heaton et al. (1986) used the Russell, Neuringer, and Goldstein (1970) Average Impairment Rating (AIR) and found that for their total sample ($n = 553$) there was a correct classification of 83.4%. For the CT the classification was 74%. However, the percentage that were correctly classified varied with age and education. When grouped by age the correct percentages for AIR were: less than 40, 96.9%; 42–59, 84.3%; 60 and over, 39%. For the CT, the corresponding percentages were 89%, 70.2%, and 31%, respectively. When grouped by years of education (1) less than 12, (2) 12–15, and (3) 16 or more, the correct AIR classifications were 58.3%, and 90%, and 93%. For CT the corresponding values were 49.2%, 76.%, 89.%, respectively. In a related study, Thompson, Heaton, Matthews, and Grant (1987) compared the relationship of preferred and nonpreferred hand performances on four neuropsychological motor tasks to age, education, sex, and lateral preference. Intermanual performance differences for Finger Tapping Test, hand dynamometer, and grooved pegboard did not appear related to age, education, or sex. Intermanual differences were related to lateral preference on the Finger Tapping Test and the hand dynamometer test. Left-handed subjects showed a smaller difference between the two hands on tapping speed and grip strength, and right-handed subjects who consistently showed right preference had the largest intermanual differences. Thompson et al. (1987) also found a large age effect on the pattern of TPT performance. Subjects under 50 improved 20.5% from trial 1 to trial 2. Subjects over 50 and those with fewer than 9 years of education on average performed more slowly on the second trial with the nonpreferred hand. The authors suggested that the reason for older persons not showing improvement might stem from a reduced rate of learning in older, normal subjects. This same reason was offered for subjects of limited education who failed to improve from trial 1 to trial 2.

Yeudall, Reddon, Gill, and Stefanyk (1987) reported small correlation coefficients, from .02 to .27, between age and HRB performance. Their subjects were male and female volunteers ($n = 225$) and restricted in age range from 15 to 40, which may have attenuated their findings.

Moehle and Long (1989) used a sample of 86 distributed over six age-cohort groups. Of six tests from the HRB, age effects were observed for five, with the most sensitive being the TPTL; they did not find an age effect for finger tapping, which may have been due to a lack of statistical power. Elias, Robbins, Walter, and Shultz (1993) ($n = 427$) found a significant linear trend across age cohorts not only for finger tapping but also for the other measures in the HRB. The standardized discriminant coefficients for the multivariable linear trends for the individual tests ranged from a high of .35 to a low of .13. The rank order for the tests was TPTL, CT, TMTA, TMTB, TPT Total Time, IFT, and TPT Memory. There was a gender difference—men tapped faster than women—on the IFT. While the Elias et al. study reported an age–gender interaction for the CT, the effect size was quite low.

Leckliter and Matarazzo (1989, p. 509) made an intensive survey of the literature and stated that demographic variables such as age, education, IQ, and gender have significant effects on the HRB performance. Among their conclusions were:

1. In the HRB performance of normal individuals, there is an interaction effect between age and education. The effects of education are more apparent in younger subjects than in elderly subjects. Among younger subjects, individuals with more education perform better on HRB measures than do individuals with less education.
2. The effects of age and IQ on HRB scores appear additive, such that older, brighter individuals perform better than older, less bright individuals, and older individuals perform less well than their younger IQ-equated cohorts.
3. Gender differences are found on the finger tapping and dynamometer subtests of the HRB and show that men perform more quickly and with

greater strength than do women. Some investigators have found gender differences on TPT Total Time (men scored better than women), Aphasia Screening, and Speech Sounds Perception tests (women scored better than men), but these results have not held up consistently across studies.

The foregoing studies are illustrative of much of the recent research with the HRB, which has been directed toward questions of refinement and precision of the battery. The studies provide empirical evidence for what experts who have long worked with the HRB know, i.e., that level of performance on a wide variety of neuropsychological tests is related to age and education.

THE HRB AND CLINICAL INTERPRETATION

In clinical interpretation, age and education are used as modifying scores, although subjectively. For example, if two patients each age 50 had a CT error score of 50, the significance given to this score will vary depending on the education. Patient A has a history of heavy alcohol consumption, has 8 years of formal education, and has always worked as a laborer. For him, 50 errors might be considered a good performance. Assume that patient B is a brilliant neurosurgeon and has achieved the rank of admiral in the Navy. This patient also has a history of heavy alcohol consumption. Fifty errors on the CT may be indicative of significant impairment of brain functions. Hence, research studies and expert clinical judgment are in agreement that the significance of impairment in level of performance on the HRB cannot be evaluated accurately independently of the age and education of the patient. One method of increasing objectivity in evaluation is through the use of demographically corrected T scores.

Traditionally, impairment on the HRB has been determined by the use of the Halstead cutoff scores (HCS) (Reitan & Wolfson, 1985). For each test in the battery, there is a cutoff beyond which the patient's performance is said to be impaired, and the percentage of tests exceeding the cutoff has been used to determine a general impairment index (II). Using HCS and the II, skilled clinicians have been able to evaluate a given patient's performance with a high degree of reliability and validity. Interpretation of the HRB scores can be enhanced by use of Adult Severity Ranges (ASR) (Reitan and Wolfson, 1985), which permits the score for each test in the battery to be rated as to degree of impairment. For example, a Category error score of 45 or less represents a normal performance, 46 to 65 errors is indicative of mild impairment, 65 or more errors represents serious impairment. Nevertheless, the use of HCS and ASR basically relies on a single set of norms, and accuracy of interpretation depends on the skill of the individual clinician, which may vary widely, depending on training and experience, from person to person. Parsons (1986) has expressed concern about the lack of uniform age and educational norms for the HRB. Similar concerns have been stated by Cullum,

Thompson, and Heaton (1989), and they have urged caution in the interpretation of the results of the HRB when based on HCS, particularly for older adults.

Heaton, Grant, and Matthews (1991) have published comprehensive norms for an extended battery of the HRB. These are tables of demographically corrected T scores for age, education, and gender. The T scores have a mean of 50 and a standard deviation of 10. Tentative guidelines for clinical application are T scores of 1–19, severe impairment; 20–24, moderate to severe impairment; 25–29, moderate impairment; 30–34, mild to moderate impairment; 35–39, mild impairment; and 40–44, below average/borderline.

The Heaton et al. (1991) tables represent an important contribution to the refinement and clinical interpretation of the scores from the HRB. However, this statement is not universally accepted, and the value of the T scores has been a matter of debate. Reitan and Wolfson (1995a) point out that the effect of age and education on the neuropsychological performances of normal subjects may differ from that of brain-damaged subjects. Hence, the use of attribute variables may be misleading. However, their argument does not negate the fact that one way to determine the extent of impairment in a person who has had, for example, a recent closed head injury is to compare that person to a cohort control group of similar age, education, and sex.

Merits and Demerits of T Scores

The value of a T or standard score is that it provides a common metric for comparing raw scores on tests of different measures, e.g., vocabulary, arithmetic, Halstead CT, TMTB, and so forth. Clearly, the use of T or other standard scores is not new in psychological practice. The adult Wechsler Scales are presented in standard scores, and comparisons can be made among the individual subtests. The Wechsler adult IQ values have been adjusted for age but not for education. Obviously, for a T score to be meaningful, the person being examined must be representative of the group on whom the T scores were derived, but this is also true for HCSs, ASRs, and for all psychological tests. It is not unique to neuropsychological tests.

The use of demographically corrected T scores, however, is only an aid to effective clinical interpretation. If they are used to assist one's thinking, they can be extremely valuable. When used as a substitute for one's thinking, they have little if any merit. Accurate interpretation of the HRB scores depends on four methods of inference: (1) level of performance, (2) intertest differences or ratio scores, (3) pathognomonic signs, and (4) comparisons and contrasts based on test performance that involve the two sides of the body (Reitan & Wolfson, 1985). Demographically corrected T scores only provide evidence of level of performance. Furthermore, the T scores in Heaton et al. (1991) do not consider the quality of the educational experience. A graduate of the local college in Podunkville has 16 years of formal education; so does the graduate of Harvard University. The two educational experiences are probably not equivalent. Brain impairment cannot be inferred only on the basis of level of performance. However, given that brain impairment can be inferred from other methods of inference and/or historical data, demographically corrected T scores can be used to infer the extent of impairment or the adequacy of the performance for a person of given age, education, and sex. Heaton et al. (1991) provide a number of caveats concerning the use of demographically corrected scores. The authors rightfully caution against an over-reliance on a purely statistical approach in clinical interpretation. They indicate, by example, how a T score can fall into the impaired range as a result of only a small deviation from a perfect performance in a variable, which, among normal subjects, has a skewed raw score distribution and a small standard deviation. For such variables the clinical interpretation should be based heavily on the patient's actual performance. The authors' caution and caveats should be taken seriously.

NEUROPSYCHOLOGICAL EVALUATION: TEST SCORES AND T SCORES

For illustrative and heuristic purposes we present the findings on a patient of two evaluations that were performed at approximately a 2-year interval (see Table 1). The purpose is to compare differences and similarities in interpretation based on clinical experience and HCS versus demographically corrected T scores. There are places where our judgment as to the degree of impairment differs markedly from the rating of the T scores. At other places, no important disparity exists. We are presenting only some of the data because our purpose is to highlight ratings based on test and T scores, rather than give an exhaustive clinical interpretation and report. We did not include findings from the Wechsler Memory Scale (WMS), because our administrative procedures differ from those in the Heaton et al. (1991) manual. We did not report on the AST, because we do not use quantitative scoring for this test. However, at the first examination, the results from both of these instruments were unremarkable and noncontributory.

Neuropsychological Evaluation 1

Name: Dr. X
Age: 70
Education: 20
Marital Status: Married
Occupation: Physician, now retired, formerly Chief of Medicine at a large hospital.
Presenting Complaint and Brief History: The patient was a 70-year-old retired male physician, who had developed complaints of brief memory losses, concentration difficulties, and minor mood swings. He had been seeking psychiatric help and was referred by his psychiatrist to help assess current functional status. The patient's primary care physician stated that there was a history of heavy drinking,

TABLE 1. HRB Test Scores and *T* Scores for Two Evaluations

Tests	Exam 1		Exam 2	
	Test score	*T* score	Test-score	*T* score
Intelligence tests				
Verbal IQ	122	37	112	28
Performance IQ	114	42	105	31
Full Scale IQ	120	37	109	25
Information	13	38	11	29
Digit Span	12	53	10	44
Vocabulary	15	48	11	30
Arithmetic	7	19	10	31
Comprehension	15	47	7	34
Similarities	12	43	8	26
Picture Completion	10	44	7	34
Picture Arrangement	6	40	9	53
Block Design	7	32	6	28
Object Assembly	10	54	6	38
Digit Symbol	7	43	5	39
Neuropsychological tests				
Category	104	36	114	25
TPT				
R	4.5	64	3.8	72
L	6.3	52	4.2	60
B	2.7	59	3.5	51
T	13.5	56	11.5	60
Memory	6	40	6	40
Location	2	49	4	40
SRT	27	53	29	62
SSPT	7	40	11	33
IFT (dominant)	61	69	42	38
IFT (nondominant)	44	46	31	26
GS (dominant) (kg)	37	42	25	27
GS (nondominant) (kg)	35	44	34	28
TMT A (sec)	59	36	61	32
TMT B (sec)	110	42	315	17

but the patient denied it and said that he did not drink anymore than his friends did, but he admitted to visiting his friends frequently.

Behavior: The patient appeared somewhat anxious during the evaluation, but he was cooperative, oriented in all spheres, and his speech was fluent and goal oriented.

Tests: Wechsler Adult Intelligence Scale, Wechsler Memory Scale, Halstead–Reitan Neuropsychological Tests, Trails A & B.

1. *How well is this patient functioning?* The WAIS IQ values have been adjusted for age and the *T* scores have been adjusted for age and education. The VIQ

and FSIQ values are above the 90th percentile rank, and the PIQ is at approximately the 85th percentile rank. The IQ values indicate that for the patient's age group he scored at a relatively high level, but they do not indicate whether impairment might be present. For the patient's age and education, the T scores indicate that the IQ values are in the range of below average/borderline to mild impairment, but they give no indication of how well or at what level the patient is functioning.

With the exception of the arithmetic subtest score, the WAIS verbal subtest scores indicate that the patient is functioning at the upper end of the average range or better. The patient is able to express himself, to communicate, and has a satisfactory understanding of social situations. The T scores, again with the exception of arithmetic, indicate borderline to mild impairment in selective areas but satisfactory performances in the remaining ones. The arithmetic score is probably spuriously low and should be disregarded. The patient made some simple calculation errors, and there was much intratest variability, i.e., he failed some of the simple questions and passed the more difficult questions. The performance did not reflect a deficiency in the calculation process; rather, it probably resulted from anxiety or nervousness. The WAIS performance subtest scores suggest mild impairment. Three of the five performance subtest scores are somewhat low. The T scores indicate below average/borderline to mild/moderate impairment on four of the five subtest scores.

2. *Is cognitive decline present?* The PIQ appears questionably low, but we would interpret the VIQ and FSIQ as adequate if not satisfactory. The T scores, however, indicate mild impairment for both VIQ and FSIQ and below average/borderline impairment for PIQ.

Among the subtest scores there is evidence of cognitive decline. The WAIS subtest scaled scores, which have a mean of 10 and a standard deviation of 3, are based on a reference group in the age range of 20–34 (Wechsler, 1955). At examination 1, 8 of the 11 WAIS scores were in the average range or below. Only three of the WAIS scores were above the average range. The patient was a successful physician, chief of a large department in a major hospital, and it is unlikely that as a younger man he would have performed in the average range or below on the majority of the tests from the WAIS. The T scores, which are corrected for gender, education, and age, provide consistent evidence of cognitive decline. Seven of the 11 scores indicate borderline impairment or worse for a 70-year-old male with 20 years of education.

3. *Is there evidence of impairment on the neuropsychological tests?* Clinically, the neuropsychological scores indicate moderate to severe impairment on the CT, moderate impairment on the location component of the TPT, and mild impairment on TMTA & B. Hence, the three scores most sensitive to presence or absence of brain impairment indicate dysfunction.

The T scores indicate only mild impairment on the CT, a normal performance on the location component of the TPT, and a borderline performance on Trails B.

On two of these three measures there is a difference between our clinical interpretation based on test scores and what is reflected by the T scores. We do not regard 104 errors on the CT as mild impairment. We would state that cognitively this man is a hollow shell of what he probably once was.

Among the remaining tests, there is no essential disagreement between clinical interpretation from the test scores and interpretation based on the T scores. For example, our interpretation of seven errors on SSPT is that it is an adequate performance. The T score value of 40 indicates borderline impairment, but that is a trivial difference.

In summary, both sets of scores indicate probable cognitive decline, and there is evidence of impairment of brain functions. However, the two data sets agree that the patient probably functions at a sufficiently high level so that it would not interfere with his lifestyle as a retired physician, which consisted mainly of playing golf, meeting with his friends, and puttering around the house.

4. *What is the basis of the impairment?* The basis of the impairment is uncertain. There was no evidence of a focal neurological disease. There were no pathognomic signs. There were no significant left–right differences. The main evidence of impairment comes from the discrepancies between the expectations based on the patient's educational history and the many impaired performances on the neuropsychological tests. The results raise the question of a possible dementing disease process, but the findings also may stem from impairment associated with chronic ethanol abuse and possible adverse vascular changes. With respect to the presenting complaint of brief memory lapses and concentration problems, the lapses appear to be symptomatic of a more general problem in information processing and storage.

5. *What are the recommendations?* The obvious recommendations are to (1) discuss the nature of the problem with the patient and to give counsel about the alternative etiologies of the impairments; (2) consider a reduction in alcohol intake; (3) recommend neurological workup to rule out reversible dementias; and (4) monitor and repeat neuropsychological evaluation in a year.

Neuropsychological Evaluation 2

A second evaluation was performed on this same patient 2 years later. The test scores and T scores are given on the right-hand side of Table 1.

The patient had a dementing disease and expired within 4 years of the original evaluation. We examined him twice more. At the fourth examination he was so impaired that most of the tests had to be discontinued. The second set of test results (Table 1), when compared with the original scores, shows the deterioration in the patient's level of functioning. The majority of the T scores reflect moderate impairment, but the decline can be seen by examining either the change in the T scores or in the test scores. It is now a matter of semantics as to whether one wants to call a score moderately impaired or severely impaired.

There was much more of an adverse change on TMTB than in the CT score. Why? There was more room for deterioration on the TMTB test. The Trails score was not limited by a ceiling effect. We initially interpreted the CT score as moderately to severely impaired. If the impairment had been more severe, the patient probably would not have been able to complete the CT. The level of impairment now reflected by the T score is more nearly consistent with the clinical interpretation than was the original.

There was no adverse change on the TPT. In fact, the second performance might be somewhat better than the first. This is indeed a surprising finding and there is no logical explanation for it, except to say that sometimes the test performances are not internally consistent.

For reiteration, the T scores show the level of performance in comparison to persons of equal age and education. VIQs and PIQs from the WAIS can be compared to persons of equal age but not education. The T scores may show areas where deterioration has occurred, but they may not reflect the patient's level of competence. At the second evaluation, the patient earned a full-scale IQ at approximately the 75th percentile rank for his age group. Both the VIQ and the PIQ were above average for the patient's age group. They indicate that the patient is still functioning at a level where he can probably adjust to routine environmental demands. On the WAIS vocabulary test, the Heaton T score was 30, which shows mild to moderate impairment for a 72-year-old man with 20 years of education. The WAIS score of 11 can be compared to the reference group, and it indicates (1) an average score on the vocabulary subtest, and (2) that the patient functions at a level where he can communicate his desires and needs to others. Test scores and T scores can both be useful in clinical interpretation.

At evaluation 1, there was a major difference between clinical judgment and the T scores concerning the degree of impairment indicated by the CT error score and the TPTL score. How does one resolve these differences? One thinks! First, there is no "right answer." The earlier-cited research has shown that among older patients HRB scores are more apt to give false positives than false negatives. Second, one recognizes that terms such as borderline, mild, moderate, severe, and so on are ratings of neuropsychological deficiency. They do not constitute a ratio scale, nor is there an isomorphic relation between these ratings and severity as listed in either *Diagnostic and Statistical Manual of Mental Disorders,* 4th edition (DSM-IV) (American Psychiatric Association, 1994) or in actual life adjustment. Third, one looks at a given score in the context of other findings. In other words, a clinical report should be based on a complete set of findings, not just one score. Still, it is not that simple. There are times when a single score, if valid, cannot be ignored.

Subjectively, on the neuropsychological tests, some T scores seem to underrate impairment. Conversely, for some of the WAIS scores, they appear to overrate impairment. Further research on these points is needed, particularly on persons at the extreme ends of the distribution. In the meantime, one balances the severity rating of *T* scores, the HCS, and ASR against each other and against one's clinical experience. The combined clinical experience with the HRB for the two authors extends over three score and ten years—the allotted time of man.

T Scores and Test Scores

It is important to understand the precise nature of *T* scores in order to use them properly. The normative data provided by Heaton et al. (1991) should add to the usefulness of the HRB, particularly among older patients. For a geriatric population, particularly, the *T* scores should provide a guard against false positives. They should also assist in determining the degree of neuropsychological impairment in the patient with lesser education: the 50-year-old laborer with 6 years of formal education who suffered a head injury, or the 67-year-old female with 5 years of formal education who has her first psychiatric admission, is disheveled, and is presenting with mild depression. Is organicity present? The *T* scores should increase objectivity and reliability of interpretation between and among clinicians. They do not guard against either a lack of understanding or misuse for what they are intended. There is no fail-safe mechanism to protect against clinical incompetence. Guarding against errors in judgment is a matter of eternal vigilance.

Tangential to the discussion of *T* scores is the question of sensitivity and specificity of the HRB, addressed to a degree by Parsons (1986) and by Heaton et al. (1991). This issue is a complicated and technical matter: sensitivity to what and specificity for what? Is the HRB sensitive to presence or absence of brain impairment? Is the HRB sensitive to type of lesion? Is it sensitive to location of lesion? For each of the foregoing questions substitute the word *specificity* for *sensitivity*. How does the false-positive rate compare with the false-negative rate? The base rate in the population must be known before quantitative answers to these questions can be provided. For each, a large number of patients needs to be tested. We do not wish to minimize the importance of the problem, but from a practical standpoint, it is almost impossible to gather the relevant data.

FIXED AND FLEXIBLE BATTERIES

The previous section showed how neuropsychology appraisal and behavioral changes can be measured with the HRB or a fixed battery. Arguments still continue over the merits of "fixed versus flexible batteries." Benton (1992) recommended combining the strengths of each in assessing the patient by developing a standard battery that could be administered in 60 to 90 minutes and following with flexible procedures, which would depend on the referring question or leads detected from the standard battery. Reitan and Wolfson (1994a) have recommended achieving flexibility by evaluating test results through comparative performances of a patient on an array of neuropsychological tests.

We did not find any studies that made a direct comparison between the HRB and flexible batteries. Within fixed batteries the main thrust has been between the merits of the HRB and the Luria–Nebraska Battery (LNB). Kane (1991) provided a comprehensive review of these issues. His findings indicated that both the HRB and LNB are sensitive measures of the integrity of the cerebral hemispheres. A substantial correlation exists between the LNB and the scores from the HRB. The hit rate for both batteries (false positive and false negative) is approximately the same. Though not stated by Kane, it is safe to say that LNB relies more on a sign approach than does the HRB. Higher cognitive functions, i.e., abstraction, mental flexibility, concept formation, and so on, are probably better assessed by the HRB than by the LNB.

Goldstein (1986) has also reviewed the similarities and differences of the HRB and LNB. The thrust of his analysis was that in many areas of assessment their efficiency was essentially the same. Differences between the two batteries exist depending on the question being asked, distinguishing between brain-damaged and chronic schizophrenic patients, test performances and the chronicity of an illness, the capacity to make precise localizations, and so on. Shelly and Goldstein (1982) did a factor analysis and compared the two batteries with respect to their psychometric relations. They found that both batteries assessed similar areas of function and there is a high correlation between them when it comes to estimating degree of impairment. They found that both batteries measure language, nonverbal cognitive abilities, and perceptual motor skills. There were, however, differences in emphasis between the two batteries in these areas. The factor loadings for the LNB on the language factor were high relative to the Halstead–Reitan, while the reverse was true for the other factors.

Kane, Parsons, Goldstein, and Moses (1987) had three experienced neuropsychologists use the HRB and the LNB to rate 92 subjects (46 control and 46 brain damaged) for presence and extent of brain impairment. With either battery the raters were accurate in judging the presence or absence of brain damage, and there was a high degree of consistency among the raters and test batteries for both presence and extent of brain impairment.

The foregoing studies show high comparability between the LNB and the HRB, but discrepant findings have been reported. Bryson, Silverstein, Nathan, and Stephen (1993) studied 55 schizophrenic and 64 affective disorder patients. Each patient was given both batteries and the overall rate of dysfunction was higher for the HRB (65%) compared to the LNB (36%). The discrepancies were in the direction of greater impairment on the HRB. In terms of impaired versus nonimpaired neuropsychological performance, the agreement for the two batteries was 65.2% for the schizophrenic patients and 67.5% for those with affective disorder. The reasons for the disjunction between this study and the previously cited investigations are unknown. The patient population may have different demographic characteristics or the ambience of the laboratory may have an effect. The majority of these studies show high agreement between HRB and LNB, and this last study may represent just an aberrant finding.

Returning to the fixed versus flexible arguments, they continue, and it is unlikely that they will be resolved. Our own view is that a fixed battery provides a standard amount of information, and after one has obtained this information, there is time to be flexible, and flexibility is frequently necessary.

The HRB provides a wide range of information, but with adults we routinely supplement it with either the WMS or the WMS-R. The final section of the CT depends on memory. Incidental memory is reflected in the memory and location scores from the TPT. However, in a geriatric population one of the most frequently mentioned complaints is memory deficiency, and one needs more data than are provided by the measurement of memory in the HRB. Furthermore, there are occasional patients with memory complaints and memory deficiencies who do not show defects on the HRB. One needs to be able to obtain enough data to describe in one or more paragraphs the practical problems that the memory presents for a given patient. The WMS-R offers possible advantages over the older version, but the downside in terms of time required to administer and score the test must be carefully considered. The Rey–Osterrieth Complex Visual Figures test in association with a verbal memory of some kind, e.g., Wechsler stories, offers another approach to flexibility.

Patients are frequently referred with a presenting complaint of attention deficit hyperactivity disorder (ADHD), and disrupted attention is frequently a concomitant of neurological disease and head injury. Formal tests or rating scales plus information from an interview and history can provide valuable information concerning ADHD. There is no unique pattern on the HRB that is specifically diagnostic of ADHD, but impaired scores on the CT, TPTL, and TMTB can indicate whether the attention deficits are associated with cortical impairment. In addition, the scores from SRT, SSPT, TMT, and the Sensory–Perceptual examination can frequently furnish useful information concerning attention problems. Good performances on those measures almost certainly rule out a significant ADHD. Furthermore, a detailed observation is recorded by the technician administering the test and can be focused to include attention and concentration as specific matters to be noted and described. Except in rare occasions, we do not believe that additional measures are needed to evaluate ADHD.

Another area where flexibility is necessary is in the evaluation of elderly patients, because for many of them the physical and mental demands of the HRB are too overwhelming, so that they negate the possibility of differential description of mental/neurological deficits. There is no specific solution to this problem, because it may require many different approaches. For some patients the administration of a dementia rating scale should be adequate. For others, a detailed history should be sufficient to identify the progression of a dementing disease process. The patients for whom IQ and educational data suggest possible congenital limitations, but for whom one is still interested in providing a differential description of neurologically based losses, the consideration of normative data that permits adjustments for age and education is essential.

Finally, it is necessary to be flexible when poor performances are encountered that may signify neurological impairment, but where it is also necessary to be sure that the performances represent reliable and dependable findings. Deviant IQ test performances can be approached by alternate tests such as the Stanford–Binet scale, the Leiter International Performance Scale, the Peabody Picture Vocabulary Test—Revised (PPVT-R), or the Raven Progressive Matrices test. The Leiter scale can be used to separate language from nonlanguage cognitive deficit. The Raven test can be used to separate mental from motor problems. The Peabody and Binet tests can be used simply as cross-checks on the Wechsler VIQ. A word of caution is in order. Among patients with validly low verbal skills, the PPVT-R may over-estimate their verbal ability, because it is more a measure of receptive or recognition ability than verbal expression. The SRT, SSPT, IFT, and dynamometer test can always be repeated, because there is not significant practice effect on these.

The preceding paragraphs indicate possible defects for shortcomings in the HRB, or at least where it may be necessary to supplement it. Perhaps we should add a parallel on defects or shortcomings or the need for flexibility in the neuro-psychologist, since those problems are undoubtedly of much greater clinical importance than are the problems in the tests and measurements part. Even very sophisticated neuropsychological judges have bad days and personal blind spots or biases. Human fallibility interacts with and enlarges upon psychometric short-comings and defects, and the foregoing considerations represent a limited approach only to the latter source of error variance. In sum, much of the argument between the fixed and flexible is superficial. In a comprehensive neuro-psychological evaluation, one obtains a standard amount of information and proceeds from there on an as needed basis.

THE HRB AND REHABILITATION

The earlier sections of this chapter were concerned with diagnostic assessment and clinical appraisal. An equally important aspect of neuropsychological evaluation is to assist in treatment planning. What is the progress and state of the HRB in rehabilitation and cognitive retraining? On the basis of face validity the HRB can contribute a significant amount to counseling and planning for rehabilitation purposes. The umbrella of the HRB covers a wide domain of cognitive functions. If a 56-year-old physician makes 100 errors on the CT, he perhaps should be counseled against continuing his practice. If an artist shows right-hemisphere impairment and secondary visual–spatial deficiencies, perhaps the artist should seek another means of employment. For a geriatric patient the level of performance on the HRB may provide useful information as to whether the patient should go to a nursing home or a rest home or whether the patient can manage at home with minimal supervision. Lezak (1987) stated that the integrity of the executive functions and the capacity for taking an abstract attitude must be evaluated in order to identify realistic treatment goals.

Goldstein (1987) compared the HRB with the LNB for use in rehabilitation, and emphasized the necessity of having a comprehensive neuropsychological evaluation. However, one example was related to determining the level at which to approach the patient, with the treatment based on behavioral therapeutic lines instead of on patterns of deficit based on the test scores. Another example showed that the neuropsychological evaluation was important in order to direct the patient into an area where he might have the capacity to succeed. In other words, the neuropsychological data provided information concerning treatment alternatives as opposed to indicating a specific plan of rehabilitation. Intuitively, it should be obvious that the HRB provides measures of integrity of the executive function, and, through pattern analysis, areas where the patient is likely to succeed and where the patient is likely to fail can be identified. The HRB can provide measures of baseline functioning, and it can be used to monitor and assess progress. In spite of these potentials, to date there has been little objective evidence as to the efficacy of the HRB in planning rehabilitation or in cognitive retraining.

Reitan and Wolfson (1988b, 1992b) have described the Reitan Evaluation of Hemispheric Abilities and Brain Improvement Training (REHABIT) program. The rationale for REHABIT is given in detail. The program is based on five tracks that stem from the Reitan–Wolfson model of brain functions. Track A contains materials designed for developing expressive and receptive language and verbal skills. Track B codes language and verbal materials and also integrates abstraction, reasoning, logical analysis, and organizational skills. Track C includes tasks that focus on reasoning, organization, planning, and abstraction skills. Track D emphasizes abstraction abilities that require visual–spatial, sequential, and manipulatory skills. Track E is devoted to fundamental aspects of visual–spatial and manipulatory abilities. There have been limited studies of the effectiveness of the REHABIT program. Encouraging results have been reported by Reitan and Sena (1983), Reitan and Wolfson (1988b), Reitan (1988), Sena (1985, 1986), and Sena and Sena (1986a,b).

Three research problems need to be addressed in cognitive retraining and remediation programs. The first is to show the relation between the assessment and the procedures used in the training program. In evaluating a dyslexic male, it is necessary to determine the extent of his sight vocabulary and whether or not he has word-attack skills. Knowing, however, that the person is deficient in sight vocabulary and word-attack does not tell one what method should be used to teach him. Second, is the problem one of transfer of training. If a patient is weak in abstraction skills and is given training on the CT, does this training transfer to other situations? Third, the evidence is indeed scanty that shows that brain-impaired patients need materials that differ from non-brain-impaired subjects. Brain impairment may affect the level that the patient may eventually achieve, or brain impairment may affect the amount of time it takes to reach a given level, but it does not follow that the laws of learning for the brain-impaired differ from the normal. A patient who is unable to read needs to develop a sight vocabulary, develop word-attack skills, differentiate between main ideas and details, and draw inferences and predict outcomes. Much is known about how to teach reading. It is unknown whether brain-impaired patients need different instructional methods and materials from the non-brain-impaired to achieve a given educational goal. The same statement applies to cognitive retraining.

Meier, Benton, and Diller (1987) edited a book on neuropsychological rehabilitation. The HRB is described in only one out of a total of 18 chapters. There are nine chapters devoted to international neuropsychological rehabilitation programs. In none of these nine chapters is there a citation either to REHABIT or the HRB. At present, and not surprisingly, the HRB is much more widely used in diagnostic and assessment areas than in rehabilitation programs. In general, whether one uses a fixed battery or a flexible battery, the relation between evaluation and retraining and/or rehabilitation needs to be clarified, and at present comprehensive research answers are lacking.

EVALUATING THE HRB TESTS

Thus far in this chapter we have emphasized the clinical application of the HRB; but to improve the clinical usefulness of a battery there must be a continuing effort to examine the individual test in order to determine its usefulness in the battery, clarify what the test measures, determine its lateralizing and/or localizing properties, or determine the test's specific value in distinguishing between brain-impaired and non-brain-impaired subjects. In this section we will review research investigations that pertain to specific HRB tests. In aggregate, the studies represent important steps in the process needed to refine neuropsychological measures.

Category Test

Abstraction, reasoning, mental flexibility, and problem-solving skills in general are processes that are impaired by brain damage. The CT is a measure of non-verbal concept formation, and its psychometric properties, validity as a measure of brain damage, and relation to neurological diseases have been widely investigated. In 1993, at the American Psychological Association annual meetings, there was a symposium on the history of the CT (Choca, Laatsch, Wetzel, Agresti, 1993). The participants displayed a bibliography of more than 200 published studies on the CT. The test has been used for more than 50 years and is relatively unchanged in content and administration since it was first introduced. Few other psychological tests have achieved this same standard.

Kane (1991) observed that among tests of abstraction—CT, Wisconsin Card Sorting Test (WCST), the abstraction section of the Shipley Institute of Living Scale, and Raven's Progressive Matrices—the correlation coefficients have been modest and it would be an error to use them interchangeably. Goldberg et al. (1988) found statistically significant correlations between CT total errors and WCST but generally low common variance. Perrine (1993) related performances on the WCST and CT to each other and to measures of concept formation drawn from the cognitive psychology literature. He reported that WCST bore a stronger relationship to attribute identification problems than to rule-learning tasks. He found the opposite for the CT. Donders and Kirsch (1991) studied a heterogeneous group of brain-damaged patients and reported a correlation between WCST and the Booklet Category Test (BCT) of .34. They recommended replication with different test batteries and especially with the traditional CT, which supports the conclusion that tests that are said to measure the same trait, e.g., abstraction, should not be used interchangeably.

Halstead (1947) believed that the CT was particularly impaired by lesions of the frontal lobe, and recent reports have also referred to the CT as a frontal lobe measure (Farmer, 1994). However, specific studies (Scheibel, Hannay, & Meyers, 1993; Reitan & Wolfson, 1995b) that compared patients with frontal lobe lesions with cerebral but not frontal lesions confirmed what Reitan (1964) found earlier: to wit, the CT is no more sensitive to frontal lobe lesions than to other cerebral lesions. The CT should be viewed as a general indicator of cerebral impairment.

Seashore Rhythm and Speech Sounds Perception Tests

These two tests traditionally have been regarded as measures of concentration and attention. Their validity for distinguishing between brain-impaired and non-brain-impaired patients has been well documented (Wheeler et al., 1963; Lezak, 1983). However, there has been disagreement concerning the lateralizing significance of the two measures and whether they are equally sensitive to lesions of either hemisphere. Reitan and Wolfson (1985) concluded that many of the beliefs concerning the SRT and SSPS with respect to lateralization, localization, and general usefulness were not supported by the results of empirical studies. It was as though the statements represented folklore as opposed to experimental evidence. Reitan and Wolfson (1989) showed that non-brain-damaged groups were effectively discriminated from brain-damaged groups by their performances on SRT. They did not find any significant differences on SRT between or among groups of left, right, or generalized cerebral dysfunction. They concluded that brain damage, regardless of lateralization, adversely affects performance on SRT.

In a similar study, Reitan and Wolfson (1990) showed that patients with left cerebral lesions performed more poorly on VIQ than did subjects with right cerebral vascular lesions, but on SSPT the lateralization effect was not demonstrated for the two groups or for patients with left and right traumatic cerebral injures. Sherer, Parsons, Nixon, and Adams (1991) also used the SSPT and SRT and compared the test performances of patients with left, right, and diffuse cerebral impairment against one another and against a pseudoneurological group. Consistent with previous findings, SSPT and SRT were found to be valid measures of brain impairment, but neither test distinguished among the three brain-damaged groups.

Sherer et al. (1991) calculated an attention index from the patient's WMS Digits Total and Mental Control scores. They found significant Pearson product-moment correlation coefficients between the attention index and SRT and SSPT, but when they controlled for the Average Impairment Rating (Russell et al., 1970), the correlation remained statistically significant but of low magnitude. They concluded that there was no evidence to suggest that SSPT and SRT were specifically associated with attention compared to other neuropsychological tests. They implied that attention and concentration were broad neuropsychological functions and likely to be impaired by brain injury, and they questioned whether these tests should be routinely administered as parts of the HRB.

The foregoing remarks overlook the difficulty in generalizing from the effects of a single test considered in isolation and a test used as part of a battery. When good scores are obtained on SRT and SSPT, failures on other parts of the battery should not then be attributed to lack of attention and concentration. Good scores on SRT and SSPT may aid in indicating the degree of recovery or the level of mental stability that a patient has reached. In the clinical evaluation of a patient, good scores on SSPT and SRT may provide more useful information than do poor scores. The argument for dropping a test or tests is neither as simple nor as straightforward as it may appear.

Tactual Performance Test

This is one of the most difficult tests in the HRB battery, and certainly it is the most physically exhausting test, particularly for geriatric patients. There is some controversy over its usefulness (Lezak, 1983) as well as its validity at different age levels. Thompson et al. (1987) found that among older normal subjects it is common on TPT not to show an improvement from trial 1 (T1) to trial 2 (T2). Thompson and Heaton (1991) compared normal persons ($n = 96$), who improved from T1 to T2, with a matched group ($n = 96$) (age within 1 year, education within 2 years), who did not improve from T1 to T2, on 19 neuropsychological measures. Statistically significant mean differences were found in favor of the improved group on AIR, WAIS FSIQ, left-hand performance on Grooved Pegboard, nonverbal measures from WAIS, and CT, but the differences were sufficiently small so that practical implications were minimal. The authors cautioned against interpreting slight decrements on TPT-1 to TPT-2 as indicating an acquired lesion of the right cerebral hemisphere. The TPTL score has been regarded as one of the most sensitive HRB measures to cerebral dysfunction. Heaton et al. (1991) reported that beyond the age of 60 the measure has little or no potential to detect neurological disorders in older subjects.

Clark and Klonoff (1988) attempted to determine whether the six-block TPT (TPT-6) might be a useful substitute for the ten-block board. They found that among older patients (mean age, 55) studied to determine the effects of coronary bypass surgery, the TPT-6 reliability coefficients and internal consistency measures were stable over time, and they reported that TPT-6 takes one half to one third the time to administer compared with TPT-10. Russell (1985) found (1) satisfactory discriminative validity for the TPT-6 in terms of differentiating brain-damaged from non-brain-damaged subjects; (2) that TPT-10 was inadequate for severe damage, but TPT-6 could be used; and (3) that TPT-10 and TPT-6 were highly correlated. However, further investigations on the TPT-6 need to be made before using it as a substitute.

The foregoing studies looked at the TPT in terms of differentiating the brain-damaged from normal subjects or in terms of its validity with respect to age and to the meaning of improvements or lack of improvement from T1 to T2. In terms of evaluating an individual patient, a more basic question is how valuable is the TPT? As previously indicated, the TPT is a stressful test, and Lezak (1983) has argued that the test creates a degree of suffering and distress that "does not warrant the use of an instrument that may give very little information in return" (p. 462).

Heilbronner and Parsons (1989) have provided an alternative point of view. In an insightful article they analyzed the TPT results of four patients who were referred for neuropsychological evaluation. They gave detailed examples of the kinds of analyses that might be made that would provide information concerning the patient's cognitive-processing skills. For example, "What steps did you go through to help you fit the blocks into the spaces?" (p. 262), or "How did you try to remember where the blocks were located on the board?" (p. 262). They indicated that the TPT can provide unique data about a person's response to an unfamiliar situation and how the location score may identify subtle difficulties in incidental recall, and they stated the necessity of developing the patient's trust and preparing the patient for a challenging task. After all, finger tapping can also be onerous if the patient views the testing situation as a hostile one. We believe the TPT is useful, particularly in terms of its psychomotor component, but there are two questions: (1) Does it add validity in a battery? and (2) Is it useful in and of itself for an individual patient?

General Neuropsychological Deficit Scale

The General Neuropsychological Deficit Scale (GNDS) is not a test. Rather, it is a measure of a patient's overall neuropsychological competency. In contrast, the impairment index is a consistency index—the percentage of tests on which a patient is impaired—not a severity index. The GNDS was developed by Reitan and Wolfson (1988a, 1993) from 42 variables from the HRB: 19 based on level of performance that tap a broad range of psychological functions; 9 variables representing motor and sensory–perceptual performances; 12 variables that provide measures of basic language and visuospatial skills, i.e., dysphasia and constructional dyspraxia; and 2 variables that represent ratio scores with a differential score approach. Thus, the scale is based on the four methods of inference, which are used in the clinical evaluation of a patient. Each of the items entering into the scale is assigned a rating between 0 (normal), 1 (mildly deviant without clinical significance), 2 (mildly to moderately impaired), and 3 (severely impaired). The cutoff score between 2 and 3 differentiates normal from brain-damaged subjects. For the total score the ratings on each item are summed; the ranges are: 0–25, normal; 26–40, mild impairment; 41–67 moderate impairment; and severe impairment over 68. Cross-validating studies for this scale have been reported by Sherer and Adams (1993) and Wolfson and Reitan (1995), and the GNDS score appears to be a valid indicator of the presence or absence of cerebral damage, but more research is needed to determine its use in clinical evaluation, as the authors have indicated.

The clinical usefulness of the GNDS can be enhanced by the use of the Left and Right Neuropsychological Deficit Scales (L-NDS and R-NDS), also developed by Reitan and Wolfson (1988a). As their name implies, these two scales permit a comparison and contrast of the integrity of the two cerebral hemispheres, and the two scales provide a means for differentiating between left and right cerebral lesions. The measures for both the L-NDS and the R-NDS are items from the HRB, which have been classified according to their lateralizing significance for either the right or left cerebral hemisphere. Reitan and Wolfson (1988a) recommend the use of the L-NDS and R-NDS in conjunction with the GNDS, "although scoring procedures of this kind can never be expected to replace clinical insight and understanding" (p. 100).

Summary of Test Studies

The foregoing studies illustrate that recent research on the HRB has been concerned with individual tests in an attempt to define more precisely what the tests are measuring and their specific contributions to the HRB. Details are being provided that help fill in the general mosaic. Unfortunately, it is not possible to determine the usefulness of a test in a battery by examining the test singly. One of the methods of clinical inference is pattern of performance or ratio scores; examining a test singly does not indicate how it fits into a pattern, but as Reitan (1988) indicated, "each test in a neuropsychological test battery must be carefully validated for its sensitivity to cerebral dysfunction" (p. 345). The major validating studies for the HRB were conducted prior to 1975. From the standpoint of clinical interpretation and clinical application, the recent research with individual tests represents progress inch by inch instead of by a long touchdown pass.

HRB AND CONTEMPORARY RESEARCH

In the previous sections we have reviewed the HRB as a clinical instrument and have directed our efforts toward studies that have influenced the HRB in clinical practice. Halstead's original conception was to develop his battery as a measure of the biological intelligence of the organism. There have been recent efforts to return to those roots (Matarazzo, 1972; Reitan, Hom, & Wolfson, 1988; Reitan & Wolfson, 1992a), but the HRB has been much more widely used in scientific research than was perhaps envisioned by Halstead's original purpose. In this section we want to consider the HRB in the *Zeitgeist* of current neuropsychological research. We will do this by indicating areas where the HRB has been used.

HRB and Neurological Disease

The HRB continues to be used in investigations pertaining to neurological disease and their neuropsychological concomitants, edifying not only from the standpoint of understanding the course of the disease but also for shedding light on the complexities of brain–behavior relationships. Hom (1991) has written a detailed and comprehensive chapter on the contributions of the HRB in the understanding of stroke. He also reported on cognitive deficits in patients with Alzheimer's disease (AD) (Hom, 1992) and relatives of AD patients (Hom, Turner, Risser, Bonte, & Tintiner, 1994) and on the relation of brain tumors and dementia (Hom, 1993). Related investigations on neuropsychological deficits associated with stroke have been reported by Hom and Reitan (1990) and on deficits associated with intrinsic cerebral neoplasms (Hom & Reitan, 1984).

Collectively, the foregoing studies show that in order to have a comprehensive understanding of the concomitants of neurological disease, measurements need to be made that include both general and specific neuropsychological functions. In addition to the generalized impairment found with serious cerebral disease there are focal neuropsychological deficits that differ from patient group to patient group. Tumor patients have shown lateralized focal deficits. AD patients show focal impairments that involved both cerebral hemispheres but there were few signs of lateralization. The effects of cerebral vascular disease on cortical neuropsychological functions were much more extensive than the deficits associated with the side or specific location of the lesion. The extent and variation of cognitive deficit associated with cerebral disease supports the desirability in patient evaluation of using a battery of tests that contains measures of both general and specific deficits. Additionally, the research findings suggest the need for a rehabilitation program that goes beyond physical therapy and speech therapy used in the treatment of motor and language deficits.

HRB and Head Injury

Neuropsychologists are in an advantageous position to evaluate behavioral and cognitive impairment as a consequence of head injury. Frequently, medical diagnostic procedures, electroencephalogram, computed tomography scan, magnetic resonance imaging, and the clinical neurological exam will not show any impairment of the brain because their diagnostic procedures do not include measures of cognitive functions such as abstract reasoning, visuospatial abilities, attention, and concentration. In other words, cognitive and behavioral impairment may exist as a consequence of cerebral dysfunction even without demonstrable structural impairment of the brain. Nevertheless, neuropsychological testing can reveal subtle as well as more major deficits.

The clinical questions that the neuropsychologist must address when evaluating head injury patients include whether neuropsychological impairment occurred as a consequence of the head injury. If so, what is the extent of the impairment? What is the prognosis for recovery? In the case of a severe head injury, questions of competency may arise such as, Is the patient competent to manage his own money? If comorbidity is present—ethanol or polysubstance abuse—what part of the impairment is head injury and what part comorbidity?

The degree of impairment that a patient will show on a neuropsychological test battery will vary with the amount of time that exists between the time of the injury and the time of the evaluation. In most head injuries where brain damage occurs, the damage is diffuse, involving both cerebral hemispheres as opposed to a strictly focal lesion, although in the context of the diffuse impairment a focal lesion may occur. It should be obvious then that the neuropsychological evaluation should tap a wide range of functions; in addition to an impaired level of performance the clinician should examine the asymmetrical motor and sensory functions, the presence of pathognomonic signs, and areas of sparing as well as impairment. The use of a neuropsychological test battery as opposed to a single-test approach should provide the most useful amount of information.

Research with the HRB has made significant contributions to the understanding of the dynamics of head injury as well as to recovery processes (Reitan & Wolfson, 1986b, 1988a). Since the mid-1970s, Dikmen and her colleagues at the University of Washington have studied the effects of head injury and the HRB has been a major tool in their investigations. The interested readers, particularly neuropsychologists with forensic interest and expertise, should acquaint themselves with this literature in order to have documentation of the validity of the HRB in head injury evaluation and to understand the pertinent variables that may affect the outcome of head trauma and the recovery process. The head injury literature is vast and only a few recent references that pertain to the HRB are suggested here (Dikmen, McLean, & Temkin, 1986; Dikmen, McLean, Temkin, & Wyler, 1986; Dikmen, Machamer, Temkin, & McLean, 1990; Dikmen, et al., 1994; Ross, Temkin, Newell, & Dikmen, 1994).

HRB and Schizophrenia

Schizophrenia is a psychiatric disease in which psychologists have had a long-term interest from the standpoint of both clinical evaluation and research. In the earlier textbooks of abnormal psychology, schizophrenia was listed as one of the "functional psychoses" (Cameron, 1944). The clinical evaluation of the schizophrenic patient when done by psychologists largely consisted of intelligence measures and projective techniques: the Rorschach, the Thematic Apperception Test, Word Association Tests, Figure Drawings, and so on. With the development of neuropsychological tests, there was the potential for relating behavioral impairment to underlying brain mechanisms, and psychologists had the opportunity to do a more comprehensive assessment on the schizophrenic patient than was afforded by the tests of Goldstein and Scheerer (1941) or the Hanfman–Kasanin (Rappaport, 1945).

In many psychiatric units today, schizophrenic patients are routinely referred for neuropsychological evaluation. The neuropsychological tests provide an indication not only of the degree of impairment in areas such as abstraction, language, visual–spatial processes, and motor and sensory functions, but also they may provide evidence as to whether there is comorbidity involving central nervous system functions. In the psychiatric setting patients are referred for a wide variety of reasons. Examples of referring questions are: Is there cognitive impairment beyond age and/or educational expectations? What is this patient's potential for living alone? Is this a dementia of depression (pseudodementia) or is it an organic dementia? Can this patient's presenting symptoms be explained on an organic basis; If an organic condition is present, is it comorbid? Frequently, the referring statement reads, "Is there any organicity? Tell me as much as you can about this patient."

The referring question is rarely to evaluate a specific syndrome; hence, a battery such as the HRB, which measures a wide range of functions from higher-level cognitive skills through psychomotor problem solving skills, visuoconstructive abilities, and down to simple motor and sensory functions, is ideally suited for use. The principles of evaluating the psychiatric or schizophrenic patient do not differ from those of any other patient. It is necessary to have the patient's cooperation. It is necessary to determine that peripheral factors, e.g., poor vision, fatigue, and, if possible, medication do not influence the results.

However, it is rare to see a psychiatric patient who is not on some form of drug, and its influence on the results of neuropsychological tests may be unknown. Obviously, if the patient is extremely drowsy, the outcome will be affected; but under such a condition the patient should not be tested. Medication effects rarely produce pathognomonic signs and they rarely will have a differential effect on the two sides of the body. However, medication itself may induce toxicity, which is an organic condition. This may occur particularly when the patient is taking several medications that are incompatible, each of which has been prescribed by a different physician. Using the four methods of inference, level of performance, ratio scores, pathognomonic signs, and right–left comparisons will go a long way to provide meaningful answers to the questions of the referring physician.

The HRB has been widely used in a number of research studies pertaining to schizophrenia and these studies contain valuable information for the neuropsychologist in a psychiatric setting. Goldstein (1991) has written a detailed and comprehensive review of the use of neuropsychological test batteries in a psychiatric setting and of the research in schizophrenia.

Psychologists who work in a psychiatric setting know that there is a great deal of variability in schizophrenic patients. Many of the patients have acute psychiatric symptoms and, on neuropsychological tests they are almost astonishingly unimpaired, given their degree of dysfunction. Other patients who also have acute psychiatric symptoms show considerable impairment on neuropsychological tests. This variability has many dimensions, and studies where the HRB has been used indicate it may be related to a schizophrenic positive and negative deficit syndrome (Braff et al., 1991; Goldstein, 1994; Harris, et al., 1991), age and education (Goldstein, Zubin, & Pogue-Geile, 1991; Heaton, Paulsen, et al., 1994), type of thought disorder (Silverstein, Marengo, & Fogg, 1991), and presence or absence of neurological dysfunction (Goldstein & Zubin, 1990). However, length of hospitalization for schizophrenia does not appear related to cognitive deterioration (Goldstein et al., 1991).

The thoughtful reader might inquire as to the stability of neuropsychological test performances among neuropsychiatric patients in general and among schizophrenic patients in particular. Goldstein and Watson (1989) provided a semi-reassuring answer. For a total sample ($n = 150$) of patients, test–retest coefficients for HRB tests (with a mean intertest interval of 105.9 weeks, range from 4 to 469 weeks) varied from .48 for TPTL to .81 for finger tapping, nondominant. For schizophrenics ($n = 33$) the coefficients ranged from .32 for TPTL to .73 for finger tapping, dominant. From a psychometric standpoint these reliability measures suggest relative stability at least for groups; but in evaluating an individual patient, especially a schizophrenic for neuropsychological deficiency, caution must be exercised in interpreting the results.

The studies cited in this section represent state of the art with respect to the HRB in schizophrenic research and application in a psychiatric setting. The research provides a solid background that should be of value to the clinician in making decisions concerning the neuropsychological status of psychiatric patients.

The HRB and Systemic Disease

In this section we are going to document studies where the HRB has been used in areas that have an indirect as opposed to a direct effect on cognitive functions. For example, head injury may directly affect and alter cognitive functions. If there is an effect from cardiac failure, the effect on cognitive functions is secondary. We have also included in this section studies that were difficult to classify elsewhere. Our purpose here is to demonstrate not only the potential for neuropsychological research, but also to provide the clinician with justification for performing a neuropsychological evaluation on a patient with a systemic disease, as well as to indicate the kinds of cognitive deficits that might be encountered. We will not comment on the experimental design, the results, or the methodological issues involved.

Farmer (1994) gave a detailed and wide-ranging review of cognitive deficits associated with major organ failure. She listed many disease entities that have an impact on cognitive abilities and how neuropsychological evaluation would be important in helping assess the functional status of the patient for quality of living and regimen compliance. Farmer referred to the TMT as the "gold standard" test for hepatic encephalopathy (1994, p. 146). Since many of the deficits resulting from organ disease may be subtle, the use of a battery of tests that tap a wide range of functions may prove desirable. As Heaton, Velin, et al. (1994) indicated, the use of only a single or a few neuropsychological measures limits the conclusions that can be made about particular deficits.

Savage et al. (1988) investigated the effects of organic pesticides and found significant deficits in AIR, Halstead II, CT, and several subtests from the WAIS in the affected group. They reported major cognitive deficits on tests and abilities that receive limited evaluation in the clinical neurological examination.

Goldstein et al. (1990) studied behavioral and cognitive functions in elderly, mild-to-moderately hypertensive men who underwent antihypertensive therapy. They used a comprehensive battery of neuropsychological tests, but from the HRB only TMTA & B and Finger Tapping were included. Their studies suggested that in elderly males with mild-to-moderate hypertension neither blood pressure reduction nor specific medication regimens produced significant adverse cognitive decline.

Skenazy and Bigler (1985) studied neuropsychological performance in diabetic patients. The level of psychological adjustment was not related to the diabetic patient's performance on most of the neuropsychological measures from the HRB. Elias, Robbins, Schultz, and Pierce (1990) found that blood pressure, age, and the multiplicative effects of blood pressure and age were significant as predictors of performance on selected tests from the HRB. However, when age, sex, and education were controlled, blood pressure's main effects were observed for AIR, CT score, and TPT-M and -L.

The HRB has been used to investigate neuropsychological deficiency in areas important for public health planning. O'Malley, Adamse, Heaton, and Gawin (1992) reported that 50% of cocaine abusers, in contrast to 15% of controls, scored in the impaired range on the Summary Index of the Neuropsychological Screening Exam. The cocaine abusers also performed more poorly on the CT and related neuropsychological measures. Filley, Heaton, and Rosenberg (1990) found that among 14 chronic toluene abusers, 3 had normal neuropsychological protocols, 3 were in a borderline range, and 8 were impaired. There was a significant relationship between neuropsychological impairment and adverse white matter changes as measured by magnetic resonance imaging. Grant and Heaton (1990) stated that patients with acquired immunodeficiency syndrome (AIDS) may show significant neuropsychological impairment in speed of information processing, abstraction, learning, and recall. Sewell et al. (1994) showed that human immunodeficiency virus (HIV) infected men who had new-onset psychosis without delirium or previous psychotic episodes differed from nonpsychotic comparison subjects in showing a trend toward greater global neuropsychological impairment. Finally, Heaton, Velin, et al. (1994) found that patients with HIV-1 were at risk for neurobehavioral impairment in later stages of the disease, but even patients who were medically asymptomatic or minimally symptomatic might show mild deficits on comprehensive neuropsychological test batteries. Furthermore, those who showed neuropsychological impairment had a significantly higher unemployment rate than did their unimpaired counterparts. Neuropsychological impairment was associated with subjective decreases in job-related abilities.

In this section on research studies we have shown a wide range of areas where the HRB has been used. The traditional areas of neurological disease and head injury were included. Intensive studies were also done on brain-related deficits associated with psychopathology. Finally, there have been explorations into a variety of conditions associated with systemic disease. These medical conditions may also produce brain impairment, and to discover their debilitating effects it is necessary to use a test battery that measures the full continuum of brain-related behaviors. It is only when the full effect of a given disease is realized that policy and social planners can develop programs for effective rehabilitation and programs for disease prevention.

PRESENT STATUS AND FUTURE OF THE HRB

In the last half of the 20th century the HRB has had a major impact on the direction of both research and practice of clinical neuropsychology. In this chapter we have emphasized developments over the last 10 years, and we have shown that there has been significant work in improving and refining the HRB. Parsons (1986) indicated three areas for future development of the HRB: methodological improvements, clinical sensitivity, and rehabilitation. We will review each of these areas from the vantage point of 10 years later, and then, as Parsons did, attempt to place the HRB in the context or perspective of today's clinical neuropsychology.

Methodological Improvements in the HRB

The most significant amount of improvement has occurred in terms of methodological changes. As we indicated, important research has been done toward refining individual tests. There has been voluminous work on the CT test, the lateralizing status of the SRT and SSPT has been clarified, and there have been investigations, of which more need to be done, on the TPT and the use of its shortened forms. Of greater, importance, however, is the research that has been done to improve the objectivity and the precision in test interpretation. Previously for each test there was a cutoff score, impaired versus nonimpaired. Now, for each test in the HRB there is an adult severity range. There is also a General

Neuropsychological Deficit Scale (Reitan & Wolfson, 1988a, 1993). This scale can be used to obtain an index of neuropsychological competency or deficiency, depending on the viewpoint one wishes to emphasize. Finally, there are comprehensive tables of demographically corrected T scores. As indicated, the scores have been adjusted for age and education. These scores permit comparing a patient to a defined population. Furthermore, when the T scores are graphed, they permit easy visualization of the patient's strengths and weaknesses in the various areas measured by the WAIS, HRB, and related neuropsychological tests.

In summary, there has been significant notable methodological improvement. Further research needs to be done to refine the norms that have been developed, and to relate the severity ratings and the deficit ratings to problems of life adjustment, employment, and rehabilitation. However, there is a wealth of material available to the clinician who wishes to improve his or her diagnostic and interpretative skills with the HRB.

The Clinical Sensitivity of the HRB

Parsons (1986) indicated two important areas: the objective actuarial discriminating power of the HRB, and improving the interpreter of the HRB test findings, i.e., the clinician. As we implied earlier in the chapter, improving the objective discriminating power or the sensitivity and specificity of the HRB has many facets to it, one of which is a large data pool. The validity of the HRB has been demonstrated through many different types of research studies, but sophisticated actuarial studies where the base rates in the population have been specified have not been done. Furthermore, for reasons that will become apparent later, it appears unlikely that they will be done.

With respect to improving the clinician, there are more postdoctoral fellowships available than previously; the clinician has a better literature base to study; the diplomate examination of the American Board of Clinical Neuropsychology has become more rigorous. All of these factors should help increase the sophistication of the individual clinician, but the fact remains that by far the single-most important factor in contributing to the clinical sensitivity of the battery is the skills of the individual neuropsychologist. To make use of the subtleties and nuances of the test findings from the HRB requires not only long experience in using the battery with a wide variety of neurologically impaired patients but also a thorough understanding of clinical neurology and neurological diseases that affect the central nervous system. Training in medicine and neurology develops the skills that are propaedeutic to being an expert in human clinical neuropsychology.

Rehabilitation

The REHABIT program was developed (Reitan & Wolfson, 1988b, 1992b), but its promise has yet to be fulfilled. The field of rehabilitation psychology is developing on its own, and the relation of clinical neuropsychology to rehabilitation psychology has yet to be clarified. As we indicated, neuropsychological evaluation has great face validity for rehabilitation. It is now a matter of transferring face validity to concurrent and predictive validity. Parsons (1986) indicated that the HRB should receive more attention in the future as a predictor of life adjustment for the brain-damaged patient, as a baseline of functioning, and as a method for determining deficit on which rehabilitative and cognitive retraining methods can be based. Definitive studies in these areas still need to be done.

The future for rehabilitation is still promising. In the past 10 years there has been major research on head injury, psychopathology, and a wide range of neurological diseases. The results of these studies should translate into a solid base for using the HRB in rehabilitative programs.

What Is the Status of the HRB Today?

To sum up, in the past 10 years a substantial amount of time, money, effort, and energy has been spent on this vehicle known as the HRB. Today, the fair conclusion is that the HRB is a well-researched battery of tests, which can be used to document, delineate, and demonstrate the behavioral effects of disease and conditions that affect the cerebral hemispheres. The diseases and conditions range from those that directly involve brain tissue, such as infiltrating tumors, cerebral vascular accidents, penetrating and closed head injuries, to mention only a few, to those systemic diseases where the effect on the brain may be secondary, such as alcoholism, hypertension, lead poisoning, electrocution, infectious diseases, and many others. The HRB can be used to assist in differential diagnosis of organic dementia versus the dementia of depression, Alzheimer's disease versus depression, malingering versus organic brain impairment, again to mention only a few. For each of the foregoing, as well as many more, there are studies in the literature that can be cited for validating evidence.

To evaluate and understand certain specific conditions, such as aphasia, memory defects, and visual–spatial problems, other test procedures are needed, and the procedures will vary depending on the nature of the problem and the question being asked. However, when one wants to measure a wide range of skills and abilities from nonverbal concept formation through psychomotor problem skills, language disturbances, visual–spatial disruptions, to the intactness of simple sensory and motor functions, the HRB can be recommended. The status of the HRB in contemporary neuropsychology is assured.

What of the Future?

If the best prediction of the future is the past and the present, the future of the HRB is bright. But behind the silver lining is there a dark cloud? Social and political policies of the past had a direct impact in terms of the availability of research grant money, fellowships, and other training opportunities for the neuropsychologist. Social and political policies still have a major impact on the activities of the neuropsychologist, including job opportunities. For better or worse, the impact today is somewhat different from that of previous years. The future of the HRB may depend more on economic and political factors than on social and scientific merit.

REFERENCES

American Psychiatric Association. (1994). *Diagnostic and statistical manual of mental disorders* (4th ed.). Washington, DC: Author.

Benton, A. (1992). Clinical neuropsychology: 1960–1990. *Journal of Clinical and Experimental Neuropsychology, 14,* 407–417.

Braff, D. L., Heaton, R., Kuck, J., Cullum, M., Moranville, J., Grant, I., & Zisook, S. (1991). The generalized pattern of neuropsychological deficits in outpatients with chronic schizophrenia with heterogeneous Wisconsin Card Sorting Test results. *Archives of General Psychiatry, 48,* 891–898.

Bryson, A. J., Silverstein, M. L., Nathan, A., & Stephen, L. (1993). Differential rate of neuropsychological dysfunction in psychiatric disorders: Comparison between the Halstead–Reitan and Luria–Nebraska batteries. *Perceptual and Motor Skills, 76,* 305–306.

Cameron, N. (1944). The functional psychoses. In J. McV. Hunt (Ed.), *Personality and the behavior disorders* (Vol. I, pp. 861–921). New York: Ronald Press.

Choca, J. P., Laatsch, L., Wetzel, L., & Agresti, A. (1993, August). *The Halstead Category Test: A fifty-year perspective.* J. P. Choca (Chair), Symposium conducted at the meeting of the American Psychological Association, Toronto, Canada.

Clark, C., & Klonoff, F. (1988). Reliability and construct validity of the six-block Tactual Performance Test in an adult sample. *Journal of Clinical and Experimental Neuropsychology, 10,* 175–184.

Cullum, C. M., Thompson, L. L., & Heaton, R. K. (1989). The use of the Halstead–Reitan battery with older adults. *Clinics in Geriatric Medicine, 5,* 595–610.

Dikmen, S., Machamer, J., Temkin, N., & McLean, A. (1990). Neuropsychological recovery in patients with moderate to severe head injury: 2 year follow-up. *Journal of Clinical and Experimental Neuropsychology, 12,* 507–519.

Dikmen, S., McLean, A., & Temkin, N. (1986). Neuropsychological and psychosocial consequences of minor head injury. *Journal of Neurology and Psychiatry, 49,* 1227–1232.

Dikmen, S., McLean, A., Temkin, N. R., & Wyler, A. R. (1986). Neuropsychologic outcome at one-month post injury. *Archives of Physical Medicine and Rehabilitation, 67,* 507–513.

Dikmen, S. S., Temkin, N. R., Machamer, J. E., Holubkou, A. L., Fraser, R. T., & Winn, R. (1994). Employment following traumatic head injuries. *Archives of Neurology, 51,* 177–186.

Donders, J., & Kirsch, N. (1991). Nature and implications of selective impairment on the Booklet Category Test and Wisconsin Card Sorting test. *The Clinical Neuropsychologist, 5,* 78–82.

Elias, M. F., Robbins, M. A., Schultz, N. R., Jr., & Pierce, T. W. (1990). Is blood pressure an important variable in research on aging and neuropsychological test performance? *Journal of Gerontology, 45,* 128–135.

Elias, M. F., Robbins, M. A., Walter, L. J., & Schultz, N. R., Jr. (1993). The influence of gender and age on Halstead–Reitan neuropsychological test performance. *Journal of Gerontology, 48,* 278–281.

Farmer, M. E. (1994). Cognitive deficits related to major organ failure: The potential role of neuropsychological testing. *Neuropsychology Review, 4,* 117–160.

Filley, C. M., Heaton, R. K., & Rosenberg, N. L. (1990). White matter dementia in chronic toluene abuse. *Neurology, 40,* 532–534.

Fitzhugh, K. B., Fitzhugh, L. D., & Reitan, R. M. (1962). Wechsler Bellevue comparisons in groups with "chronic" and "current" lateralized diffuse brain lesions. *Journal of Consulting Psychology, 26*, 303–310.

Gardner, E. (1947). *Fundamentals of neurology.* Philadelphia: Saunders.

Goldberg, T. E., Kelsoe, J. R., Weinberger, D. R., Pliskin, N. H., Kirwin, P. D., & Berman, K. F. (1988). Performance of schizophrenic patients on putative neuropsychological tests of frontal lobe function. *International Journal of Neuroscience, 42*, 51–58.

Goldstein, G. (1986). An overview of similarities and differences between the Halstead–Reitan and Luria–Nebraska neuropsychological batteries. In T. Incagnoli, G. Goldstein, & C. J. Golden (Eds.), *Clinical application of neuropsychological test batteries* (pp. 235–275). New York: Plenum Press.

Goldstein, G. (1987). Neuropsychological assessment batteries for rehabilitation: Fixed batteries, automated systems and non-psychometric methods. In M. Meier, A. Benton, & L. Diller (Eds.), *Neuropsychological rehabilitation* (pp. 18–40). New York: Guilford Press.

Goldstein, G. (1991). Comprehensive neuropsychological test batteries and research in schizophrenia. In S. R. Steinhauer, J. H. Gruzelier, & J. Zubin (Eds.), *Handbook of Schizophrenia: Vol. 5. Neuropsychology, psychophysiology, and information processing* (pp. 525–551). New York: Elsevier.

Goldstein, G. (1994). Neurobehavioral heterogeneity in schizophrenia. *Archives of Clinical Neuropsychology, 9*, 265–276.

Goldstein, G., Materson, B. J., Cushman, W. C., Reda, D. J., Freis, E. D., Ramirez, E. A., Talmers, F. N., White, T. D., Nunn, S., Chapman, R. H., Khatri, I., Schnaper, H., Thomas, J. R., Henderson, W. C., & Fye, C. (1990). Treatment of hypertension in the elderly: II. Cognitive and behavioral function. *Hypertension, 15*, 361–369.

Goldstein, G., & Watson, J. R. (1989). Test–retest reliability of the Halstead–Reitan battery and the WAIS in a neuropsychiatric population. *The Clinical Neuropsychologist, 3*, 265–273.

Goldstein, G., & Zubin, J. (1990). Neuropsychological differences between young and old schizophrenics with and without associated neurological dysfunction. *Schizophrenia Research, 3*, 117–126.

Goldstein, G., Zubin, J., & Pogue-Geile, M. F. (1991). Hospitalization and the cognitive deficits of schizophrenia. The influences of age and education. *Journal of Nervous and Mental Disease, 179*, 202–206.

Goldstein, K., & Scheerer, M. (1941). Abstract and concrete behavior: An experimental study with special tests. *Psychological Monographs, 53* (2, Serial No. 239).

Grant, I., & Heaton, R. K. (1990). Human immunodeficiency virus-type 1 (HIV-1) and the brain. *Journal of Consulting and Clinical Psychology, 58*, 22–30.

Halstead, W. C. (1947). *Brain and intelligence: A quantitative study of the frontal lobes.* Chicago: University of Chicago Press.

Harris, M. J., Jeste, D. V., Krull, A., Montague, J., & Heaton, R. K. (1991). Deficit syndrome in older schizophrenic patients. *Psychiatry Research, 39*, 285–292.

Heaton, R. K., Grant, I., & Matthews, C. G. (1986). Differences in neuropsychological test performance associated with age, education, and sex. In I. Grant & K. M. Adams (Eds.), *Neuropsychological assessment in neuropsychiatric disorders: Clinical methods and empirical findings* (pp. 100–120). New York: Oxford University Press.

Heaton, R. K., Grant, I., & Matthews, C. G. (1991). *Comprehensive norms for an expanded Halstead–Reitan battery. Demographic corrections, research findings, and clinical applications.* Odessa, FL: Psychological Assessment Resources.

Heaton, R. K., Paulsen, J. S., McAdams, L. A., Cuck, J., Zisook, S., Graff, B., Harris, M. J., & Jeste, E. V. (1994). Neuropsychological deficits in schizophrenia. *Archives of General Psychiatry, 51*, 469–476.

Heaton, R. K., Velin, R. A., McCutchan, J. A., Gulevich, S. J., Atkinson, J. H., Wallace, M. R., Godfrey, H. P., Kirson, D. A., & Grant, I. (1994). Neuropsychological impairment in human immunodeficiency virus–infection: Implications for employment. *Psychosomatic Medicine, 56*, 8–17.

Heilbronner, R. L., & Parsons, O. A. (1989). Clinical utility of the Tactual Performance Test: Issues of lateralization and cognitive style. *The Clinical Neuropsychologist, 3,* 250–264.

Hom, J. (1991). Contributions of the Halstead–Reitan battery in the neuropsychological investigation of stroke. In R. A. Bornstein & L. C. Brown (Eds.), *Neurobehavioral aspects of cerebrovascular disease* (pp. 165–181). New York: Oxford University Press.

Hom, J. (1992). General and specific cognitive dysfunction in patients with Alzheimer's disease. *Archives of Clinical Neuropsychology, 7,* 121–133.

Hom, J. (1993). Brain tumors and dementia. In R. W. Parks, R. F. Zec, & R. S. Wilson (Eds.), *Neuropsychology of Alzheimer's disease and other dementias* (pp. 210–233). New York: Oxford University Press.

Hom, J., & Reitan, R. M. (1984). Neuropsychological correlates of rapidly vs. slowly growing intrinsic cerebral neoplasms. *Journal of Clinical Neuropsychology, 3,* 303–324.

Hom, J., & Reitan, R. M. (1990). Generalized cognitive function after stroke. *Journal of Clinical and Experimental Neuropsychology, 12,* 644–654.

Hom, J., Turner, M. B., Risser, R., Bonte, F. J., & Tintiner, R. (1994). Cognitive deficits in asymptomatic first-degree relatives of Alzheimer's disease patients. *Journal of Clinical and Experimental Neuropsychology, 16,* 568–576.

Kane, R. L. (1991). Standardized and flexible batteries in neuropsychology: An assessment update. *Neuropsychology Review, 2,* 281–339.

Kane, R. L., Parsons, O. A., Goldstein, G., & Moses, J. A. (1987). Diagnostic accuracy of the Halstead–Reitan and Luria–Nebraska Neuropsychological batteries: Performance of clinical raters. *Journal of Consulting and Clinical Psychology, 55,* 783–784.

Leckliter, I. N., & Matarazzo, D. (1989). The influence of age, education, IQ, gender, and alcohol abuse on Halstead–Reitan Neuropsychological Test Battery performance. *Journal of Clinical Psychology, 45,* 484–512.

Lezak, M. D. (1983). *Neuropsychological assessment* (2nd ed.). New York: Oxford University Press.

Lezak, M. D. (1987). Assessment for rehabilitation planning. In M. Meier, A. Benton, & L. Diller (Eds.), *Neuropsychological rehabilitation* (pp. 41–58). New York: Guilford Press.

Mahalanobis, P. C. (1936). On the generalized distance function in statistics. *International Science Congress, India, XII,* 49–55.

Matarazzo, J. D. (1972). *Wechsler's measurement and appraisal of adult intelligence.* Baltimore: Williams and Wilkins.

Meier, M., Benton, A., & Diller, L. (Eds.). (1987). *Neuropsychological rehabilitation.* New York: Guilford Press.

Meyerink, L. H. (1982). Intellectual functioning: The nature and patterns of change with aging. (Doctoral dissertation, University of Arizona, 1982). *Dissertation Abstracts International, 43,* 855B.

Moehle, K. A., & Long, C. J. (1989). Models of aging and neuropsychological test performance decline with aging. *Journal of Gerontology, 44,* 176–177.

O'Malley, S., Adamse, M., Heaton, R. K., & Gawin, F. H. (1992). Neuropsychological impairment in chronic cocaine abusers. *American Journal of Drug and Alcohol Abuse, 18,* 131–44.

Parsons, O. A. (1986). Overview of the Halstead–Reitan battery. In T. Incagnoli, G. Goldstein, & C. J. Golden (Eds.), *Clinical application of neuropsychological test batteries* (pp. 155–192). New York: Plenum Press.

Perrine, K. (1993). Differential aspects of conceptual processing in the Category and Wisconsin Card Sorting Test. *Journal of Clinical and Experimental Neuropsychology, 15,* 447–626.

Preiss, J., & Hynek, K. (1991). The Halstead–Reitan neuropsychology battery. Initial experience with its use in Czechoslovakia. *Ceskoslovenska Psychiatrie, 87*(5–6), 249–54.

Rappaport, D. (1945). *Diagnostic psychological testing* (Vol. 1). Chicago: Yearbook Publications.

Reed, H. B. C., & Reitan, R. M. (1963). Change in psychological test performance associated with the normal aging process. *Journal of Gerontology, 18,* 271–274.

Reed, J. C. (1984). The contribution of Ward Halstead, Ralph Reitan, and their associates. *International Journal of Neuroscience, 25*, 289–293.

Reitan, R. M. (1955a). Certain differential effects of left and right cerebral lesions in human adults. *Journal of Comparative and Physiological Psychology, 48*, 474–477.

Reitan, R. M. (1955b). An investigation of the validity of Halstead's measures of biological intelligence. *Archives of Neurology and Psychiatry, 73*, 28–35.

Reitan, R. M. (1959). The comparative effects of brain damage on the Halstead Impairment Index and the Wechsler–Bellevue Scale. *Journal of Clinical Psychology, 15*, 281–285.

Reitan, R. M. (1964). Psychological deficits resulting from cerebral lesions in man. In J. M. Warren & K. A. Akert (Eds.), *The frontal granular cortex and behavior* (pp. 295–312). New York: McGraw Hill.

Reitan, R. M. (1984). *Aphasia and sensory perceptual deficits in adults.* Tucson, AZ: Neuropsychology Press.

Reitan, R. M. (1988). Integration of neuropsychological theory, assessment, and application. *The Clinical Neuropsychologist, 2*, 331–349.

Reitan, R. M. (1994). Ward Halstead's contribution to neuropsychology and the Halstead–Reitan Neuropsychological Test Battery. *Journal of Clinical Psychology, 50*, 47–80.

Reitan, R. M., & Davison, L. A. (Eds.). (1974). *Clinical neuropsychology: Current status and applications.* Washington, DC: V. H. Winston & Sons.

Reitan, R. M., Hom, J., & Wolfson, D. (1988). Verbal processing by the brain. *Journal of Clinical and Experimental Neuropsychology, 10*, 400–408.

Reitan, R. M., & Sena, D. (1983, August). *The efficacy of the REHABIT techniques in remediation of brain-injured people.* Paper presented at the meeting of the American Psychological Association, Anaheim, CA.

Reitan, R. M., & Wolfson, D. (1985). *The Halstead–Reitan Neuropsychological Test Battery.* Tucson, AZ: Neuropsychology Press.

Reitan, R. M., & Wolfson, D. (1986a). The Halstead–Reitan Neuropsychological Test Battery and aging. *Clinical Gerontologist, 5*, 39–61.

Reitan, R. M., & Wolfson, D. (1986b). *Traumatic brain injury:* Vol. I. *Pathophysiology and neuropsychological evaluation.* Tucson, AZ: Neuropsychology Press.

Reitan, R. M., & Wolfson, D. (1988a). *Traumatic brain injury:* Vol. II. *Recovery and rehabilitation.* Tucson, AZ: Neuropsychology Press.

Reitan, R. M., & Wolfson, D. (1988b). The Halstead–Reitan Neuropsychological Test Battery and REHABIT: A model for integrating evaluation and remediation of cognitive impairment. *Cognitive Rehabilitation, 6*, 10–17.

Reitan, R. M., & Wolfson, D. (1989). The Seashore Rhythm Test and brain functions. *The Clinical Neuropsychologist, 3*, 70–78.

Reitan, R. M., & Wolfson, D. (1990). The significance of the Speech Sounds Perception Test for cerebral functions. *Archives of Clinical Neuropsychology, 5*, 265–272.

Reitan, R. M., & Wolfson, D. (1992a). Conventional intelligence measures and neuropsychological concepts of adaptive abilities. *Journal of Clinical Psychology, 48*, 521–529.

Reitan, R. M., & Wolfson, D. (1992b). *Neuropsychological evaluation of older children.* Tucson, AZ: Neuropsychology Press.

Reitan, R. M., & Wolfson, D. (1993). *The Halstead–Reitan Neuropsychological Test Battery: Theory and clinical interpretation* (2nd ed.). Tucson, AZ: Neuropsychology Press.

Reitan, R. M., & Wolfson, D. (1994a). Dissociation of motor impairment and higher-level brain deficits in strokes and cerebral neoplasms. *The Clinical Neuropsychologist, 8*, 193–208.

Reitan, R. M., & Wolfson, D. (1994b). A selective and critical review of neuropsychological deficits and the frontal lobes. *Neuropsychology Review, 4*, 161–198.

Reitan, R. M., & Wolfson, D. (1995a). Influence of age and education on neuropsychological test results. *The Clinical Neuropsychologist, 9*, 151–158.

Reitan, R. M., & Wolfson, D. (1995b). The Category Test and the Trail Making Test as measures of frontal lobe functions. *The Clinical Neuropsychologist, 9,* 50–56.

Ross, B. L., Temkin, N. R., Newell, D., & Dikmen, S. S. (1994). Neuropsychological outcome in relation to head injury severity. *American Journal of Physical Medicine and Rehabilitation, 73,* 341–347.

Russell, E. W. (1985). Comparison of the TPT ten and six hole formboard. *Journal of Clinical Psychology, 41,* 68–81.

Russell, E. W., Neuringer, C., & Goldstein, G. (1970). *Assessment of brain damage.* New York: Wiley.

Savage, E. P., Keefe, T. J., Mounce, L. M., Heaton, R. K., Lewis, J. A., & Burcar, P. J. (1988). Chronic neurological sequelae of acute organophosphate pesticide poisoning. *Archives of Environmental Health, 43,* 38–45.

Scheibel, R. S., Hannay, H. J., & Myers, C. A. (1993, February). *The Category Test in patients with lateralized frontal and nonfrontal gliomas.* Poster session presented at the meeting of the International Neuropsychological Society, Galveston, TX.

Sena, D. A. (1985). The effectiveness of cognitive retraining for brain impaired individuals. *The International Journal of Clinical Psychology, 7,* 62.

Sena, D. A. (1986). The effectiveness of cognitive rehabilitation for brain-impaired patients. *Journal of Clinical and Experimental Neuropsychology, 8,* 142.

Sena, H. M., & Sena, D. A. (1986a). The comparison of subject characteristics between treatment and non-treatment patients. *Archives of Clinical Neuropsychology, 1,* 74.

Sena, H. M., & Sena, D. A. (1986b). A quantitative validation of the effectiveness of cognitive retraining. *Archives of Clinical Neuropsychology, 1,* 74.

Sewell, D. D., Jeste, D. V., Atkinson, J. H., Heaton, R. K., Hesselink, J. R., Wiley, C., Thal, L., Chandler, J. L., & Grant, I. (1994). HIV-associated psychosis: A study of 20 cases. *American Journal of Psychiatry, 151,* 237–242.

Sheikh, M., Nagdy, S., Townes, B. D., & Kennedy, M. C. (1987). The Luria Nebraska and Halstead–Reitan Neuropsychological Test batteries: A cross-cultural study in English and Arabic. *International Journal of Neuroscience, 32*(3–4), 757–764.

Shelly, C., & Goldstein, G. (1982). Psychometric relations between the Luria–Nebraska and Halstead–Reitan Neuropsychological batteries in a neuropsychiatric setting. *Clinical Neuropsychology, 4,* 128–133.

Sherer, M., & Adams, R. L. (1993). Cross-validation of Reitan and Wolfson's Neuropsychological Deficit Scales. *Archives of Clinical Neuropsychology, 8,* 429–435.

Sherer, M., Parsons, O. A., Nixon, S. J., & Adams, R. L. (1991). Clinical validation of the Speech-Sounds Perception Test and the Seashore Rhythm Test. *Journal of Clinical and Experimental Psychology, 13,* 741–751.

Silverstein, M. L., Marengo, J. T., & Fogg, L. (1991). Two types of thought disorder and lateralized neuropsychological dysfunction. *Schizophrenia Bulletin, 17,* 679–687.

Skenazy, J. A., & Bigler, E. D. (1985). Psychological adjustment and neuropsychological performance in diabetic patients. *Journal of Clinical Psychology, 41,* 391–396.

Thompson, L. L., & Heaton, R. K. (1991). Pattern of performance on the Tactual Performance Test. *The Clinical Neuropsychologist, 5,* 322–328.

Thompson, L. L., Heaton, R. K., Matthews, C. G., & Grant, I. (1987). Comparison of preferred and nonpreferred hand performance on four neuropsychological motor tasks. *The Clinical Neuropsychologist, 1,* 324–334.

Wechsler, D. (1955). *Manual for the Wechsler Adult Intelligence Scale.* New York: The Psychological Corporation.

Wheeler, L. (1964). Complex behavioral indices weighted by linear discriminant functions for the prediction of cerebral damage. *Perceptual and Motor Skills, 19,* 907–923.

Wheeler, L., Burke, C. J., & Reitan, R. M. (1963). An application of discriminant functions to the problem of predicting brain damage using behavioral variables. *Perceptual and Motor Skills, 16,* 417–440.

Wheeler, L., & Reitan, R. M. (1962). The presence and laterality of brain damage predicted from response to a short Aphasia Screening test. *Perceptual and Motor Skills, 16,* 681–701.

Wheeler, L., & Reitan, R. M. (1963). Discriminant functions applied to the problem of predicting cerebral damage from behavior tests: A cross-validation study. *Perceptual and Motor Skills, 16,* 681–701.

Wolfson, D., & Reitan, R. M. (1995). Cross-validation of the General Neuropsychological Deficit Scale (GNDS). *Archives of Clinical Neuropsychology, 10,* 125–131.

Yeudall, L. T., Reddon, J. R., Gill, P. M., & Stefanyk, W. O. (1987). Normative data for the Halstead–Reitan neuropsychological tests stratified by age and sex. *Journal of Clinical Psychology, 43,* 346–367.

5

The Evolution of the Luria–Nebraska Neuropsychological Battery

JAMES A. MOSES, JR., AND ARNOLD D. PURISCH

INTRODUCTION

The Luria–Nebraska Neuropsychological Battery (LNNB) (Golden, Purisch, & Hammeke, 1985) is a standardized neuropsychological instrument that provides a broadscale evaluation of sensorimotor, linguistic, academic, memorial, and conceptual reasoning ability domains. Since the first published description of the LNNB appeared in 1978 (Golden, Hammeke & Purisch, 1978), there has been continuing, intense interest in its applicability and limitations across a wide variety of neuropsychiatric clinical settings and patient samples. The LNNB has been the subject of extensive and intensive psychometric scrutiny and critical discussion since its public appearance. Such intense investigation of a new instrument has been rare in the field of psychological assessment in recent years, but it is reminiscent of reactions to the original appearance of the Minnesota Multiphasic Personality Inventory (MMPI). The MMPI provided an alternative actuarial model for assessment of personality and mental status characteristics that stood in contrast to the subjectively interpreted Rorschach, which was the prevailing mental status diagnostic technique at that time.

While most of the theoretical controversy surrounding the public appearance of the LNNB has raised more questions than it has answered, the various critiques of the LNNB clearly have provided an impetus for the conduct of a large number of empirical studies. Although significant criticism of the LNNB continues to be offered by some prominent neuropsychologists (e.g., Lezak, 1995, pp. 717–722), the vast majority of these criticisms are empirically unfounded and likely are the

JAMES A. MOSES, JR. • Department of Veterans Affairs Medical Center, Stanford University, Palo Alto, California 94304-1207   ARNOLD D. PURISCH • Irvine, California 92718 result of personal and theoretical bias. The reliability, concurrent validity, and construct validity of the LNNB now have been empirically demonstrated. The sensitivity and limitations of the LNNB to evaluation of cognitive dysfunction in a wide variety of clinical syndromes also has been empirically proven. Multiple published review articles have summarized trends that were involved in the early theoretical and psychometric development, clinical applications, and empirical evaluations of the LNNB (Franzen, 1985, 1986; Golden, 1981; Purisch & Sbordone, 1986). A series of exhaustive critical reviews of the LNNB literature through 1988 also was published by Moses and Maruish (1987, 1988a–f, 1989a–c, 1990a,b, 1991a,b).

In this chapter we will present an expanded rationale for some of the major theoretical and empirical principles that have guided development of the LNNB. This material has not been published previously. Additions and changes to the LNNB since it was first commercially published in its original form (Golden, Hammeke, & Purisch, 1980) also will be clarified. An updated critical review of the literature of the past decade, since the publication of the most recent LNNB manual (Golden et al., 1985), also will be included. Practitioners who may be interested in details of the early LNNB literature may consult the test manual as well as the more extensive, detailed, and critically oriented series of reviews by Moses and Maruish that have been cited above. A brief discussion of background information on the development of the LNNB is provided in this chapter to serve as a foundation for the discussion of the recent developments in the LNNB literature. This review also will address only literature that deals with the adult versions of the LNNB.

Item Scaling and Selection

Golden et al. (1978) mentioned their methodology for LNNB item selection and scaling only briefly in their initial published article on the LNNB. At that time the instrument was known as the Luria–South Dakota Neuropsychological Battery and it consisted of 285 items. It was later shortened to the current 269 items and the name of the instrument was changed to the Luria–Nebraska Neuropsychological Battery (Form I).

The LNNB actually consists of over 700 discrete tasks that have been combined into logical groupings to arrive at 269 individual item scores. Many items rate performance on only a single question or task, while others have multiple subparts in which individual components are added to arrive at a global score. For example, item 99 on the fourth clinical scale requires one to perceptually rotate squares in different spatial orientations to a standard position without moving the stimulus figure from its presentation position. While each of these responses are scored separately, the final item score consists of the total number of errors that are made across all eight of these subtasks. Furthermore, given the varied nature of the sensorimotor, linguistic, and conceptual skills that are assessed across the LNNB item pool, it was necessary to utilize a number of different dimensions to convert qualitative performance observations into reliably quantified scores.

The general quality or accuracy of the performance was quantified in many ways, depending on the nature of the task. Many items lent themselves to a simple scoring method based on response accuracy that could be scored as correct or incorrect. For many other tasks, however, the adequacy of the performance was not an obvious performance level phenomenon, nor were the performance criteria discrete or operationally well defined. Specific scoring criteria were developed to quantify these performance patterns based on the quality, comprehensiveness, and abstraction level aspects of the response. Clinical characteristics of other performances included response speed as well as response accuracy. Depending on the item features, the adequacy of the performance was rated according to parameters such as response accuracy, frequency, latency, and duration.

The significant variability in the number of response subtasks and scoring parameters posed a problem of how to scale items psychometrically so that performance patterns could be compared across items. How, for example, is the level of performance on an item that measures the number of times that an individual can touch each finger with the thumb in 10 seconds to be compared with the quality with which that person is able to copy a triangle? An objective, standardized rating system was developed so that raw score performances for each item could be compared on a common ordinal scale. These ratings were accomplished by cross-tabulating the frequency distributions of raw scores for each of the 285 items of the original Luria–South Dakota Neuropsychological Battery in samples of 50 neurologically impaired patients and 50 control subjects. Performance levels on approximately one third of the items were clearly correct or incorrect, but the remainder of the items presented a performance continuum in both the neurological and the control groups. Raw score ranges that were primarily distinctive of the neurological group were used to anchor one end of the scoring continuum, whereas score ranges that were predominantly characteristic of the normal subjects anchored the other end of the scoring continuum. The frequency distributions of the neurological and control groups frequently overlapped and created an intermediate score zone between these anchor points.

Ultimately a three-point scoring system was chosen to provide a common metric for comparison of ordinal scoring levels across all of the test items. Since the majority of LNNB items are scored for errors, an ordinal rating score of zero (absence of deficit) was assigned to the raw scores that were typical of the performances of control subjects, and an ordinal rating score of two (definite presence of deficit) was assigned to raw scores that were typical of the performances of the neurologically impaired subjects. An intermediate score of one (questionable deficit) was assigned to raw scores that fell into the overlapping middle score range that was not typical for performance by either the neurological or the control subjects. Optimal discrimination between performance levels of the neurological and control subjects was the primary criterion that was used to establish rank-ordered score ranges for each LNNB item. In addition, care was taken to balance the frequency of false-positive and false-negative classification errors when these scoring values were chosen.

There appears to be some loss of information when scoring units for items are translated from continuous distribution raw scores to an ordinal two- or three-point scaling system (Russell, 1981). This situation is perhaps best exemplified by item 234, which requires the immediate recall of a short story that is scored for 14 details that may be recalled. On this item a raw score of three or less story elements recalled receives a scaled score of two (definitely impaired). A raw score of four or five story elements recalled receives a scaled score of one (questionably impaired). The ability to recall six or more story elements receives a scaled score of zero (normal performance). Clearly an individual who recalls 13 details is demonstrating a level of recall efficiency that is superior to that of a person who recalls only six or seven details. Yet both of these individuals would receive the same scaled score of zero.

The purpose of translating raw scores to scaled scores is to provide a common ordinal metric scale for all LNNB items across a variety of item types. In this way all responses can be classified and compared with each other according to a uniform, categorical, performance level criterion (impaired–questionable–normal). The LNNB item scoring system is not designed to provide fine gradations of performance level. When expanded systems of four (0–3) and five (0–4) points were tested during the development of the LNNB scoring system, these more complex scoring methods failed to provide additional discriminative accuracy for differentiation between neurological and control patients for the vast majority of LNNB items. In addition, the more complex scoring methods were abandoned because of the greater complexity that they introduced to the calculation of global scale scores and ipsative item scoring comparisons.

The clinician or research investigator who uses the LNNB is urged to consider both the general classification of impaired versus nonimpaired functional status that is provided by the three-point scale and the actual raw score on the item when individual item performances are interpreted. Supplementing this quantitative analysis with consideration of the qualitative aspects of the patient's performance can greatly increase the information that is yielded by any given item. Such qualitative analysis lies at the heart of Luria's clinical approach to syndrome analysis. It is also a critical component that contributes substantially to the full understanding of the meaning of the itemized or summary LNNB scale scores. Such an itemized qualitative approach to syndrome analysis also is embodied in the Boston Process Approach (Milberg, Hebben, & Kaplan, 1986). The rationale, development, and scoring criteria for a standardized qualitative scoring system for the LNNB is thoroughly described in the most recent LNNB manual (Golden et al., 1985, pp. 23–34) and therefore will not be resummarized here.

Golden et al. (1978) briefly described their item selection procedure utilizing itemized *t* tests to compare performance levels on each of the LNNB items between groups of neurological and control subjects. They reported statistically significant differences between the groups on 253 of these items. Sixteen of the remaining 32 items distinguished group performance levels between the .06 and the .20 levels. These items were retained in the battery, whereas the 16 items that did not differentiate between the neurological and control groups at even the .20 level were eliminated from the final LNNB item pool. The use of the t-test methodology for analysis of the LNNB ordinal item scores has been criticized; a nonparametric test should have been used to make these comparisons (Adams, 1985, p. 879).

Given the liberal .05 level of significance that was used to select items for the LNNB across the 285 comparisons, it is probable that many items met the inclusion criteria based on chance capitalization alone. The chance capitalization effect was increased with the decision to accept 16 more items that met the very liberal statistical criterion of reaching at least the .20 significance level for group discrimination. This overly liberal acceptance criterion also has been criticized. The LNNB developers chose this liberal statistical significance criterion because they wished to preserve any item that demonstrated reasonable potential to discriminate impaired from nonimpaired performance. It also was recognized that the performance levels of the groups on which the items were selected represented only a limited sample of the full range of all control and neurological populations. Different items might prove to be more or less discriminating of performance level differences between these heterogeneous groups as a function of the setting and population in which the test was administered. Statistical conservatism was therefore sacrificed to this logical criterion to optimize the potential utility of the LNNB across a broad range of differential diagnostic applications.

Scale Label Changes

The original LNNB consisted of 11 clinical scales and 3 summary scales that were derived from the clinical scale item pool. The original names of each of the 11 clinical scales were descriptive of the major functional system domains that each scale was designed to assess according to the diagnostic model of A. R. Luria (1966, 1973, 1980). These 11 scales were respectively labeled Motor, Rhythm, Tactile, Visual, Receptive Speech, Expressive Speech, Writing, Reading, Arithmetic, Memory, and Intellectual Processes. The 269 LNNB items are divided among these scales in groups of 12 (Rhythm scale) to 51 (Motor scale) items. The Pathognomonic scale consists of 34 items that were empirically selected to be maximally sensitive to cognitive dysfunction associated with the presence of acquired brain dysfunction. The Left Hemisphere and Right Hemisphere scales each consist of 21 items that were rationally selected to identify the presence of lateralized sensorimotor impairment.

The original names that were assigned to each of these scales were meant to identify the common component of a group of related functional systems rather than a single underlying process or skill. For example, items on the Motor scale are a heterogeneous grouping of tasks that are designed to identify the conditions that are necessary for integrated motor function and the specific functions than may be disrupted in motor disorder. It does not provide a unitary assessment of global motor skill on any one item. An example of a more traditional, unitary type of scale would be the Block Design subtest of the Wechsler Adult Intelligence Scale—Revised (WAIS-R). On this measure each item demonstrates at least a face validity assessment of the same nonverbal cognitive reasoning skill. According to a Lurian functional system analysis, however, one could separate constructional ability, visual–spatial analysis, visual pattern recognition, fine motor coordination, foresight, planning, and other cognitive component skills that contribute to performance on this "unitary" measure.

Many users of the LNNB have attempted to apply the unitary or unidimensional reasoning concept to the interpretation of the LNNB clinical scales such that an elevated (abnormal) score on the Motor scale was considered to be evidence of a primary impairment in global motor functioning. Critics of the LNNB inferred on this basis that the absence of frank paresis, dystonia, ataxia, incoordination, or other motor signs was considered to be evidence of the lack of construct validity of the Motor scale. Analogously, an elevation on the MMPI Depression scale in the absence of an obvious depressive syndrome would putatively invalidate the interpretation of that measure. Clearly this is not the case, since in clinical practice most clinical syndromes are multidimensional. A summary measure may be elevated owing to impairment on a variety of syndrome features that may be enhanced or attenuated in the individual case.

To lessen the tendency toward oversimplified generalizations and interpretations of the LNNB scales, the test authors changed the original descriptive labels for the scales to alphanumeric acronyms that were similar to the numeric labels that now are standardly used instead of syndrome names for the MMPI clinical scales. The 11 LNNB clinical scales now are referred to as scales C1 through C11, which refers to their categorization as clinical (C) LNNB scales in their original scale order. Thus, the Arithmetic scale, which is the ninth clinical scale in order of administration, is referred to as scale C9. The summary scales were given similar acronyms with an S preceding their ordinal scale number. Thus, the Pathognomonic scale now is designated as the S1 scale. The original names of the LNNB clinical and summary scales and their current acronyms are as follows: C1 (Motor), C2 (Rhythm), C3 (Tactile), C4 (Visual), C5 (Receptive Language), C6 (Expressive Language), C7 (Writing), C8 (Reading), C9 (Arithmetic), C10 (Memory), C11 (Intellectual Processes), C12 (Intermediate Memory) (LNNB-Form II only), S1 (Pathognomonic), S2 (Left Hemisphere), S3 (Right Hemisphere), S4 (Profile Elevation), and S5 (Impairment).

Cognitive Skill Coverage

Although the LNNB assesses many major domains of neuropsychological functioning, like any broad scope instrument it does not comprehensively assess all sensorimotor, linguistic, and cognitive skill areas. The most significant deficiencies that limit the broad applicability of the original battery are in the assessment of recent and delayed memory, higher-level visual–spatial perceptual and related constructional skills, and complex integrative intellectual skills. In the 1985 LNNB manual (Golden et al., 1985), the test authors presented experimental procedures to attempt to remedy some of these shortcomings.

An eight-item Delayed Memory scale was developed to assess the individual's ability to retain visual and verbal information approximately 20 minutes after the initial presentation. The effect of memorial recognition and cuing procedures are systematically analyzed. This scale also includes an item that requires the delayed reproduction of a complex visual design that was added for initial presentation and immediate recall at the end of scale C10 (Memory). This item was added to extend the LNNB's assessment of higher-level visual–spatial skills. Use of this complex visual figure item as a memorial task may limit its usefulness as a measure of constructional ability per se. The intact ability to accurately reproduce the figure from memory would confirm the normality of constructional skills, but failure on the item would not allow one to differentiate memorial from constructional difficulty. The subject could be asked to copy the figure to assess these skills as a testing-the-limits procedure. Assessment of higher-level constructional skills, therefore, remains a significant gap in the evaluation provided by the LNNB items. Depending on the nature of the syndrome analysis in the individual case, the clinician may supplement the LNNB with other appropriate psychometric measures.

There have been no additions or modifications to the LNNB to increase its intellectual challenge with regard to higher-level complex integrative executive skills since it was first designed. Thus, individuals with only mild right hemispheric disorders or individuals with high premorbid intellectual functioning levels who present with only mild, well-compensated cognitive disorder may not be optimally challenged by the LNNB item content. Currently, additional procedures are recommended to supplement the LNNB so that a more thorough evaluation of constructional and higher-level complex integrative skills can be provided. Addition of selected subtests from the WAIS-R, the Rey–Osterreith Complex Figure, the Wisconsin Card Sorting Test, or the Halstead Category Test often is sufficient to supplement the LNNB to extend the desired range of task difficulty and syndrome analytic coverage in the individual case without adding a great deal of time to the overall testing process.

Two forms of the LNNB currently are commercially available for clinical and experimental use. While the LNNB-Form II (LNNB-2) was designed to measure the same theoretical and item content areas as the original LNNB-Form I (LNNB-1), the test authors introduced systematic changes into the LNNB-2 test materials to make them more suitable for use with an American audience. Scoring of some items in LNNB-2 also was changed relative to LNNB-1. The preceding introductory comments that refer to the "LNNB" without reference to one or the other form are equally applicable to both forms. Research findings based on LNNB-1 or LNNB-2 are relevant only to the form of the test on which they have been developed, since the two forms of the test are not equivalent (Moses & Chiu, 1993). The literature concerning the two forms of the LNNB therefore will be discussed in separate sections of our literature review.

LNNB-1 LITERATURE REVIEW, 1985–1994

This critical review of the LNNB-1 literature for the decade since 1985 has been designed to supplement and update the descriptive literature reviews that appeared in the most recent LNNB test manual (Golden et al., 1985). For more detailed reviews and critical evaluations of the complete LNNB literature from 1977 through 1988, one may consult the series of topically organized review articles by Moses and Maruish (1987, 1988a–f, 1989a–c, 1990a,b, 1991a,b).

Reliability

Internal Consistency

Moses (1985) demonstrated that all of the LNNB-1 clinical scales exceeded the optimal .80 level of internal consistency according to Cronbach's coefficient alpha statistic (scale range .82–.91). Nunnally (1978) recommended use of this psychometric standard, since it reduces error variance to a practical minimum. Most of the LNNB-1 localization scales also met or closely approximated this criterion (range, .75–.90). Failure of the Right Frontal and Right Sensorimotor localization scales to meet this criterion was due to their relative brevity.

Item-to-Scale Correlations

Nunnally (1978) also recommended demonstration of a moderate correlation (with a minimum correlational value of .25) between an item and the total score of the scale to which it had been assigned. According to this criterion, each item should contribute in a significant but nonredundant manner to the total scale score. This psychometric index complements the internal consistency criterion that is tested by calculation of coefficient alpha. Moses (1987) demonstrated that 257 of the 269 LNNB-1 items met or exceeded the minimum value item-to-scale score criterion for the LNNB-1 clinical scales. The item–total scale correlations met the optimal criterion for all but two items of the S1 and S5 scales; all items of the S2–S4 scales met this criterion.

Interrater Reliability

Moses and Schefft (1985) investigated the interrater reliability of the LNNB-1 in a sample of diagnostically mixed, consecutive neuropsychiatric patient clinical referrals to a diagnostic neuropsychology unit. The two authors served as raters who differed markedly in their experience with administration, scoring, and interpretation of the LNNB at the time of the study. The senior author had had personal experience with approximately 1200 LNNB-1 cases, whereas the junior author had completed only five LNNB-1 cases at the time the study began.

Despite this large practice effect difference, the interrater reliability of the two authors was extremely high. At the item level the two raters agreed exactly on approximately 96% of the LNNB-1 items, and scoring differences on the remaining items were minor. Interrater scoring correlations for the LNNB-1 clinical and summary scales ranged from .97 to .99; the corresponding range for the LNNB-1 localization scales was .96 to .99. Clearly, the LNNB-1 scoring criteria are explicit and objective so that both novitiate and experienced raters are able to produce comparable itemwise and scalewise scoring results.

Construct Validity

Scale Construct Uniformity

Blackerby (1985) made use of the multivariate statistical technique of item response theory to investigate the unidimensionality of constructs underlying each of the LNNB-1 scales. He concluded that each of the LNNB-1 scales exemplified a single underlying psychometric dimension and that the quality of measurement was accurate across a wide range of item difficulties. He also made the important point that latent trait unidimensionality is a function of how the testees typically *respond* to the items of the scale rather than to the face validity content uniformity of the items that compose the scale. Thus, construct validity of a scale can be accurately and objectively assessed only by a statistical analysis of item response patterns and not simply by rational item inspection.

Multitrait–Multimethod Matrix Analyses

Macciocchi, Fowler, and Ranseen (1992) pooled scores from the LNNB-1 C1 scale score with the Finger Tapping and Grooved Pegboard scores from the Halstead–Reitan Neuropsychological Battery (HRNB) as tests of motor functions, the LNNB-1 C10 scale score with the Wechsler Memory Scale Visual Memory subtest and the Buschke Selective Reminding Test as measures of nonverbal and verbal memory functions, and the LNNB-1 C11 scale score with the WAIS Verbal and Performance IQ scores as measures of intellectual functioning. These nine measures were submitted to maximum likelihood confirmatory factor analysis, and load-ings showed strong and specific associations for each of the LNNB-1 C1, C10, and C11 scales with the marker variables for the respective motoric, memorial, and in-tellectual factorial constructs. Macciocchi et al. (1992, p. 548) concluded that these LNNB-1 measures showed both "convergent and discriminant validity."

LNNB-1 Replicated Factor Structure

The orthogonal factor structure of the LNNB-1 clinical and summary scales was established in diagnostically mixed samples in a series of early papers by Moses (1983b, 1984a–c). Moses (1986) subsequently pooled the items of the C1–C4 or sensorimotor scale band, the C5–C8 or linguistic scale band, and the C9–C11 or conceptual scale band to search for item-to-scale factorial correspon-dence and possible cross-scale factors. These bandwise factor scale constructs were very similar to the scalewise solutions.

Stambrook (1983) subsequently raised the important question of whether the factorial structure of the LNNB-1 would be invariant among different diagnostic groups. Large groups of patients with neurological disorder only or psychiatric disorder only who had been tested with the LNNB-1 were assembled. Factorial structure of the LNNB-1 was established for each group independently, and full factor scales (with all weighted scale items included) were composed separately for the neurological and psychiatric samples. The factor scales for each LNNB-1 clinical and summary scale were refactored as a group. There was very robust cor-respondence between the factorial dimensions of the LNNB-1 scales for the neuro-logical and psychiatric samples. Detailed results of these analyses are presented in a series of papers by Moses (1990a–c, 1991a–d).

In previously unpublished work, Moses (1994a–e) extended these analyses to compare the scalewise LNNB-1 factor patterns of the neurologic and psychiatric groups with a mixed sample of subjects that included those groups and a much larger group of diagnostically mixed neuropsychiatric patients. These studies were conducted to test the robustness and specificity of the LNNB-1 factorial dimen-sions across a wide range of diagnostic groups whose members typically are re-ferred for clinical evaluation. The itemized factor structure of the entire LNNB-1 sample ($N = 1922$) that was available to the first author at the time of the study was computed and complete factor scales were calculated for all of these factorial constructs as had been done in the previous studies. The factor scales for the neu-rologic subjects only, the psychiatric subjects only, and the total sample (including the neurologic and psychiatric subjects) were refactored for each LNNB-1 clinical and summary scale. Again, the factor scale correspondence results were robustly isomorphic across diagnostic samples. Clinicians are encouraged to analyze per-formance patterns within these item groupings since they represent rigorously de-fined functional system components that are central to the concept of Lurian syndrome analysis. A summary of the item listings and interpretive labels is presented in Table 1 for the factor analytic results that are based on the total sample.

LNNB-1 and WAIS-R Subtest Relationships

The LNNB-1 and WAIS-R scale scores are globally interrelated as performance level measures, but the specific scaled scores of either of these measures cannot be accurately predicted from the other measure (Koffler & Zehler, 1986). Zarantonello, Munley, and Milanovich (1993) also attempted to predict WAIS-R IQ scores from LNNB-1 scale scores. They rationally modified the regression equations reported by Prifitera and Ryan (1981) and by McKay, Golden, Moses, Fishburne and Wisniewski (1981) that were designed to predict WAIS IQ scores from the LNNB scale scores. To adjust for the level of performance difference between the WAIS and the WAIS-R, Zarantonello et al. (1993) subtracted 7.5 IQ points from the regression equations of Prifitera and Ryan (1981) and those of McKay et al. (1981). The adjusted regression equations of Prifitera and Ryan (1981) for prediction of WAIS-R Full-Scale IQ from the LNNB-1 scale scores were accurate within 10 points in 76% of cases. The comparable classification accuracy for the modified McKay et al. (1981) regression equation was 89% for prediction of WAIS-R Full-Scale IQ. Predicted WAIS-R Verbal and Performance IQ values were consistently inaccurate with either set of modified regression equations. None of the regression equations approached clinically useful classification accuracy rates when a five-point prediction accuracy window was used as the criterion.

The WAIS-R and LNNB-1 measures are better conceptualized as complementary indices that also are related as performance level measures. Moses (1989) has demonstrated a series of factorially complex relationships among the subtests of the LNNB-1 and those of the WAIS-R. For clinical interpretive purposes, several subtest groupings are particularly important. The WAIS-R and LNNB-1 sensorimotor band subtests (C1–C4) are very closely related measures of nonverbal conceptual and sequential reasoning. These scales therefore should be interpreted as a single group of measures. The C6 through C8 LNNB-1 scales are closely related to each other as measures of basic, overlearned verbal information processing. They are dimensionally independent of the WAIS-R Verbal and Performance IQs, which require primarily original conceptual verbal and nonverbal reasoning, respectively. The C9 through C11 conceptual reasoning group of LNNB-1 scales are related dimensionally to the WAIS-R Verbal and Performance IQs. Patterns of conceptual reasoning strength and deficit on the WAIS-R subtests and the LNNB-1 item factor groupings (see Table 1) may be particularly useful to consider in functional system analyses among these measures.

Silverstein, McDonald, and Fogg (1990) investigated the construct validity of the LNNB-1 S5 scale relative to the WAIS Full-Scale IQ (FSIQ) as a criterion performance level variable. There was a strong association of the S5 scale to FSIQ

TABLE 1. Factor Scale Exemplars for Complete Neuropsychiatric and Control Sample

Factor scale	LNNB-1 scale	LNNB-1 items
LNNB-1 clinical scales		
Drawing speed	C1	37, 39, 41, 43, 45, 47
Manual motor dexterity	C1	1, 2, 3, 4, 21, 22, 23
Spatial-based movement, left hand	C1	10, 12, 16, 20
Spatial-based movement, right hand	C1	9, 11, 13, 15, 19
Basic drawing accuracy, square and triangle	C1	38, 40, 44, 46
Manual kinesthesia	C1	5, 7, 8
"Optic-spatial movement," crossed	C1	17, 18
Oral motor sequencing	C1	25, 31, 32
Verbally cued alternative motor response	C1	48, 49, 50, 51
Basic drawing accuracy: circle	C1	36, 42
Complex praxes	C1	26, 27
Oral–facial praxis	C1	29, 34, 35
Lingual praxis	C1	30
Rhythm and pitch discrimination	C2	52, 53, 54, 55, 58, 59, 60, 61, 62, 63
Singing	C2	56, 57
Stereognosis	C3	82, 83, 84, 85
Pinprick/pressure sensation	C3	66, 67, 69
Kinesthetic sensation, right	C3	64, 74, 76
Kinesthetic sensation, left	C3	65, 75, 77
Proprioception	C3	80, 81
Literal graphesthesia	C4	78, 79
Visual–spatial analysis	C4	94, 95, 96, 97, 98
Visual naming	C4	86, 90, 91
Visual concept formation	C4	88, 89, 93
Phonemic comprehension	C5	100, 101, 102, 103, 104, 105
Syntactical comprehension: related forms	C5	117, 119, 120, 123, 129
Verbal concept recognition	C5	110, 112, 113, 115, 116
Sequential verbal analysis	C5	107, 109, 132
Elementary auditory comprehension: single step commands	C5	111, 114, 118
Syntactical analysis: concept formation	C5	108, 121, 126
Syntactical analysis: contrasted forms	C5	122, 127, 128, 131
Complex verbal decoding	C6	138, 140, 144, 148, 149, 151
Simple sight reading	C6	146, 147, 150, 152, 153
Repetition	C6	133, 134, 135, 137, 142
Syntactical reorganization	C6	173, 174
Overlearned-automatic language	C6	156, 160, 161, 162, 163
Verbal response latency	C6	164, 166
Naming	C6	143, 157, 158
Verbal fluency	C6	165, 167, 169
Sequential grammatical analysis	C6	139, 170, 171
Lexical analysis	C7	175, 176, 179, 183, 184, 185, 186, 187

TABLE 1. (*Continued*)

Factor scale	LNNB-1 scale	LNNB-1 items
Overlearned motor writing	C7	177, 178, 180, 181, 182
Complex reading	C8	188, 190, 192, 195, 196, 199, 200
Simple reading	C8	190, 194, 197, 198
Serial step calculation	C9	212, 215, 216, 217, 219, 220, 221, 222
Number structure analysis	C9	207, 208, 209
Number writing	C9	201, 203, 204, 205
Numerical quantity analysis	C9	206, 210, 211, 214
Immediate verbal memory	C10	223, 224, 225, 230, 231, 232, 233, 234
Immediate visual memory	C10	226, 229, 235
Sequential step reasoning	C11	247, 256, 262, 264, 268
Verbal abstraction	C11	244, 245, 246, 248, 249, 250
Mental calculation efficiency	C11	263, 265, 266, 267, 269
Verbal conceptual reasoning	C11	251, 252, 253, 255
Simple mental calculation	C11	258, 259, 260, 261
Nonverbal conceptual reasoning	C11	236, 237, 242, 243
Nonverbal sequential reasoning	C11	238, 239, 240, 241
LNNB-1 summary scales		
Elementary drawing speed	S1	37, 39, 43, 45
Phonemic analysis	S1	101, 102, 103, 139
Complex—sequential verbal analysis	S1	175, 184, 185, 196
Stereognosis	S1	82, 83, 85
Spatial-based movement	S1	9, 19, 64, 108
Verbally mediated visual analysis	S1	42, 89, 157, 227
Graphesthesia	S1	77, 79
Verbal fluency	S1	166, 169, 241, 267
"Optic–spatial movement," right hand	S2	9, 11, 13, 15
Kinesthetic and cutaneous sensation, right hand	S2	5, 64, 66, 68, 70, 72, 80
Kinesthetically mediated movement, right hand	S2	1, 3, 82, 83
Kinesthetically cued sensation, right hand	S2	7, 17, 76, 78
"Optic–spatial movement," left hand	S3	10, 12, 14, 16, 20
Kinesthetic and cutaneous sensation, left hand	S3	65, 67, 69, 71, 73, 75, 81
Kinesthetically mediated movement, left hand	S3	2, 4, 84, 85
Kinesthetically cued sensation, left hand	S3	18, 77, 79
Strategic problem solving	S4	59, 92, 218, 223, 230, 256
Verbal analysis	S4	178, 185, 199, 215
Sensory stimulus naming	S4	75, 82, 84, 91
Number structure analysis	S4	113, 209, 210, 214, 258
Serial mental calculation	S5	217, 220, 222, 264, 266, 268
Immediate verbal recall	S5	224, 225, 234, 235
Syntactical verbal analysis	S5	166, 185, 199, 200
Visual–spatial analysis	S5	7, 24, 46, 77, 95

($r = -.82$ overall; $r = -.82$ for schizophrenic and schizoaffective disordered patients; $r = -.77$ for depressives; $r = -.84$ for manics). They concluded that S5 appears to bear a comparable and robust linear performance level relationship to WAIS FSIQ across the psychiatric diagnostic groups that they studied.

Halstead–Reitan Neuropsychological Battery

The LNNB-1 repeatedly has been shown to be actuarially and clinically comparable to the Halstead–Reitan Neuropsychological Battery (HRNB). A variety of approaches have been taken to demonstrate this correspondence. The LNNB-1 and HRNB have been shown to be clinically equivalent sets of measures based on exemplary case reports (Goldstein & Incagnoli, 1986), theoretical analyses of item content (Goldstein, 1986), blind ratings by clinicians (Kane, Parsons, Goldstein, & Moses, 1987), and actuarial intertest comparison and prediction analyses (for reviews, see Moses & Maruish, 1988b; Kane, 1986, 1991).

Mini-Mental State Examination

Horton and Alana (1990) validated the Mini-Mental State Examination (MMSE) with the LNNB-1 clinical scales as criterion measures in a diagnostically mixed, neurologically impaired sample. After partial correlational control for age effects they reported significant ($p < .01$ or greater) correlations of the MMSE with the LNNB-1 C1, C3, C6 ($p < .001$), and C7 scales. These results are sensible in that the MMSE contains both sensorimotor (C1, C3) and overlearned linguistic (C6, C7) items.

Memorial Indices

Pheley and Klesges (1986) validated the LNNB-1 C10 scale against a variety of clinical and experimental attentional and memorial psychometric measures in a sample of 40 college undergraduates. The C10 scale was not significantly correlated with the Digit Span measure ($r = -.14$), which is a standard measure of attention span. The C10 scale also showed a nonsignificant correlation to a rote consonant trigram memory task with a distractor condition (for details, see Pheley & Klesges, 1986, p. 234). The C10 scale *did* correlate significantly ($p < .01$) with multiple measures of visual–verbal associative recall and paired associate verbal recall with and without "filled interval" delay conditions. These results support the construct validity of the LNNB-1 C10 scale as a measure of short-term associative memory function. The C10 scale appears to be relatively insensitive to attentional nuances, and it also appears to be primarily sensitive to learning and recall that requires active rather than passive (rote) strategic verbal encoding and recall.

Motoric Skills

Gruber, Hall, McKay, Humphries, and Krysclo (1989) attempted to study the relationship of the LNNB-1 clinical and selected summary scales (14 measures) to the Bruininks–Oseretsky Motor Proficiency Test (12 measures) in a sample of only 22 adolescents. Their use of multiple regression to predict the scores of one set of variables from the other is inappropriate. This study illustrates a very common experimental design error. The analysis includes all available predictor variables of interest without a theoretical rationale, and the sample size is very small. When multivariate techniques are used in such conditions, there is great capitalization on chance, and the results that appear at first to be actuarially impressive in fact are statistically artifactual (Nunnally, 1978).

Concurrent Validity

Computerized Diagnostic Classification

Horton, Vaeth, and Anilane (1990) developed and preliminarily validated a computerized actuarial interpretive system for LNNB-1. They grouped their archival LNNB-1 data into broad categories of patients with and without apparent brain damage according to the medical history. The neurologically "normal" group included control patients and diagnostically mixed psychiatric cases. The correct classification rate for identification of the presence or absence of global neurological deficit with their algorithm was 80% (52 of 65 cases). Actuarial assessment of the degree of cognitive deficit using their method was 60% (12 of 20 cases) based on a four-level classification system (no deficit through severe deficit). The accuracy of identification of a unilaterally lesioned cerebral hemisphere was 71% (10 of 14 cases). Based on their review of the literature, Horton et al. (1990) concluded that their actuarial classification algorithm was comparable to similar procedures that had been developed for actuarial interpretation of the HRNB.

Ecological Validity

Heinrichs (1989) predicted concurrent employment status from the mean global performance level on LNNB-1 scales C1 through C11 and S1 in addition to age, educational level, and global neurological status (normal/abnormal brain function). Age, educational level, and categorical neurological diagnostic status jointly predicted 21% of the variance in global employment status. Addition of the mean LNNB *T* score to the regression equation accounted for an additional 8% of unique variance. Crosstabulation analysis showed a significant ($p < .01$) relationship of global neuropsychological status (normal/impaired) to employment status (employed/unemployed). In contrast, a similar analysis of normal versus abnormal neurological status relative to employment status showed no significant relationship between these two indices. Thus, it appears that global neuropsychological status is related significantly to employment status, while global neurological status is not. These important but preliminary findings require replication in independent samples.

McCue, Rogers, and Goldstein (1990) investigated the relationship of performance on the Performance Assessment of Self-Care Skills (PASS) to their short form of the LNNB-1 (LNNB-S) that was designed for use with the elderly (McCue, Shelly, & Goldstein, 1985; for review, see Moses & Maruish, 1989b, p. 106). Their sample consisted of elderly (age: mean = 74.5, SD = 7.9) neuropsychiatric patients. The LNNB-S C1, C3, C10, and C11 scales showed significant ($p < .01$) correlations with PASS personal self-care indices, but the LNNB-S measures explained little variance (10–15%) in the PASS measures. The LNNB-S showed generally low correlations with the PASS mobility measures. Sensorimotor, memorial, and intellectual competence on the LNNB-S C1 through C4, C10, and C11 scales showed moderate correlational relationships (15–20% of explained variance) to PASS indices of physically oriented instrumental self-care (household chores). All of the LNNB-S measures were moderately related (14–37% of explained variance) to PASS measures of cognitively oriented instrumental self-care (routine practical problem-solving tasks). The LNNB-S sensorimotor measures predicted competence on tasks that required those skills specifically (beyond basic mobility), but all of the LNNB-S measures were relevant to the prediction of performance ability on tasks that required problem solving ability.

Falk-Kessler and Quittman (1990) investigated the relationship of performance level on the LNNB-1 S1 scale, other psychometric measures, and demographic variables to performance level competence in social, occupational, and leisure activities. They reported chance differences on the quality of life activity indices between their subgroups of subjects with normal and impaired S1 scale scores. The quality of performance on complex sociobehavioral indices appears to be too complex a criterion to predict with the S1 scale alone.

Silverstein, Fogg, and Harrow (1991) attempted to examine related predictive validational issues using the 11 LNNB-1 clinical scales to predict social adjustment, employment competence, and likelihood of rehospitalization in a psychiatric patient sample. Unfortunately, they employed multivariate techniques with a sample of only 51 subjects, which produced theoretically plausible but statistically artifactual results. The ratio of subjects to variables should be on the order of 10-to-1 to prevent substantial chance capitalization in such studies (Nunnally, 1978).

Schizophrenia and Related Disorders

Syndrome Analyses

A series of innovative papers by Silverstein and his colleagues (Frazier, Silverstein, & Fogg, 1989; Silverstein & McDonald, 1988; Silverstein, McDonald, & Meltzer, 1988; Silverstein, Strauss, & Fogg, 1990) have actuarially investigated

LNNB-1 performance patterns among schizophrenic, depressed, manic, and schizoaffective disorder patients. Unfortunately, each of these studies has been flawed methodologically, since the groups of subjects were demographically mismatched. In each case the depressives were significantly older than the schizophrenics on the average. In general, it also would be preferable in syndrome analytic studies to study diagnostically homogeneous or at least closely related groups of subjects rather than diagnostically mixed samples, so that syndrome-specific conclusions might be drawn.

When cross-group comparisons are made and there is a consistent finding of significant demographic intergroup differences, it is best to match the subjects in individual pairs and to avoid inclusion of outliers in the matching process, so that the groups will be demographically comparable and representative. Such demographic mismatching differences cannot be adjusted by means of analysis of covariance (for discussion, see Adams, Brown, & Grant, 1985, 1992; Berman & Greenhouse, 1992).

Silverstein, Harrow, and Marengo (1993) investigated the relationship of LNNB-1 performance to concreteness and bizarre–idiosyncratic types of thought process disorder. They classified their psychiatric patient samples using rigorous diagnostic criteria, but they then pooled relatively small samples of schizophrenic, schizoaffective disorder, manic, and psychotically depressed patients into the same sample. This procedure will obscure syndrome analytic findings. Various multivariate analyses in this study employed the entire sample ($n = 99$) and schizophrenic spectrum disorder cases ($n = 58$). Analyses based on the entire sample in this study are diagnostically confounded by categorically different medication regimens and symptomatology. Multivariate analyses of the schizophrenic spectrum subjects is unfortunately seriously compromised by insufficient sample size. Use of the LNNB-1 localization scales as criterion marker variables for left- and right-hemispheric function also is not advisable, since there are no published validational studies to support their use for that purpose in a psychiatric patient sample. These points are made to illustrate common errors in the experimental design of LNNB-1 research.

Dickerson, Ringel, and Boronow (1991) found that the LNNB-1 Left Frontal localization scale and the C10 and C11 clinical scales were the best predictors of Brief Psychiatric Rating Scale (BPRS) psychopathology measures in their chronic schizophrenic sample. The LNNB-1 measures were most strongly related to BPRS-positive symptomatic indices of conceptual disorganization, hallucinations, and disorientation. Negative symptoms were not significantly related to performance on the LNNB-1 measures in their sample.

Schizophrenic Subtype

Langell, Purisch, and Golden (1987) found greater cognitive deficit among their sample of nonparanoid schizophrenics than among their sample of paranoid schizophrenics. Their schizophrenic subjects were not neurologically examined, although efforts were taken to eliminate subjects with any medical history of head trauma or symptomatology that was suggestive of neurological disorder. Moses (1991e) replicated and extended the Langell et al. (1987) study. He studied LNNB-1 intergroup differences at the item level in groups of paranoid and nonparanoid schizophrenics with proven normal neurological status. He reported comparable performance patterns between the paranoid and nonparanoid schizophrenic groups, with occasional intergroup differences that were consistent with chance alone. Paulman et al. (1990) also reported no performance level differences between their paranoid and nonparanoid schizophrenic samples on the LNNB-1 clinical and summary scales.

Faustman, Moses, and Csernansky (1988) studied the performance of a group of carefully diagnosed, unmedicated, neurologically normal schizophrenics on selected scales of the LNNB-1, the BPRS, and multiple demographic variables. They chose two summary indices from the LNNB-1: the global deficit score (number of scales exceeding critical level) and the mean of the C2–C10–C11 scales (that are known to be sensitive to cognitive deficit in schizophrenia). Negligible correlational values were found between each of these LNNB-1 summary variables and a variety of symptomatic measures that were derived from the BPRS: total negative (schizophrenic) symptoms, total positive (schizophrenic) symptoms, the global BPRS psychopathology score, and measures of emotional withdrawal, psychomotor retardation, blunted affect, hallucinatory behavior, conceptual disorganization, and unusual thought content. Age at time of testing, age at disorder onset, and duration of disorder also showed negligible correlations with the LNNB-1 global cognitive deficit measures.

Neuroradiological Studies

Kemali et al. (1986) compared schizophrenic subgroups with normal sized and enlarged cerebral ventricles on the LNNB-1 scales and a variety of symptomatic measures. The schizophrenic subgroup with enlarged cerebral ventricles typically showed longer illness duration, a longer period of hospitalization, and greater impairment on the measures of alogia, affective flattening, and attentional impairment from the Schedule for Assessment of Negative Symptoms. Their performance on the Disability Assessment Schedule showed lessened ability to manage self-care, to participate in household chores, to work productively, and to manage adaptively in personal crises. On the LNNB-1, the schizophrenic subgroup with enlarged ventricles showed greater impairment on the C2, C7, C8, C9, and S2 scales, and on the WAIS they showed relatively greater impairment on the Digit Span, Digit Symbol, and Block Design subtests.

Rossi et al. (1990) reported that a small subgroup of their schizophrenic sample could not comprehend the instructions for the LNNB-1 tasks, even after repeated instruction and explanations were offered. Several of these patients also showed enlarged cerebral ventricles on brain-imaging studies and met diagnostic criteria for Krapelin's original dementia praecox syndrome. The global inability to understand the LNNB-1 directions thus may be a useful screening method for preliminary identification of a severely cognitively impaired schizophrenic subgroup whose cognitive deficit may have a physical basis related to periventricular brain atrophy.

Paulman et al. (1990, p. 388) found different patterns of correlation between LNNB-1 scales and forebrain regional cerebral flow rates in paranoid and nonparanoid schizophrenics. In paranoid schizophrenics they reported significant inverse correlations of regional cerebral blood flow (rCBF) rate in the left frontal area with the total number of elevated LNNB-1 scales ($r = -.58$), the C1 scale ($r = -.77$), and the C11 scale ($r = -.63$). In nonparanoid schizophrenics they found significant inverse correlations between the C2 scale and rCBF rate in the right temporal ($r = -.51$) and right frontal ($r = -.49$) areas.

DiMichele et al. (1992) investigated relationships between findings on magnetic resonance imaging (MRI) brain scans and cognitive performance on the LNNB-1. They found no significant univariate correlational relationships between the MRI structural brain indices and scale scores on the LNNB-1. Correlations between the LNNB-1 scales and the scales of the BPRS also were consistent with chance differences between the groups. When the sample was divided into subgroups of cognitively normal and abnormal subjects based on the LNNB-1 performance, however, significant differences in temporal lobe anatomy were found between these groups on the MRI measures. DiMichele et al. (1992, p. 487) concluded that the effect of temporal lobe dysgenesis in the cognitively impaired group was manifested in cognitive performance level deficit (as assessed by the LNNB-1), but that it was not associated with psychopathological symptomatology on the BPRS indices.

Left-Handedness

Faustman, Moses, Ringo, and Newcomer (1991) investigated the finding of other investigators that mixed handedness and left-handedness frequency was increased in schizophrenia. They contrasted the LNNB-1 C2, C10, and C11 scale performance levels in samples of left- and right-handed schizophrenics and left- and right-handed controls. They found a specific association of left-handedness to impairment on the LNNB-1 C2 and C10 scales but not on the C11 scale among schizophrenics. The effect of handedness on LNNB-1 performance was absent in the control group. They concluded that there appeared to be a specific relationship of handedness to schizophrenic status and that it might be a marker variable related to early cerebral insult and specific patterns of cognitive deficit.

Winter Birth

Faustman, Bono, Moses, and Csernansky (1992) investigated a reported putative relationship of increased incidence of schizophrenia associated with winter birth. They employed several indices of winter birth in their study. Faustman et al. (1992) failed to find any significant relationship of birth season to the incidence of schizophrenic disorder.

Specific Linguistic Deficit

Condray, Steinhauer, and Goldstein (1992) made use of the Relational Concepts Factor Scale (RCFS) of the LNNB-1 as a marker variable to identify specific syntactical language disturbance in pairs of brothers who were discordant for schizophrenic disorder. RCFS abnormal scores were similar among schizophrenics and their brothers who suffered from other schizophrenic spectrum disorders. The schizophrenic-spectrum-disordered brothers showed significantly poorer RCFS scores relative to unaffected brothers and normal controls. This LNNB-1 marker variable thus may be a useful psychometric screening variable for identification of a continuum of disturbed complex language functioning in schizophrenic spectrum patients. The severity of schizophrenic spectrum disorder and the level of cognitive performance (on selected WAIS and Wisconsin Card Sorting Test variables) was not related to the severity of linguistic deficit on the RCFS measure.

Violent Behavior

Adams, Meloy, and Moritz (1990) investigated the relationship of violent behavior to global cognitive deficit level on the LNNB in inpatient and outpatient schizophrenics. Outpatient but not inpatient violent behavior was significantly related to global cognitive deficit on the LNNB-1. A history of extremely violent acts was uniquely associated with global cognitive deficit on the LNNB-1. Within the cognitively impaired group, however, extreme and mild acts of violence occurred with approximately equal frequency. There is no evidence of a direct link of violent behavior to cognitive deficit based on these preliminary results.

Depression

Newman and Silverstein (1987) employed a specific set of LNNB-1 indices to analyze cognitive characteristics of diagnostic subgroups of depressed patients (endogenous–nonendogenous, psychotic–nonpsychotic, primary–secondary, retarded–nonretarded, agitated–nonagitated, unipolar–bipolar). They employed the LNNB-1 S4 and S5 scales, the eight localization scales, the empirically derived left (L*) and right (R*) hemispheric lesion lateralization scales, and a global speed score based on the 33 response latency scores for the LNNB-1 item pool. Our reanalysis of their data with statistical correction for the number of score comparisons made shows that their occasional intergroup differences are consistent with chance.

Miller, Faustman, Moses, and Csernansky (1991) compared demographically matched, neurologically normal groups of patients diagnosed with major depression to normal controls on each of the LNNB-1 clinical and summary scales. Performance levels of the two groups were comparable on all of the LNNB-1 measures. When the subjects who were most severely depressed were compared with their demographically matched control group peers, again the intergroup differences were not significant on any LNNB-1 measure. The Hamilton Rating Scale for Depression was correlated with each of the LNNB-1 scale measures and none of these values was significant.

Mixed Neuropsychiatric Syndromes

Actuarial Group Classification

Nizamie, Nizamie, and Shukla (1992) reported from India on the use of a translated (Hindi) version of the LNNB-1 to study performance level differences between groups of patients with schizophrenia ($n = 40$), mixed brain damage ($n = 30$), and normal mental and neurologic status ($n = 30$). The groups were well matched for age, but they differed significantly in educational level (schizophrenic sample: mean = 15.5 years; neurological sample: mean = 10.4 years; normal controls: mean = 12.0 years). The schizophrenics were reported to perform at a significantly better level than the neurological patients, but their performance was inferior to that of the controls. Unfortunately, in these data there is confounding of a powerful predictor variable (educational level) with diagnostic category, so that it is unclear whether the demographic or the diagnostic variable set accounts for the level of performance level differences.

Goldstein, Shelly, McCue, and Kane (1987) employed hierarchical cluster analysis and ipsative profile analytic techniques in an attempt to identify patterns of performance among subgroups of subjects with learning disability, left-hemispheric brain lesions, and right-hemispheric lesions. Their diagnostic groups were actuarially categorized by level rather than by pattern of performance. The actuarially identified subgroups were not reliably associated with externally determined diagnostic subtypes. Based on these results, Goldstein and his colleagues questioned the utility of the LNNB-1 for actuarial categorical syndrome analysis.

Subsequent work by Moses, Pritchard, and Faustman (1994) applied the multivariate statistical classification technique of modal profile analysis (MPA) to a more varied and diagnostically specific set of syndromes: cerebral concussion, dementia, bipolar disorder, paranoid schizophrenia, undifferentiated schizophrenia, major depression, neurologically normal medical patients, and normal volunteers. A particular advantage of MPA is that it analyzes profile patterns independently of profile elevation. These MPA analyses identified a total of 22 modal LNNB-1 profiles across all of the diagnostic groups. Approximately one third of the modal profile patterns occurred in more than one diagnostic group. Eighty-two percent of all subjects in the derivation sample were assigned to a modal profile pattern group according to rigorous actuarial statistical classification criterion. Seventy-seven percent of the subjects in the cross-validation sample also were actuarially classified correctly. A considerably higher percentage of subjects could have been classified with a minor relaxation of the MPA classification criterion. A strict criterion was chosen to test the robustness of the classification algorithm.

Clearly, LNNB-1 profile analysis is enhanced by statistical methods such as MPA that actuarially remove the effect of profile elevation, so that specific profile patterns can be identified. It also appears from these analyses that multiple subtypes of cognitive performance may occur within a single clinical diagnostic group and that there may be commonalities of LNNB-1 profile type across some diagnostic groups. Empirical analyses of syndromes and subtypes may benefit from MPA-based typological analysis of commonalities and differences within and between clinical diagnostic groups rather than among clinical subtypes alone.

Posttraumatic Stuttering

Rousey, Arjunan, and Rousey (1986) reported a case of stuttering that began after closed-head injury. The patient was administered the LNNB-1 as part of the neuropsychological evaluation of cognitive effects that were associated with his brain injury. The LNNB-1 profile showed elevation of the C6 and S1 scales only. The authors noted the coincidence of the isolated symptom of speech dysfluency and the concomitant selective elevation of the C6 scale of the LNNB-1. These results support the concurrent validity of the C6 scale as a measure of expressive language.

Posttraumatic Mania

Nizamie, Nizamie, Borde, and Sharma (1988) reported from India about two cases of secondary mania with a characteristic LNNB-1 profile. Both individuals developed their manic symptomatology as a side effect of closed-head injury. In both cases there was no pretraumatic personal or familial history of psychiatric symptomatology. The LNNB-1 pattern included elevations on the C1, C4, C9, C10, and C11 scales. Nizamie et al. interpreted their findings as being consistent with a nonfocal lesion syndrome with some suggestion of greater right-hemispheric involvement. The electrocencephalographic results and the LNNB-1 profile both remained abnormal 18 months after the head injury in the individual who returned for follow-up evaluation.

Mixed Emotional Disturbance

Stephens, Clark, and Kaplan (1990) compared scalewise LNNB-1 performance levels of emotionally disturbed adolescents with performance levels of LNNB-1 standardization sample subjects. They failed to account for the demographic mismatch in terms of age and educational level between their sample and the standardization sample. All of the LNNB-1 intergroup performance level differences that they reported are strongly influenced by this demographic mismatch, since both age and educational level are powerful predictors of cognitive performance level on LNNB-1 (Golden et al., 1985).

Mental Retardation

Bogner (1990) compared the LNNB-1 profile patterns of 19 adult patients with Down's syndrome and 18 adult patients with mental retardation of unknown origin. The level of intellectual deficit was mild to moderate overall (IQ range = 50–70). The subjects were matched across diagnostic groups for age, sex, handedness, and IQ level. Most of the profiles showed deficit on scales C2, C5, C6, and C11. Deficits in sustained attention (C2), verbal mediation (C5, C6), and cognitive reasoning (C11) are predictable in these individuals. Almost every individual showed deficit on the C2 scale. The C4 scale was characteristically best performed by the Down's syndrome patients, whereas the C3 scale typically was best performed by the etiologically mixed group subjects. The profile patterns were more consistent in the Down's syndrome group than in the etiologically mixed group.

Learning Disability Syndromes

Lewis and Lorion (1988) compared LNNB-1 performance levels between groups of learning disabled and normally achieving adolescents who were matched for age, grade placement, and intelligence level. The groups were compared on the 11 LNNB-1 clinical scales and the S1 scale, but no correction was made to adjust the significance level for multiple comparisons of means. After such correction, significant intergroup differences ($p < .01$) remain on eight LNNB-1 scales: C2, C6, C7, C8, C9, C10, C11, and S1. In each case the measures of mean performance and variability were greater in the learning disabled student group.

Lewis and Lorion then attempted to make use of discriminant analysis to predict group membership actuarially and to determine the relative contribution of each of the LNNB-1 scales to group membership. This portion of the analysis is invalidated and the classification results are artifactual due to chance capitalization, since the number of variables (12) is excessive for the sample size (60). The sample size also should be larger to meet distributional assumptions for multivariate analysis (Nunnally, 1978).

Goldstein, Katz, Slomka, and Kelly (1993) investigated LNNB-1 profile patterns in subgroups of learning disabled subjects with specific reading, arithmetic, or global deficit syndromes. They reported that the LNNB-1 differentiated these groups on the basis of level rather than pattern of performance. Unfortunately, their statistical classification procedures did not allow for control of profile elevation as a variable that commonly confounds analysis of profile patterns among diagnostic subgroups.

Lewis, Hutchens, and Garland (1993) attempted to cross-validate the effectiveness of the LNNB-1 for diagnostic classification of learning disabled adolescents relative to control subjects. Unfortunately, they made use of discriminant analysis with 16 predictor variables in a sample of only 62 subjects. This ratio of subjects to variables is insufficient to prevent great chance capitalization and inflation of classification rates. Their classification results are, while actuarially impressive, unfortunately artifactual.

Specific Neurological Syndromes

Headache

Tsushima and Tsushima (1993) evaluated the effect of frequency of headache (daily, frequent, infrequent, or absent) on LNNB-1 performance. Comparison of the LNNB-1 performance of those with various frequencies of headache occurrence showed no intergroup differences relative to each other or controls. Comparison of patients who suffered headache during the LNNB-1 administration was not significantly different from that of headache-free, demographically matched controls. These results reinforce the robustness of the LNNB findings and their relative insensitivity to nonspecific extratest factors.

Limbic Epilepsy

Moses, Csernansky, and Leiderman (1988) reported 75% correct classification accuracy of patients with limbic epilepsy using the standard LNNB-1 profile elevation decision rules that are provided in the test manual (Golden et al., 1985). The presence of generalized seizures did not significantly increase the frequency or severity of cognitive deficit on the LNNB-1 relative to that which occurred in patients without generalized seizures.

Dementia Assessment

McCue, Goldstein, and Shelly (1989) employed their LNNB-1 short form (for review, see Moses & Maruish, 1989b, p. 106) to investigate performance level and pattern differences between demographically matched groups of elderly patients with Alzheimer's-type dementia and elderly depressed patients. They demonstrated large performance level differences between these two diagnostic groups on all 10 of their LNNB-1 short-form scales.

MacInnes et al. (1990) compared the relative sensitivity of the LNNB-1, LNNB-2, and independent clinical reading (by four radiologists) of computerized tomographic (CT) brain scans as indices of presence or absence of cognitive deficit in normal controls and patients with Alzheimer's disease. Patients were classified as cognitively normal or abnormal based on their global LNNB-1 performance level. The sample of normal volunteers averaged less than one LNNB-1 clinical scale score over their critical level, whereas the demented patients averaged approximately four clinical scale scores over their critical level.

Relative to this classification criterion, the radiologists were 80% accurate in identifying the absence of cognitive deficit based on impressionistic reading of CT scans of the normal subjects. They performed at less than a chance level, however, in attempts to identify the presence of cognitive deficit from sight reading of CT scans among the sample of demented patients (accuracy range = 0–18.2%). While the LNNB-1 was accurate in predicting the presence or absence of cognitive deficit among demented patients, expert reading of the CT scan findings was not. Many patients showed cognitive signs of dementia without structural change in the brain that could be recognized by expert radiological reading of the CT scan results.

Normal Aging Effects

Menich and Baron (1987) compared the performance level of younger (age 18–26) and older (age 62–76) men on the LNNB-1. Unfortunately, these two age cohort groups were demographically mismatched with regard to educational level; the older group was significantly better educated than the younger group (16.0 years vs. 14.4 years). Both age groups performed well within normal limits when a T-score impairment criterion of 60 was chosen (91% of younger group, 97% of older group). Age differences also were minimal at the 50 T-score level. When the impairment criterion was made absolute (at T-score 40, minimal error criterion), age group differences became significant, but the clinical relevance of this finding is at best moot. Clearly, there was no direct relationship of normal aging to impaired performance level on the LNNB-1. The magnitude of the cross-age-group comparison, however, was influenced by the educational level mismatch between the two comparison groups. Less well-educated elderly subjects very likely would have shown a more frequently impaired level of performance at the more stringent deficit criterion levels.

Abbreviated LNNB-1 Forms

Odd–Even LNNB-1 Short Form

Horton, Anilane, Puente, and Berg (1988) divided the LNNB-1 item pool into halves by grouping the even-numbered and odd-numbered items into separate categories. The global psychometric characteristics of these two item subgroups were comparable. Subjects performed at very similar levels on the total number of scales that exceeded critical level and on the frequency of scores that occurred in 1- to 10-point ranges above or below the critical level. The correlations of the odd- and even-numbered items for each LNNB-1 scale were uniformly high (range = 0.80–0.95). Similarly, the correlations of each split-half short form to the total item pool also was consistently high (odd items to full-scale score range = 0.82–0.89; even items to full-scale score range = 0.81–0.90). Comparison of estimated scale scores between odd and even item short forms, however, showed significant differences on three clinical scales: C4 ($p < .01$), C8 ($p < .05$), and C10 ($p < .05$). The odd- and even-numbered items for many LNNB-1 scales measure complementary aspects of performance speed and accuracy on the same tasks, so that the correlational correspondence without the consistent predictive accuracy between these measures is understandable.

Golden LNNB-1 Short Form

Golden (1989) published a rationally derived, decision-tree administration procedure to shorten LNNB-1 administration time for assessment of patients with serious cognitive deficit. The administration procedure details are complex, and they are described in detail in the original article. Correlational correspondence between the clinical and localization scales of the full LNNB-1 and estimated scores on those measures that are derived from these procedures are anecdotally noted by the author to exceed .93, although the specific data were not reported in the article. The reported correspondence between the long- and short-form scaled scores also was reported to be extremely close, but again, specific data were not reported. Golden (1989) reported that use of this short form of LNNB-1 could approximately halve the administration time that is required for administration of the full LNNB-1. This experimental procedure requires independent validation in a variety of normal and clinical groups.

LNNB-1 Greek Language Revision

Donias, Vassilopoulou, Golden, and Lovell (1989) reported results of a rigorous study that established the reliability and validity of a Greek language revision of the LNNB-1 (LNNB-G). The various components of this complex investigation will be presented serially.

LNNB-G Item Scoring

Donias (1985) empirically adjusted scoring values for 117 LNNB-1 items to make them normatively appropriate for use with a native Greek population.

LNNB-G S1 (Pathognomonic) Scale

Donias (1985) empirically constructed a 10-item S1 scale for the LNNB-G based on results from a native Greek population. This revised S1 scale is composed of items with maximal value for differentiation between brain-lesioned and control subject groups. The internal consistency of this revised S1 scale may be compromised, however, due to its relative brevity. Its internal consistency level should be empirically established by computation of coefficient alpha.

LNNB-G Interrater Reliability

The LNNB-G has been shown to have extremely high interrater reliability (scalewise range = .97–.99) (Donias et al., 1989, p. 131).

LNNB-G Split-Half Reliability

The LNNB-G clinical scales show moderate-to-high internal consistency according to the split-half method (range = .63–.90). These values would have been better estimated by coefficient alpha, which is the mean of all possible split-half values for a given item pool (Nunnally, 1978).

LNNB-G Critical Level

Donias et al. (1989, p. 131) also developed a critical level formula and decision rules for the LNNB-G. These procedures were 78% accurate in actuarial identification of brain-lesioned patients and 82% accurate in identification of controls.

LNNB-G Discriminant Validity

Donias et al. (1989) reported consistently high ($p < .005$) levels of scalewise intergroup performance level difference between their neurologic and control groups. These results were based on scalewise t tests, but they were not corrected for the number of correlated comparisons that were made. The intergroup differences remain significant at the .05 level of statistical significance after the Bonferroni correction is made to adjust for the number of comparisons.

LNNB-1 METHODOLOGY: CRITIQUES AND REBUTTALS

Mapou (1988) noted results from Kane, Parsons, and Goldstein (1985) that demonstrated performance level estimation equivalence of the LNNB-1, WAIS, and the HRNB. Mapou questioned whether "testing to detect brain damage" was an outmoded practice goal for clinical neuropsychologists, since "brain damage" is not a unitary syndrome. Mapou questioned whether the functional–organic differential diagnostic distinction was clinically meaningful in view of our current level of knowledge of neuropsychiatric disorder and associated cognitive deficit. Neurologic patients may develop secondary psychiatric syndromes and psychiatric patients may show associated neurobehavioral deficit. He objected to level of performance rather than pattern of performance evaluation of cognitive deficit, since the former is not prescriptive, whereas the latter is diagnostically and rehabilitatively more specific. Mapou also called for construction of tests that measure unitary functions at the syndrome analytic level. He overlooked the important caveat that any such measure of a theoretical construct necessarily involves multiple components of a functional system (Luria, 1966, 1973, 1980), so that an attempt to construct a unidimensional test is oversimplified.

Kane, Goldstein, and Parsons (1989) replied to Mapou (1988) to rebut his major premises. Kane et al. (1989) noted that the detection of the presence of cognitive deficit remains an important clinical question in psychiatric settings, in forensic assessment, in geriatric treatment centers, and in screening large numbers of patients for more detailed neurological and neuropsychological test procedures. They noted that exposure to toxic substances or minor head trauma often raises the medical referral question of the presence of acquired cognitive deficit that may not be demonstrable by other means. There remain characteristic symptoms that typically are impaired in brain dysfunction due to varied etiologies, so that detection of the presence of cognitive deficit associated with neurological disorder also can provide preliminary guidelines for identification of specific deficits. Extensive testing also may be necessary to identify a specific area of cognitive deficit reliably, and an assessment of global brain function may be a necessary initial step in narrowing the range of cognitive deficit areas, so that specific syndrome analysis may proceed productively and systematically. While Mapou (1988) called for rigorous development of psychometric instruments, Kane et al. (1989) noted that he had overlooked the extensive and rigorous test validation procedures that already had been used for the WAIS, HRNB, and LNNB-1 at the time that he wrote. In essence, the acceptability of a neuropsychological instrument to a given clinician is a function of the assessment question that one wishes to answer.

Howieson and Lezak (1992, p. 143) inveighed against clinical use of the LNNB-1 as a "fixed battery" on theoretical grounds. They referenced similar, now outdated, nonempirical commentaries in the literature that were critical of the early LNNB-1 studies, but they disregarded a large body of recent empirical work that supports the reliability and validity of the test (for review of theoretical and psychometric issues, see in particular Moses, 1983a; Moses & Maruish, 1989c, 1990a).

LNNB-FORM II DEVELOPMENTS

Origins of LNNB—Form II

Perhaps the most significant single addition to the LNNB literature has been the development of an alternative form of the test. The psychometric construction the theoretical rationale for the LNNB—Form II (LNNB-2) is well described in the test manual (Golden et al., 1985) and will not be discussed in detail here. Briefly, the LNNB-2 was designed to overcome some of the item domain sampling, administrative, and scoring limitations of the LNNB-1. The test authors introduced systematic variations into the LNNB-2 test materials and into the content and scoring of many of the test items to achieve these ends and to make the LNNB-2 test stimuli more familiar to an American audience.

A major improvement in the LNNB-2 was the addition of a new clinical scale, which was labeled Intermediate Memory (C12). The C12 items are not directly comparable to the experimental Delayed Memory Scale (DMS) that was developed for LNNB-1 (see Golden et al., 1985, pp. 300–303, for administrative details), but the DMS and C12 measures are intended to serve similar clinical purposes for LNNB-1 and LNNB-2, respectively. An advantage of the C12 scale is that the items and the norms for scoring them were derived on the same reference sample that was used to norm the other LNNB-2 clinical scales. In contrast, the LNNB-1 DMS was standardized after the other clinical scales were developed and normed. Different samples were used to establish performance level classification values for the LNNB-1 clinical scales and the DMS. Since the LNNB-2 C1 through C12 scales are normed on the same reference population, however, ipsative comparisons of C12 scale performance to the other LNNB-2 clinical scale measures are metrically comparable. This is not the case with the LNNB-1 DMS relative to the LNNB-1 clinical scales, since these measures were normed on different reference samples.

LNNB-2 Interrater Reliability

Kashden and Franzen (1996) trained university students without previous exposure to the LNNB-2 to be raters of videotaped LNNB-2 administrations. These students received a total of 20–22 hours of didactic instruction in a series of training sessions. This experimental procedure should model the manner in which college-educated professionals typically learn the quantitative LNNB-2 scoring procedures through exposure to a didactic workshop or a similar brief introductory training course. Excellent interrater agreement was reported for quantitative scoring of the LNNB-2 items. On average, the raters differed by one point or less in scoring the 12 LNNB-2 clinical scales. The mean coefficients of interrater agreement also were excellent (multiple kappa for both tapes = .82, range = .72–.87). For most LNNB-2 items there was perfect interrater agreement (perfect interrater agreement range = 61–71% across taped sessions). High interrater reliability was achieved with responses that were routine as well as with other responses that were made in a deliberately ambiguous manner.

LNNB-2 Norm Development

Wong, Schefft, and Moses (1990) developed a normative database for LNNB-2 in a sample of relatively young (mean = 38.5, SD = 14.7) and relatively well-educated (mean = 14.0, SD = 2.67) subjects. Age and educational level jointly showed a moderate correlational relationship to the mean LNNB-2 performance level (r = .58). While these norms are suitable for use with relatively young and well-educated groups, they are not applicable to the patients who typically are seen in neuropsychological practice.

Wong, Schefft, and Moses (1992) compared their empirical LNNB-2 norms with the predicted normative values of Golden et al. (1985) in the LNNB test manual. They reported systematic performance level differences between their empirically derived norms and the predicted LNNB-2 score values for their normative sample on 8 of 11 LNNB-2 clinical scales (C1, C2, C3, C4, C5, C6, C9, and C11). Wong et al. (1992) recommended empirical development of a larger, demographically more representative normative database for LNNB-2.

Moses, Schefft, Wong, and Berg (1992, 1993) subsequently expanded the normative database of Wong et al. (1990) for LNNB-2 to make it more relevant to clinical practice. All of the data from the Wong et al. (1990) study were included as part of a much larger sample of medical controls and normal volunteers. Their mean age was 36.09 years (SD = 13.67) and their mean educational level was 12.79 years (SD = 2.50). Uniformly scaled LNNB-2 clinical scale T-score norms were developed for this sample. Normative tables based on these data are provided in the published article.

LNNB-2 Multiple Scaling Models

Moses et al. (1992) showed that there were consistent and highly significant differences in performance level between the uniform (normative) T-score values and the linear (nonuniform) T scores for the LNNB-2 clinical scales. The uniform T-score norms also were shown to be consistently different at a high significance level (p < .0005) relative to the norms of Wong et al. (1990) and the predicted norms that were recommended for clinical use by Golden et al. (1985). Only the uniform T-score norms are widely representative and have a common scaling metric, so they are the only available LNNB-2 norms that we can recommend for clinical use.

LNNB-2 Critical Level

Moses et al. (1992) developed a critical level formula for the LNNB-2, but a typographical error was made in reporting the formula. The corrected formula was published as an erratum statement by Moses et al. (1993). Users of these norms are advised to pay careful attention to use only the corrected LNNB-2 critical level formula.

Use of the critical level with the uniform T-score norms for LNNB-2 produced an overall correct classification rate of 86.36% (95/110) for neurologic and control subjects jointly with a cognitive impairment criterion of five or more scales exceeding critical level (excluding C7 and C9, and including C12 in the summary index).

LNNB-2 Construct Validity

Nagel (1990) reported a close dimensional correspondence of the scalewise exploratory factor structure for LNNB-2 relative to previously published scale-wise factorial results for LNNB-1. The results of confirmatory factor analysis, however, did not support the exploratory factor analytic results. The replicable factor structure of LNNB-2 thus remains moot at present. The inconsistency of these results, however, underlines the importance of cross-validation of this important aspect of the construct validational process. Nagel's confirmatory factorial results may be biased by the relatively small size of his sample ($n = 102$) and by the lack of variance in response patterns of his subjects (45 items were performed error-lessly by most of his subjects).

Wong and Gilpin (1993) investigated the construct validity of the LNNB-2 C10 (Memory) scale relative to the subtests of the Wechsler Memory Scale—Revised (WMS-R) as part of a larger investigation of relationships between the LNNB-2 and the WMS-R subscale measures. They studied a demographically mixed sample of normal community volunteers and undergraduate college students. On the basis of correlational and hierarchical cluster analyses they showed a significant relationship of the LNNB-2 C10 scale to the Logical Memory verbal recall subtest of the WMS-R ($r = .48, p < .001$). There was only a weak correlational relationship of the LNNB-2 C10 scale to the WMS-R Visual Reproduction subtest ($r = .30, p < .05$). The WMS-R Visual Reproduction subtest, however, has poor internal consistency (Wechsler, 1987, p. 60), so it is as yet unclear whether the LNNB-2 C10 scale actually has a remarkable visual recall or recognition component.

LNNB-2 Concurrent Validity

Garmoe (1990) demonstrated large scalewise mean performance level differences between samples of neurologically impaired and normal subjects on the LNNB-2. In a supplementary analysis he demonstrated that addition of the C12 scale to the other 11 LNNB-2 clinical scales contributed significantly to the level of group discriminability. The C12 scale successfully complemented the C10 scale as a combined measure of immediate and intermediate memory. Age and educational level were strongly correlated with LNNB-2 scalewise performance in the control group but not in the neurologically impaired group.

Becker (1991) also attempted to differentiate neurological and normal control samples using discriminant analysis in the manner of Garmoe (1990). Unfortunately, Becker's total sample of 53 subjects (neurological patients) was far too small to allow for use of this multivariate technique. While his actuarial group classification rates were impressively high, they are artifactual, since the ratio of subjects to variables was not sufficient to prevent substantial chance capitalization.

LNNB Interform Nonequivalence

Moses and Chiu (1993) administered LNNB-1 and LNNB-2 to 78 diagnostically mixed neuropsychiatric patients. Fifty-eight of the 185 corresponding items between LNNB-1 and LNNB-2 differed significantly when they were compared by means of the Wilcoxon matched pairs signed ranks test. All clinical scales except C2 showed significant interform differences at the item level. At the scale score level, significant interform differences were found on scales C1, C6, C10, and C11.

Comparison of the number of elevated scales between LNNB-1 and LNNB-2 also showed highly significant ($p < 0.005$) differences between the two test forms on scales C1, C6, C10, and C11. The global number of LNNB-2 clinical scales that exceeded critical level was consistently greater than the corresponding global score value for the LNNB-1 clinical scales. The correlations of the corresponding LNNB-1 and LNNB-2 clinical scales that differed by at least five items also are only moderate (mean rho = 0.69; rho range = 0.54–0.78).

While the corresponding LNNB-1 and LNNB-2 clinical scales appear to be related to each other as performance level measures, clearly there are systematic differences between them. The assertion of the test authors (Golden et al., 1985) that the two forms of the LNNB are interchangeable was based on similarity of central tendency and variability values, but this assertion has not been supported by subsequent findings.

These results unfortunately were not known at the time that MacInnes, Paull, Uhl, and Schima (1987) performed an ambitious study of long-term test–retest profile stability in a normal elderly sample. They administered LNNB-1 at baseline and LNNB-2 4 years later to the same subjects based on the supposition that the two forms of the LNNB were interchangeable, but this is not the case. As expected, the central tendency similarities of the two forms of the test were demonstrated over the 4-year period. The expected finding of no necessary decline in performance level with normal aging was also redemonstrated. Those who may wish to replicate and improve on this study would do well to give both forms of the LNNB at baseline and follow-up to compare their relative test–retest reliabilities over a much shorter interval, say 2 weeks. Longer-term stability coefficients need not exceed 6 months for the intertest interval period. Too many uncontrolled variables are free to change without experimental control over a 4-year intertest period.

LNNB-2 Supplementary Scales

Klein (1993) appropriately criticized the simplistic interpretive misuse of LNNB-1 summary scales with LNNB-2 data in an important forensic case. Based on the preceding discussion in which we have shown that LNNB-1 and LNNB-2 are nonequivalent test forms, clearly it is inappropriate to generalize derived scales for LNNB-1 to LNNB-2. The localization scales for LNNB-1 also still are psychometrically experimental, and should not be used clinically.

There are no summary or localization or factor scales for LNNB-2 that have been empirically validated or shown to be reliable. Any use of such scales with LNNB-2 that is based solely on research with LNNB-1 is very likely to be inaccurate on a pattern of performance basis, if not also on a level of performance (normative) basis. Summary indices and clinical interpretive principles must be developed independently for LNNB-2, and this work has only recently begun to be conducted in a systematic manner.

SUMMARY

The LNNB-1 provides a standardized, reliable, well-validated set of measures that have proved to be very useful in the objective cognitive assessment of higher cortical function integrity. Basic and applied psychometric research on the test in the past decade has continued to extend and clarify the scope and limitations of its sensitivity and specificity for identification of cognitive deficit in a wide variety of neuropsychiatric syndromes. Recent preliminary ecological validation findings using the LNNB-1 to predict employment status and functional competence in the elderly have been promising. Progress in syndrome analyses of diverse disorders including schizophrenia, depression, mental retardation, learning disability, dementia, limbic epilepsy, and normal aging effects also have continued to be made.

The LNNB-1 scale indices have shown excellent construct validational properties relative to the WAIS-R subtests and the HRNB measures. The isomorphism of the LNNB-1 factorial structure across neurological and psychiatric samples has been remarkable. It provides a common basis for cognitive syndrome analysis in a wide variety of disorders. A Greek language version of the LNNB-1 has been developed that meets rigorous psychometric standards for validity and reliability. Short forms of the LNNB-1 continue to be developed and validated, with the most recent efforts being directed toward procedures to suit those who are elderly or who are in frail health.

The LNNB-2 indices now have been empirically normed and investigators have begun to report excellent concurrent validational support for those measures. It is important to emphasize that the two forms of the LNNB are not equivalent, and that while they are related as level of performance measures, they must be studied and validated independently. Clearly, simplistic interpretation of either form of the LNNB is inadvisable (Klein, 1993).

Critics of the LNNB continue to base their arguments against it solely on theoretical or personal preference, but no empirically based, objective evidence has been produced to cast doubt on the validity or reliability of either form of the

LNNB as a psychometric instrument. Data from the LNNB can augment and supplement a wide variety of other impressionistic clinical and standardized psychometric findings. In the hands of a theoretically sophisticated and interpersonally sensitive clinician, the LNNB can provide invaluable information about cognitive functional competence and the integrity of higher cortical functions in the individual patient with general medical illness or specific neuropsychiatric disorder.

REFERENCES

Adams, J. J., Meloy, J. R., & Moritz, M. S. (1990). Neuropsychological deficits and violent behavior in incarcerated schizophrenics. *The Journal of Nervous and Mental Disease, 178,* 253–256.

Adams, K. M., Brown, G. G., & Grant, I. (1985). Analysis of covariance as a remedy for demographic mismatch of research subject groups: Some sobering simulations. *Journal of Clinical and Experimental Neuropsychology, 7,* 445–462.

Adams, K. M., Brown, G. G., & Grant, I. (1992). Covariance is not the culprit: Adams, Brown, and Grant reply. *Journal of Clinical and Experimental Neuropsychology, 14,* 983–985.

Adams, R. L. (1985). Review of the Luria–Nebraska Neuropsychological Battery. In J. V. Mitchell (Ed.), *The ninth mental measurements yearbook* (pp. 877–881). Lincoln, NE: The Buros Institute of Mental Measurements.

Becker, H. J. (1991). Consequences of closed head injury as measured by the Luria–Nebraska Neuropsychological Battery, Form II. *Dissertation Abstracts International, 52,* 3284B. (University Microfilms No. DA91-33,234).

Berman, N. C., & Greenhouse, S. W. (1992). Adjusting for demographic covariates by the analysis of covariance. *Journal of Clinical and Experimental Neuropsychology, 14,* 981–982.

Blackerby, W. F., III. (1985). A latent-trait investigation of the Luria–Nebraska Neuropsychological Battery. *Dissertation Abstracts International, 46,* 342B. (University Microfilms No. 85-05,223).

Bogner, J. A. (1990). Neuropsychological assessment: Application to mental retardation. *Dissertation Abstracts International, 51,* 421B. (University Microfilms No. DA90-14,398).

Condray, R., Steinhauer, S. R., & Goldstein, G. (1992). Language comprehension in schizophrenics and their brothers. *Biological Psychiatry, 32,* 790–802.

Dickerson, F. B., Ringel, N. B., & Boronow, J. J. (1991). Neuropsychological deficits in chronic schizophrenics: Relationship with symptoms and behavior. *The Journal of Nervous and Mental Disease, 179,* 744–749.

DiMichele, V., Rossi, A., Stratta, P., Schiazza, G., Bolino, F., Giordano, L., & Casacchia, M. (1992). Neuropsychological and clinical correlates of temporal lobe anatomy in schizophrenia. *Acta Psychiatrica Scandinavica, 85,* 484–488.

Donias, S. H. (1985). *The Luria–Nebraska Neuropsychological Battery: Standardization in a Greek population and transcultural observations.* Unpublished doctoral dissertation, Aristotelian University, Thessaloniki, Greece.

Donias, S. H., Vassilopoulou, E. O., Golden, C. J., & Lovell, M. R. (1989). Reliability and clinical effectiveness of the standardized Greek version of the Luria–Nebraska Neuropsychological Battery. *The International Journal of Clinical Neuropsychology, IX,* 129–133.

Falk-Kessler, J., & Quittman, M. S. (1990). Functional ability performance on neuropsychological indices in chronic psychiatric outpatients. *Occupational Therapy in Mental Health, 10*(2), 1–17.

Faustman, W. O., Bono, M. A., Moses, J. A., Jr., & Csernansky, J. G. (1992). Season of birth and neuropsychological impairment in schizophrenia. *Journal of Nervous and Mental Disease, 180,* 644–648.

Faustman, W. O., Moses, J. A., Jr., & Csernansky, J. G. (1988). Luria–Nebraska performance and symptomatology in unmedicated schizophrenic patients. *Psychiatry Research, 26,* 29–34.

Faustman, W. O., Moses, J. A., Jr., Ringo, D. L., & Newcomer, J. W. (1991). Left-handedness in male schizophrenic patients is associated with increased impairment on the Luria–Nebraska Neuropsychological Battery. *Biological Psychiatry, 30,* 326–334.

Franzen, M. D. (1985). The Luria–Nebraska Neuropsychological Battery. In D. J. Keyser & R. C. Sweetland (Eds.), *Test critiques: Vol. 3* (pp. 402–414). Kansas City, MO: Test Corporation of America.

Franzen, M. D. (1986). The Luria–Nebraska Neuropsychological Battery, Form II. In D. J. Keyser & R. C. Sweetland (Eds.), *Test critiques: Vol. 4* (pp. 382–386). Kansas City, MO: Test Corporation of America.

Frazier, M. F., Silverstein, M. L., & Fogg, L. (1989). Lateralized cerebral dysfunction in schizophrenia and depression: Gender and medication effects. *Archives of Clinical Neuropsychology, 4,* 33–44.

Garmoe, W. S. (1990). Evaluation of the diagnostic utility of the Luria–Nebraska Neuropsychological Battery, Form II. *Dissertation Abstracts International, 51,* 427B–428B. (University Microfilms No. DA90-20,039).

Golden, C. J. (1981). A standardized version of Luria's neuropsychological tests: A quantitative and qualitative approach to neuropsychological evaluation. In S. B. Filskov & T. J. Boll (Eds.), *Handbook of clinical neuropsychology: Vol. 1* (pp. 608–642). New York: Wiley.

Golden, C. J. (1989). Abbreviating administration of the LNNB in significantly impaired patients. *The International Journal of Clinical Neuropsychology, XI,* 177–181.

Golden, C. J., Hammeke, T. A., & Purisch, A. D. (1978). Diagnostic validity of a standardized neuropsychological battery derived from Luria's neuropsychological tests. *Journal of Consulting and Clinical Psychology, 46,* 1258–1265.

Golden, C. J., Hammeke, T. A., & Purisch, A. D. (1980). *The Luria–Nebraska Neuropsychological Battery manual.* Los Angeles: Western Psychological Services.

Golden, C. J., Purisch, A. D., & Hammeke, T. A. (1985). *The Luria–Nebraska Neuropsychological Battery Forms I and II manual.* Los Angeles: Western Psychological Services.

Goldstein, G. (1986). An overview of similarities and differences between the Halstead–Reitan and Luria–Neuropsychological Batteries. In T. Incagnoli, G. Goldstein, & C. J. Golden (Eds.), *Clinical application of neuropsychological test batteries* (pp. 235–275). New York: Plenum Press.

Goldstein, G. & Incagnoli, T. (1986). A comparison of the Halstead–Reitan, Luria–Nebraska, and flexible batteries through case presentations. In T. Incagnoli, G. Goldstein, & C. J. Golden (Eds.), *Clinical application of neuropsychological test batteries* (pp. 303–327). New York: Plenum Press.

Goldstein, G., Katz, L., Slomka, G., & Kelly M. A. (1993). Relationships among academic, neuropsychological, and intellectual status in subtypes of adults with learning disability. *Archives of Clinical Neuropsychology, 8,* 41–53.

Goldstein, G., Shelly, C., McCue, M., & Kane, R. L. (1987). Classification with the Luria–Nebraska Neuropsychological Battery: An application of cluster and ipsative profile analysis. *Archives of Clinical Neuropsychology, 2,* 215–235.

Gruber, J. J., Hall, J. W., McKay, S. E., Humphries, L. L., & Krysclo, R. J. (1989). Motor proficiency and neuropsychological function in depressed adolescent inpatients: A pilot investigation. *Adapted Physical Activity Quarterly, 6,* 32–39.

Heinrichs, R. W. (1989). Neuropsychological test performance and employment status in patients referred for assessment. *Perceptual and Motor Skills, 69,* 899–902.

Horton, A. M., Jr., & Alana, S. (1990). Validation of the Mini-Mental State Examination. *International Journal of Neuroscience, 53,* 209–212.

Horton, A. M., Jr., Anilane, J., Puente, A. E., & Berg, R. A. (1988). Diagnostic parameters of an odd–even item short-form of the Luria–Nebraska Neuropsychological Battery. *Archives of Clinical Neuropsychology, 3,* 375–381.

Horton, A. M., Jr., Vaeth, J., & Anilane, J. (1990). Computerized interpretation of the Luria–Nebraska Neuropsychological Battery: A pilot study. *Perceptual and Motor Skills, 71,* 83–86.

Howieson, D. B., & Lezak, M. D. (1992). The neuropsychological evaluation. In S. C. Yudofsky & R. E. Hales (Eds.), *The American Psychiatric Press textbook of neuropsychiatry* (pp. 127–150). Washington, DC: American Psychiatric Association.

Kane, R. L. (1986). Comparison of Halstead–Reitan and Luria–Nebraska Neuropsychological Batteries: Research findings. In T. Incagnoli, G. Goldstein, C. J. Golden (Eds.), *Clinical application of neuropsychological test batteries* (pp. 277–301). New York: Plenum Press.

Kane, R. L. (1991). Standardized and flexible batteries in neuropsychology: An assessment update. *Neuropsychology Review, 2,* 281–339.

Kane, R. L., Goldstein, G., & Parsons, O. A. (1989). A response to Mapou. *Journal of Clinical and Experimental Neuropsychology, 11,* 589–595.

Kane, R. L., Parsons, O. A., & Goldstein, G. (1985). Statistical relationships and discriminative accuracy of the Halstead–Reitan, Luria–Nebraska and Wechsler IQ scores in the identification of brain damage. *Journal of Clinical and Experimental Neuropscyhology, 7,* 211–223.

Kane, R. L., Parsons, O. A., Goldstein, G., & Moses, J. A., Jr. (1987). Diagnostic accuracy of the Halstead–Reitan and Luria–Nebraska Neuropsychological batteries: Performance of clinical raters. *Journal of Consulting and Clinical Psychology, 55,* 783–784.

Kashden, J., & Franzen, M. D. (1996). An interrater reliability study of the Luria–Nebraska Neuropsychological Battery—Form II quantitative scoring system. *Archives of Clinical Neuropsychology, 11,* 155–163.

Kemali, D., Maj, M., Galderisi, S., Salvati, A., Starace, F., Valente, A., & Pirozzi, R. (1986). Clinical, biological, and neuropsychological features associated with lateral ventricular enlargement in *DSM-III* schizophrenic disorder. *Psychiatry Research, 21,* 137–149.

Klein, S. H. (1993). Misuse of the Luria–Nebraska localization scales—Comments on a criminal case study. *The Clinical Neuropsychologist, 7,* 297–299.

Koffler, S., & Zehler, D. (1986). Correlation of the Luria–Nebraska Neuropsychological Battery with the WAIS-R. *International Journal of Clinical Neuropsychology, VIII,* 68–71.

Langell, M. E., Purisch, A. D., & Golden, C. J. (1987). Neuropsychological differentiation between paranoid and nonparanoid schizophrenics on the Luria–Nebraska Battery. *International Journal of Clinical Neuropsychology, IX,* 88–94.

Lewis, R. D., Hutchens, T. A., & Garland, B. L. (1993). Cross-validation of the discriminative effectiveness of the Luria–Nebraska Neuropsychological Battery for learning disabled adolescents. *Archives of Clinical Neuropsychology, 8,* 437–447.

Lewis, R. D., & Lorion, R. P. (1988). Discriminative effectiveness of the Luria–Nebraska Neuropsychological Battery for LD adolescents. *Learning Disability Quarterly, 11,* 62–70.

Lezak, M. D. (1995). *Neuropsychological assessment* (3rd ed.). New York: Oxford University Press.

Luria, A. R. (1966). *Higher cortical functions in man* (1st ed.). New York: Basic Books.

Luria, A. R. (1973). *The working brain: An introduction to neuropsychology.* New York: Basic Books.

Luria, A. R. (1980). *Higher cortical functions in man* (2nd ed.). New York: Basic Books.

Macciocchi, S. N., Fowler, P. C., & Ranseen, J. D. (1992). Trait analyses of the Luria–Nebraska intellectual processes, motor functions, and memory scales. *Archives of Clinical Neuropsychology, 7,* 541–551.

MacInnes, W. D., Paull, D., Uhl, H. S. M., & Schima, E. (1987). Longitudinal neuropsychological changes in a "normal" elderly group. *Archives of Clinical Neuropsychology, 2,* 273–282.

MacInnes, W. D., Rysavy, J. A., McGill, J. E., Mahoney, P. D., Wilmot, M. D., Frick, M. P., & Elyaderani, M. K. (1990). The usefulness and limitations of CT scans in the diagnosis of Alzheimer's disease. *International Journal of Clinical Neuropsychology, XII,* 127–130.

Mapou, R. L. (1988). Testing to detect brain damage: An alternative to what may no longer be useful. *Journal of Clinical and Experimental Neuropsychology, 10,* 271–278.

McCue, M., Goldstein, G., & Shelly, C. (1989). The application of a short form of the Luria–Nebraska Neuropsychological Battery to discrimination between dementia and depression in the elderly. *International Journal of Clinical Neuropsychology, XI*, 21–29.

McCue, M., Rogers, J. C., & Goldstein, G. (1990). Relationships between neuropsychological and functional assessment in elderly neuropsychiatric patients. *Rehabilitation Psychology, 35*, 91–99.

McCue, M., Shelly, C., & Goldstein, G. (1985). A proposed short form of the Luria–Nebraska Neuropsychological Battery oriented toward assessment of the elderly. *International Journal of Clinical Neuropsychology, VII*, 96–101.

McKay, S. E., Golden, C. J., Moses, J. A., Jr., Fishburne, F., & Wisniewski, A. (1981). Correlation of the Luria–Nebraska Neuropsychological Battery with the WAIS. *Journal of Consulting and Clinical Psychology, 49*, 940–946.

Menich, S. R., & Baron, A. (1987). Behavioral slowing and neuropsychological signs in a sample of active older men. *Experimental Aging Research, 13*, 23–27.

Milberg, W. P., Hebben, N., & Kaplan, E. (1986). *The Boston process approach to neuropsychological assessment.* In I. Grant & K. M. Adams (Eds.), *Neuropsychological assessment of neuropsychiatric disorders* (pp. 65–86). New York: Oxford University Press.

Miller, L. S., Faustman, W. O., Moses, J. A., Jr., & Csernansky, J. G. (1991). Evaluating cognitive impairment in depression with the Luria–Nebraska Neuropsychological Battery: Severity correlates and comparisons with nonpsychiatric controls. *Psychiatry Research, 37*, 219–227.

Moses, J. A., Jr. (1983a). "Man versus mean" revisited: A review of Lezak's second edition of *Neuropsychological Assessment. Clinical Neuropsychology Resource Supplement, 5*(3), 3–4.

Moses, J. A., Jr. (1983b). An orthogonal factor solution of the Luria–Nebraska Neuropsychological Battery items: I. Motor, rhythm, tactile, and visual scales. *Clinical Neuropsychology, V,* 181–185.

Moses, J. A., Jr. (1984a). An orthogonal factor solution of the Luria–Nebraska Neuropsychological Battery items: II. Receptive speech, expressive speech, writing, and reading scales. *The International Journal of Clinical Neuropsychology, VI*, 24–28.

Moses, J. A., Jr. (1984b). An orthogonal factor solution of the Luria–Nebraska Neuropsychological Battery items: III. Arithmetic, memory, and intelligence scales. *The International Journal of Clinical Neuropsychology, VI*, 103–106.

Moses, J. A., Jr. (1984c). An orthogonal factor solution of the Luria–Nebraska Neuropsychological Battery items: IV. Pathognomonic, right hemisphere, and left hemisphere scales. *The International Journal of Clinical Neuropsychology, VI*, 161–165.

Moses, J. A., Jr. (1985). Replication of internal consistency values for the Luria–Nebraska Neuropsychological Battery summary, localization, factor and compensation scales. *The International Journal of Clinical Neuropsychology, VII*, 200–203.

Moses, J. A., Jr. (1986). Factor analysis of the Luria–Nebraska Neuropsychological Battery by sensorimotor, speech, and conceptual item bands. *The International Journal of Clinical Neuropsychology, VIII*, 26–35.

Moses, J. A., Jr. (1987). Item analysis of the Luria–Nebraska Neuropsychological Battery clinical and summary scales. *The International Journal of Clinical Neuropsychology, IX*, 149–157.

Moses, J. A., Jr. (1989). Construct validation of the Luria–Nebraska Neuropsychological Battery clinical and summary scales with the WAIS-R subtests. *The International Journal of Clinical Neuropsychology, XI*, 80–89.

Moses, J. A., Jr. (1990a). Comparative factor structure of the Luria–Nebraska Neuropsychological Battery C1 and C2 scales for neurological and psychiatric samples. *The International Journal of Clinical Neuropsychology, XII*, 60–73.

Moses, J. A., Jr. (1990b). Comparative factor structure of the Luria–Nebraska Neuropsychological Battery C3 and C4 scales for neurological and psychiatric samples. *The International Journal of Clinical Neuropsychology, XII*, 116–126.

Moses, J. A., Jr. (1990c). Comparative factor structure of the Luria–Nebraska Neuropsychological Battery C5 and C6 scales for neurologic and psychiatric samples. *The International Journal of Clinical Neuropsychology, XII,* 147–165.

Moses, J. A., Jr. (1991a). Comparative factor structure of the Luria–Nebraska Neuropsychological Battery C7 through C9 scales for neurologic and psychiatric samples. *The International Journal of Clinical Neuropsychology, XIII,* 13–23.

Moses, J. A., Jr. (1991b). Comparative factor structure of the Luria–Nebraska Neuropsychological Battery C10 and C11 scales for neurologic and psychiatric samples. *The International Journal of Clinical Neuropsychology, XIII,* 35–46.

Moses, J. A., Jr. (1991c). Comparative factor structure of the Luria–Nebraska Neuropsychological Battery S1 through S3 scales for neurologic and psychiatric samples. *The International Journal of Clinical Neuropsychology, XIII,* 113–130.

Moses, J. A., Jr. (1991d). Comparative factor structure of the Luria–Nebraska Neuropsychological Battery S4 and S5 scales for neurologic and psychiatric samples. *The International Journal of Clinical Neuropsychology, XIII,* 153–164.

Moses, J. A., Jr. (1991e). Schizophrenic subtype differences on the Luria–Nebraska Neuropsychological Battery? A failure to replicate Langell, Purisch and Golden. *The International Journal of Clinical Neuropsychology, XIII,* 139–142.

Moses, J. A., Jr. (1994a). *Replicated factor structure of the Luria–Nebraska Neuropsychological Battery C1 through C4 scales.* Unpublished manuscript.

Moses, J. A., Jr. (1994b). *Replicated factor structure of the Luria–Nebraska Neuropsychological Battery C5 through C8 scales.* Unpublished manuscript.

Moses, J. A., Jr. (1994c). *Replicated factor structure of the Luria–Nebraska Neuropsychological Battery C9 through C11 scales.* Unpublished manuscript.

Moses, J. A., Jr. (1994d). *Replicated factor structure of the Luria–Nebraska Neuropsychological Battery S1 through S3 scales.* Unpublished manuscript.

Moses, J. A., Jr. (1994e). *Factor structure replication and construct validation of the Luria–Nebraska Neuropsychological Battery S4 and S5 scales.* Unpublished manuscript.

Moses, J. A., Jr., & Chiu, M. L. (1993, October). *Nonequivalence of Forms I and II of the Luria–Nebraska Neuropsychological Battery for Adults.* Paper presented at the meeting of the National Academy of Neuropsychology, Phoenix, Arizona.

Moses, J. A., Jr., Csernansky, J. G., & Leiderman, D. B. (1988). Neuropsychological criteria for identification of cognitive deficit in limbic epilepsy. *The International Journal of Clinical Neuropsychology, X,* 106–112.

Moses, J. A., Jr., & Maruish, M. E. (1987). A critical review of the Luria–Nebraska Neuropsychological Battery literature: I. Reliability. *The International Journal of Clinical Neuropsychology, IX,* 149–157.

Moses, J. A., Jr., & Maruish, M. E. (1988a). A critical review of the Luria–Nebraska Neuropsychological Battery literature: II. Construct validity. *The International Journal of Clinical Neuropsychology, X,* 5–11.

Moses, J. A., Jr., & Maruish, M. E. (1988b). A critical review of the Luria–Nebraska Neuropsychological Battery literature: III. Concurrent validity. *The International Journal of Clinical Neuropsychology, X,* 12–19.

Moses, J. A., Jr., & Maruish, M. E. (1988c). A critical review of the Luria–Nebraska Neuropsychological Battery literature: IV. Cognitive deficit in schizophrenia and related disorders. *The International Journal of Clinical Neuropsychology, X,* 51–62.

Moses, J. A., Jr., & Maruish, M. E. (1988d). A critical review of the Luria–Nebraska Neuropsychological Battery literature: V. Cognitive deficit in miscellaneous psychiatric disorders. *The International Journal of Clinical Neuropsychology, X,* 63–73.

Moses, J. A., Jr., & Maruish, M. E. (1988e). A critical review of the Luria–Nebraska Neuropsychological Battery literature: VI. Neurologic cognitive deficit parameters. *The International Journal of Clinical Neuropsychology, X,* 130–140.

Moses, J. A., Jr., & Maruish, M. E. (1988f). A critical review of the Luria–Nebraska Neuropsychological Battery literature: VII. Specific neurologic syndromes. *The International Journal of Clinical Neuropsychology, X,* 178–188.

Moses, J. A., Jr., & Maruish, M. E. (1989a). A critical review of the Luria–Nebraska Neuropsychological Battery literature: VIII. New summary indices. *The International Journal of Clinical Neuropsychology, XI,* 9–20.

Moses, J. A., Jr., & Maruish, M. E. (1989b). A critical review of the Luria–Nebraska Neuropsychological Battery literature: IX. Alternate forms. *The International Journal of Clinical Neuropsychology, XI,* 97–110.

Moses, J. A., Jr., & Maruish, M. E. (1989c). A critical review of the Luria–Nebraska Neuropsychological Battery literature: X. Critiques and rebuttals. Part one. *The International Journal of Clinical Neuropsychology, XI,* 145–162.

Moses, J. A., Jr., & Maruish, M. E. (1990a). A critical review of the Luria–Nebraska Neuropsychological Battery literature: XI. Critiques and rebuttals. Part two. *The International Journal of Clinical Neuropsychology, XII,* 37–45.

Moses, J. A., Jr., & Maruish, M. E. (1990b). A critical review of the Luria–Nebraska Neuropsychological Battery literature: XII. New developments, 1987–1988. Part one. *The International Journal of Clinical Neuropsychology, XII,* 191–205.

Moses, J. A., Jr., & Maruish, M. E. (1991a). A critical review of the Luria–Nebraska Neuropsychological Battery literature: XIII. New developments, 1987–1988. Part two. *The International Journal of Clinical Neuropsychology, XIII,* 89–103.

Moses, J. A., Jr., & Maruish, M. E. (1991b). A critical review of the Luria–Nebraska Neuropsychological Battery literature: XIV. Retrospect and prospect. *The International Journal of Clinical Neuropsychology, XIII,* 178–188.

Moses, J. A., Jr., Pritchard, D. A., & Faustman, W. O. (1994). Modal profiles for the Luria–Nebraska Neuropsychological Battery. *Archives of Clinical Neuropsychology, 9,* 15–30.

Moses, J. A., Jr., & Schefft, B. K. (1985). Interrater reliability analyses of the Luria–Nebraska Neuropsychological Battery. *The International Journal of Clinical Neuropsychology, VI,* 31–38.

Moses, J. A., Jr., Schefft, B. K., Wong, J. L., & Berg, R. A. (1992). Revised norms and decision rules for the Luria–Nebraska Neuropsychological Battery, Form II. *Archives of Clinical Neuropsychology, 7,* 251–269.

Moses, J. A., Jr., Schefft, B. K., Wong, J. L., & Berg, R. A. (1993). Erratum. *Archives of Clinical Neuropsychology, 8,* 184.

Nagel, J. A. (1990). Exploratory and confirmatory factor analysis of the clinical scales of the Luria–Nebraska Neuropsychological Battery, Form II. *Dissertation Abstracts International, 51,* 2630B–2631B. (University Microfilms No. 90-27,725).

Newman, P. J., & Silverstein, M. L. (1987). Neuropsychological test performance among major clinical subtypes of depression. *Archives of Clinical Neuropsychology, 3,* 115–125.

Nizamie, S. H., Nizamie, A., Borde, M., & Sharma, S. (1988). Mania following head injury: Case reports and neuropsychological findings. *Acta Psychiatrica Scandinavica, 77,* 637–639.

Nizamie, A., Nizamie, S. H., & Shukla, T. R. (1992). Performance on Luria–Nebraska Neuropsychological Battery in schizophrenic patients. *Indian Journal of Psychiatry, 34,* 321–330.

Nunnally, J. C. (1978). *Psychometric theory* (2nd ed.). New York: McGraw-Hill.

Paulman, R. G., Devous, M. D., Sr., Gregory, R. R., Herman, J. H., Jennings, L., Bonte, F. J., Nasrallah, H. A., & Raese, J. D. (1990). Hypofrontality and cognitive impairment in schizophrenia:

Dynamic single-photon tomography and neuropsychological assessment of schizophrenic brain function. *Biological Psychiatry, 27,* 377–399.

Pheley, A. M., & Klesges, R. C. (1986). The relationship between experimental and neuropsychological measures of memory. *Archives of Clinical Neuropsychology, 1,* 231–241.

Prifitera, A., & Ryan, J. J. (1981). Validity of the Luria–Nebraska intellectual processes scale as a measure of adult intelligence. *Journal of Consulting and Clinical Psychology, 49,* 755–756.

Purisch, A. D., & Sbordone, R. J. (1986). The Luria–Nebraska Neuropsychological Battery. In G. Goldstein & R. A. Tarter (Eds.), *Advances in clinical neuropsychology: Vol. 3* (pp. 291–316). New York: Plenum Press.

Rossi, A., Galderisi, S., DiMichele, V., Stratta, P., Ceccoli, S., Maj, M., & Casacchia, M. (1990). Dementia in schizophrenia: Magnetic resonance and clinical correlates. *Journal of Nervous and Mental Disease, 178,* 521–524.

Rousey, C. G., Arjunan, K. N., & Rousey, C. L. (1986). Successful treatment of stuttering following closed head injury. *Journal of Fluency Disorders, 11,* 257–261.

Russell, E. W. (1981). The pathology and clinical examination of memory. In S. B. Filskov & T. J. Boll (Eds.), *Handbook of clinical neuropsychology: Vol. 1* (pp. 287–319). New York: Wiley.

Silverstein, M. L., Fogg, L., & Harrow, M. (1991). Prognostic significance of cerebral status: Dimensions of clinical outcome. *Journal of Nervous and Mental Disease, 179,* 534–539.

Silverstein, M. L., Harrow, M., & Marengo, J. T. (1993). Disordered thinking and cerebral dysfunction: Laterality effects, language, and intellectual functions. *Archives of Clinical Neuropsychology, 8,* 497–509.

Silverstein, M. L., & McDonald, C. (1988). Personality trait characteristics in relation to neuropsychological dysfunction in schizophrenia and depression. *Journal of Personality Assessment, 52,* 288–296.

Silverstein, M. L., McDonald, C., & Fogg, L. (1990). Intelligence and neuropsychological functioning in psychiatric disorders. *Archives of Clinical Neuropsychology, 5,* 317–323.

Silverstein, M. L., McDonald, C., & Meltzer, H. Y. (1988). Differential patterns of neuropsychological deficit in psychiatric disorders. *Journal of Clinical Psychology, 44,* 412–415.

Silverstein, M. L., Strauss, B. S., & Fogg, L. (1990). A cluster analysis approach for deriving neuropsychologically based subtypes of psychiatric disorders. *The International Journal of Clinical Neuropsychology, XII,* 7–13.

Stambrook, M. (1983). The Luria–Nebraska Neuropsychological Battery: A promise that *may* be partially fulfilled. *Journal of Clinical Neuropsychology, 5,* 247–269.

Stephens, C. W., Clark, R. D., & Kaplan, R. D. (1990). Neuropsychological performance of emotionally disturbed students on the LNNB and LNNB-C. *Journal of School Psychology, 28,* 301–308.

Tsushima, W. T., & Tsushima, V. G. (1993). Relation between headaches and neuropsychological functioning among head injury patients. *Headache, 33,* 139–142.

Wechsler, D. (1987). *Wechsler Memory Scale—Revised manual.* San Antonio, TX: The Psychological Corporation & Harcourt Brace Jovanovich, Inc.

Wong, J. L., & Gilpin, A. R. (1993). Verbal vs. visual categories on the Wechsler Memory Scale—Revised: How meaningful a distinction? *Journal of Clinical Psychology, 49,* 847–854.

Wong, J. L., Schefft, B. K., & Moses, J. A., Jr. (1990). A normative study of the Luria–Nebraska Neuropsychological Battery, Form II. *The International Journal of Clinical Neuropsychology, XII,* 175–179.

Wong, J. L., Schefft, B. K., & Moses, J. A., Jr. (1992). Comparison of empirically derived and predicted standard scores for Form II of the Luria–Nebraska Neuropsychological Battery. *Perceptual and Motor Skills, 75,* 731–736.

Zarantonello, M. M., Munley, P. H., & Milanovich, J. (1993). Predicting Wechsler Adult Intelligence Scale—Revised (WAIS-R) IQ scores from the Luria–Nebraska Neuropsychological Battery (Form I). *Journal of Clinical Psychology, 49,* 225–233.

6

The Boston Process Approach

A Brief History and Current Practice

ROBERTA F. WHITE AND FREDRIC E. ROSE

HISTORICAL BASIS OF THE BOSTON PROCESS APPROACH

The Boston process approach to clinical neuropsychological assessment embodies a philosophical ideal concerning the optimal means of examining patients with suspected brain damage or cognitive disabilities. The term "process" was applied to the approach by its founder and earliest proponent, Edith Kaplan, during her tenure at the Boston Veterans Administration Hospital. A great deal of the impetus and basis of methods applied to the approach arose from investigators in the fields of aphasiology and behavioral neurology with whom Kaplan worked on clinical assessment and research at the Boston VA throughout the 1960s to 1990s. Efforts by Kaplan, her colleagues in these fields, and students trained in the process approach have resulted in a tradition of formal test measures, techniques for qualitative observation of test behavior, and clinical interpretation. This tradition has been extensively applied to both assessment of individual patients and research methodology throughout the world and continues to represent the predominant approach to neuropsychological assessment used in the Boston area. In addition, many of the tests developed based on the tradition are used by practitioners who primarily employ techniques emanating from other neuropsychological traditions.

ROBERTA F. WHITE • Department of Neurology, Boston University School of Medicine, and Department of Veterans Affairs Medical Center, Boston, Massachusetts 02130   FREDRIC E. ROSE • Department of Veterans Affairs, Decatur, Georgia 30033

The Notion of Process

Kaplan's graduate training was in developmental psychology, and she applied principles from this field to the problem of evaluating cognitive–behavioral dysfunction in patients with brain damage. She was especially interested in the effects of focal cortical brain lesions on behavior and the specific syndromes of behavioral deficits that accompanied such lesions. When evaluating these focal lesion patients, she worked closely with aphasiologists, speech pathologists, and behavioral neurologists. She is known among her colleagues in these fields for her special ability to exquisitely describe highly specific anomalies in the styles of cognitive processing and the particular types of errors made by focal lesion patients in completing challenging cognitive tasks. In her analysis of the behavior of patients completing cognitive tasks, she applied Heinz Werner's (1937) distinction between "process" and "achievement" in human development to the observation of patients' performance on cognitive–behavioral tests (Milberg, Hebben, & Kaplan, 1986).

This distinction implies that "achievement" (i.e., performing well on a test) or "failure" (earning a poor score on a test) can occur for many reasons; very different problem-solving strategies or deficits in the ability to problem solve can lead to the same score on a behavioral test. Therefore, the patient's methods of processing a task or the specific types of errors made in carrying out a task are crucial data sources in the evaluation of the patient.

The systematic observation of process led Kaplan and colleagues in many directions. These included the development of methods for observing the flow of behavior exhibited by patients in completing tasks, detailed descriptions of the types of qualitative findings seen among patients on specific tests, and the development of tests specifically designed to address processing issues. Another outgrowth of the detailed observation of process is that of "inquiry" into test performance; these procedures are aimed at uncovering the processing problems that cause a patient to fail a test (or to pass it despite cognitive impairment) and are described in later in this chapter.

Related Traditions in the Early Development of the Approach

At the time Kaplan was first developing her ideas concerning specific processing deficits in patients with brain damage, several other forces were affecting her work and that of colleagues at the Boston VA. Nationally, these included the rapid development of the field of neuropsychology as a specialty and the application of psychometric methods to the quantification of many types of behaviors. In Boston, these particularly included the systematic investigation of aphasic disorders, the development of the field of behavioral neurology, and the initiation and growth of investigations in the field of cognitive neuroscience.

Neuropsychological techniques were increasingly applied during the 1960s and early 1970s, specifically to the problem of lesion localization. This was an important issue at that time because of the lack of brain-imaging techniques for identification of lesions and lesion sites. In addition, there was increasing interest in the study of cerebral specialization and cerebral lateralization as a basis for better understanding how the brain works. While other investigators and clinicians were developing techniques for the quantification of behaviors (especially motor and sensory abilities), Kaplan and colleagues were pursuing the study of higher cortical function.

The application of psychometric methodology to the study of brain function was of enormous importance to the development of neuropsychology in general and the process approach in particular. Kaplan early on became interested in the processing components associated with completion of standard psychological tests such as the Wechsler Intelligence Scale tasks (Wechsler, 1946, 1955, 1981), the Wechsler Memory Scale (Wechsler, 1987; Wechsler & Stone, 1945), and other tests such as the Hooper Visual Organization Test (Hooper, 1958). While she utilized test scores in considering levels of performance on tests, she was far more interested in qualitative findings on the tasks than she was in patterns of test scores. Her insights concerning the association between focal brain damage and qualitative findings on these tasks became a basis for her teachings concerning cerebral specialization. One of her favorite tests for such analysis was the Block Design subtest of the Wechsler Adult Intelligence Scale (WAIS) (see Milberg et al., 1986, for a detailed description of this analysis).

At the time Kaplan developed her methodology at the Boston VA, she worked extensively with Harold Goodglass, who was carrying out detailed analysis on the phenomenology of the subtypes of aphasia. Such analyses included cerebral localization of aphasic symptoms, syndromes, and subtypes and elucidation of the mechanisms subserving the deficits observed in aphasics (alexia, agraphia, anomia, agrammatism, etc.). This work, done also in collaboration with Nancy Helm-Estabrook in speech pathology, led to the development of tests assessing the components of aphasic syndromes, such as the Boston Diagnostic Aphasia Examination (Goodglass & Kaplan, 1976, 1983), and to the design of the Boston Naming Test, a test widely used to assess naming ability (Kaplan, Goodglass, & Weintraub, 1976, 1983).

Simultaneously, the field of behavioral neurology became extremely active in the Boston VA, resulting in collaborations among neuropsychologists and behavioral neurologists such as Norman Geschwind, Frank Benson, and Martin Albert. Neuropsychological techniques using the process orientation were utilized extensively in collaborative research elaborating specific neurobehavioral syndromes (see Research section below).

During the same era, research neuropsychologists at the Boston VA developed highly specialized techniques in order to investigate the specific cognitive-processing abnormalities accompanying different types of brain damage, including alcoholic syndromes and dementing disorders. This work is integral to the historical basis of the field of cognitive neuroscience. Standard tests were adapted and other tests developed in order to describe these cognitive-processing abnormalities and to attempt to discern underlying mechanisms (both cognitive and neuropathological). Memory function was a particular focus of this work, which was pursued most notably by Nelson Butters, Marilyn Albert, and Marlene Oscar-Berman. These discoveries concerning subprocesses and abnormalities of memory function led directly to the development of process-oriented memory tests such as Albert's Famous Faces (Albert, Butters, & Levin, 1979), the California Verbal Learning Test (Delis, Kramer, Kaplan, & Ober, 1987), and the Delayed Recognition Span Test (Moss, Albert, Butters, & Payne, 1986). The discoveries of these investigators also provided essential insights for clinicians using the process approach into particular aspects of memory function that allow differential diagnosis of specific dementias and neurological syndrome (White, 1992).

Recent Applications of the Process Approach

In the past several years, the process approach has been applied to test development and revision of existing tests. Cognitive neuroscience-based constructs describing the components of memory processing were embodied in the Wechsler Memory Scale—Revised (WMS-R) (Wechsler, 1987), which is very similar to the Boston revision of the original Wechsler Memory Scale (Wechsler & Stone, 1945). In addition, Kaplan and colleagues provided detailed manuals for administering tests such as the Wechsler Adult Intelligence Scale—Revised (WAIS-R) (Kaplan, Fein, Morris, & Delis, 1991). Operationalization of these procedures not only allows for greater standardization of process-oriented assessment as it is applied outside of Boston, it also forms the basis for the quantification of process-oriented observations.

In addition, students of the process approach have applied process-based ideas to the study of neurological disorders extending well beyond the classic focal lesion–neurobehavioral syndrome investigations. These include explorations of the cognitive deficits associated with multiple sclerosis (White, Nyenhuis, & Sax, 1992), progressive supranuclear palsy (Albert, Feldman, & Willis, 1974), cerebrovascular dementia (Wolfe, Linn, Babikian, Knoefel, & Albert, 1990), and Alzheimer's disease (AD) (Albert & Moss, 1988). In addition, a manual for assessment and diagnosis based on process principles and tests has appeared (White, 1992).

THE PROCESS APPROACH TO CLINICAL
NEUROPSYCHOLOGICAL ASSESSMENT

Qualitative Assessment of Process

In the quest to understand patients' approaches to the challenges posed by neuropsychological tasks, students of the process approach have focused on several key aspects of test performance. These include the strategy or style of processing employed by the patient for task completion, the dissection of common tests into processing components that can be successfully or unsuccessfully carried out in completing the task, "pushing the limits" of patient processing capacities, the qualitative evaluation of error types, and systematic clinical observation and characterization of patient behavior during assessment. These aspects of clinical assessment are embodied in the process approach and will appear repeatedly in the descriptions of the tests most commonly used by process practitioners that will follow later in this chapter. However, a concrete description of each of these aspects of assessment will be presented here, along with examples of test applications.

Assessment of strategies or processing styles used in task completion can be carried out with flow sheets that allow the clinician to record the steps followed by the patient in completing a task. An example of this is the grid sheet used for following the patient's completion of WAIS-R Block Designs (see WAIS-R/NI, in Kaplan et al., 1991). These sheets allow the clinician to record the order in which blocks are placed (as well as errors in block placement) in order to facilitate description of the patient's strategy. The most common approaches taken by patients in completing Block Designs include the gestalt approach (in which blocks are pushed together to form the design as a whole), the analytic approach (in which the patient appears to divide the design into a grid and to fill in the parts of the grid with individual blocks), and the trial-and-error strategy (in which the patient places the block in the design and turns it until it appears to fit the stimulus example). The recording of the flow charts and the clinical notes kept during assessment allow the clinician to characterize the style of approach used for each design and the approach most prominently displayed by the patient being tested. The evaluation of the patient's strategy provides some clues to underlying brain pathology. For example, a patient using the analytic approach may be relying heavily on left hemisphere processing (implying impaired or weaker right hemisphere function), while the patient who relies completely on trial and error may have frontal lobe pathology (see Milberg et al., 1986). Another method of evaluating approach can be seen in the answer sheet developed by Boston VA neuropsychologists for recording answers to the Hooper Visual Organization Test (Hooper, 1958). For each item, responses commonly given by patients are listed by type of strategy the patient may have used (e.g., generalization from an isolate feature of the visual array). A final example is that of the recorder's sheet for the Cancellation Task (Weintraub & Mesulam, 1988), which allows the clinician to record the "trail" of responses provided by the patient. This trail can be systematic, haphazard, vertical, horizontal, perseverative, and so on.

Dissection of the task into cognitive-processing components was an early contribution of the process approach to the clinical evaluation of patients. The dissection can be part of the task itself. For example, an anterograde memory test may include several learning trials, immediate and delayed recall conditions, and both spontaneous recall and multiple choice response paradigms in order to assess several different processes of memory function (attention, learning, storage, retrieval, recognition), as is the case with the California Verbal Learning Test (Delis et al., 1987).

The investigation of processing components is also sometimes carried out through inquiry procedures in which the patient's test performance is examined in more detail. Inquiry procedures were incorporated extensively in the Wechsler Adult Intelligence Scale—Revised as a Neuropsychological Instrument (WAIS-R/NI) (Kaplan et al., 1991) answer sheets and supplementary test instruments. Examples of the inquiry technique include the investigation of the patient's Digit Symbol score by testing the contribution of memory function to the patient's performance (determining how many symbols and digit–symbol pairs the patient can recall without viewing the key) or by examining motor speed as a separate component (by determining how quickly the patient can copy the symbols alone without having to refer to a key). Similarly, the investigation of word retrieval deficit as an explanation for a lower than expected score on the WAIS-R Information subtest can be explored through the use of multiple choice response formats. Through examining the specific types of processing deficits revealed by testing, the clinician can draw inferences about specific brain structures or neural systems that appear to be dysfunctional.

"Pushing the limits" of patients performance also allows the clinician to assess patient abilities in completing different processing tasks. If a patient has a suspected deficit that does not show up on a task, the task can be made harder to determine whether a precipitous change occurs in processing capacity. For example, the patient may be able to learn material that has an internal structure (narrative material) but be totally unable to learn material low in structural associations (unrelated word pairs). Likewise, the patient may learn new information under ordinary test circumstances, but may have great difficulty if any kind of distraction is introduced. In this situation, standard memory testing such as the WMS-R (Wechsler, 1987) can be supplemented by additional testing with tasks such as the Peterson word or consonant triads (Peterson & Peterson, 1959), for which the patient must retain words or consonants in memory while carrying out a distraction task such as counting backward. By pushing the limits, it is possible to detect subtle focal brain dysfunction in patients who are very bright or who have developed strong compensatory mechanisms in adjusting to acquired deficits.

Qualitative observation of error types is a hallmark of the process approach and focuses on the observation of "pathognomonic signs" of specific types of brain damage that may be observed during testing. Some of these qualitative signs include micrographia in writing and drawing; "pull to stimulus example" when copying material; specific types of perseveration ("stuck-in-set," recurrent, continuous); specific types of errors in spontaneous speech, writing, and reading (e.g., semantic substitutions, phonemic substitutions, neologisms, agrammatism); unilateral neglect or inattention (spatial, tactile, auditory); competing hand or alien hand syndromes; errors in praxis; tremor and chorea; and specific kinds of errors made in completing tasks such as clock drawings or visual constructions. These qualitative signs are often extremely helpful clues in detecting the localization and/or underlying disorder from which the patient may be suffering and are seen as a powerful adjunct to both differential diagnosis and the development of treatment plans.

Systematic observation and characterization of patient behavior is also inherent to the process approach. Careful observation of spontaneous speech is carried out in order to characterize volume, clarity, specific types of motor deficits, linguistic characteristics, content, grammatical structure, and style. Visuospatial processing is carefully observed in regard to size of constructions, orientation of constructions in space, laterality of approach to drawing (e.g., beginning on the left or the right), effectiveness of strategic approach to drawings (does the patient complete the Rey–Osterreith by working from the outside in or from the inside out?), motor or sensory neglect in constructions, style of completing constructions, and quality of motor performance (tremor, overdrawing, light drawings, perseveration). Motor performance is observed for speed and strength throughout testing, especially in regard to lateralized performance and quality of coordination. Handwriting is observed in writing samples for evidence of motor, spatial, and linguistic processing difficulties. Functional memory is also assessed observationally by noting whether the patient remembers the examiner from one test date to another and by examining memory for patient's room placement, prior testing experience, recent events in the patient's life or in the news, contacts with other clinic caretakers, and even test instructions.

Informal Examination Techniques

In general, clinicians using the process approach carry out formal neuropsychological assessments with the steps outlined below. However, the process tradition arose in a clinical/academic setting in which interdisciplinary teams of psychologists, neurologists, and speech pathologists examine patients together for informal bed rounds and more formal grand rounds. In these settings and when working with patients for whom formal testing techniques are impossible (because the patient is severely impaired, cannot speak, does not want to "take tests"), process techniques are easily applied. This is especially true of some of the tasks described in the section below on neuropsychological test instruments that are informal and highly qualitative in terms of the information they gather. These include such tasks as the Boston Visuospatial Quantitative Battery, for which the patient draws objects and works with clocks and maps; the use of the Cookie Theft picture to obtain a writing or speech sample; and various methods of sampling language, constructional skills, and praxis derived from the Boston Diagnostic Aphasia Examination (Goodglass & Kaplan, 1983).

Formal Examinations

The process approach emphasizes interaction between the clinician and the patient. In fact, this is true to such an extent that some clinicians utilizing this approach object to the use of non-PhD technicians for the collection of neuropsychological data (though most will allow students to participate in assessment). Even among those practitioners who involve psychometricians or technicians in the collection of formal test data, however, there is a strong emphasis on knowing and interviewing the patient. The interview is generally focused on listening to the patient's primary complaints, collecting data on cognitive, psychiatric, and neurological symptoms experienced by the patient, reviewing relevant medical and academic history, and collecting data on relevant familial history (handedness, educational/academic history, medical, psychiatric, etc.). An interview based on the process approach designed for neuropsychological assessment has been published (White, 1992).

In general, the clinician will use the interview data, observation of the patient's functional status, specifically stated referral questions, and history revealed by records and charts in order to develop a testing strategy and in order to begin the testing. Currently, at the Boston Department of Veterans Affairs Medical Center (DVAMC), we sometimes add a Mini-Mental State Examination (Folstein, Folstein, & McHugh, 1975) immediately after interview in order to decide on the functional level at which testing should be aimed (e.g., do we need to give challenging tests to uncover subtle problems). In addition to level of function, it may be necessary to adjust tests for patient limitations (diminished visual acuity, aphasia, alexia, motor deficits, spatial neglect, etc.). Before formal testing begins, the use of a group of specific tests is generally contemplated. These tests might be augmented or limited as necessary as the testing proceeds and the need for inquiry occurs or if issues being assessed are answered unexpectedly quickly. Although some proponents of the process approach argue that the procedure should follow the clinician's instincts or focus narrowly on neurobehavioral syndromes, we have recently argued in favor of a broad sampling of behavioral domains with virtually all patients (White, 1992). This can eliminate some serious errors (e.g., identifying the deficits associated with a known focal stroke, but failing to observe that the patient actually shows evidence of multi-infarct dementia). It also allows the clinician to observe functional strengths that can be invoked in treatment planning and in helping the patient to develop compensatory strategies for overcoming functional deficits.

Given the above considerations, it is clear that clinicians using the process approach do not generally invoke set batteries for testing patients; every patient is not administered exactly the same group of tests. Rather, the group of tests used at any single assessment will reflect the needs of the patient being seen and the specific type of assessment required for that patient's situation. However, despite the avoidance of predetermined batteries, there is a group of tests that are commonly used in the process approach, including core tests that tend to be given to every patient who can manage the task. The commonly used tests are listed in Table 1. In addition to these tasks, many other tests will be applied as needed. For example, a case of suspected learning disability might result in the application of

TABLE 1. Neuropsychological Test Instruments

Current/premorbid patterns of intellectual and academic ability
   Wechsler Adult Intelligence Scale—Revised[a] (Wechsler, 1981)
   Mini-Mental Status Examination (Folstein et al., 1975)
   Wide Range Achievement Test—III (Wilkinson, 1993)
   Ravens Progressive Matrices (Raven, 1958, 1962)
   Peabody Picture Vocabulary Test (Dunn & Dunn, 1981)
   Stanford Binet Test of Intelligence Scale (Thorndike et al., 1986)
   Woodcock–Johnson Psycho-Educational Battery—Revised (Woodcock & Johnson, 1989, 1990)
   Gates—MacGinite Reading Test (MacGinitie, 1978)
   National Adult Reading Test (Nelson, 1982)
Attention and executive function
   WAIS-R: Digit spans, Arithmetic [Similarities, Comprehension, Picture Completion, Picture
      Arrangement][a]
   Wechsler Memory Scale (WMS, WMS-R) (Wechsler, 1987; Wechsler & Stone, 1945) [Digit Spans,
      Mental Control, Visual Spans, Attention Index][a]
   Corsi Blocks (Milner, 1971)
   Trail-making Test[b] (Halstead, 1947)
   Recurrent Series Writing, Multiple Loops[b] (see White, 1992)
   Luria 3-step[b] (Luria, 1982)
   Continuous Performance Test[c] (Rosvold et al., 1956)
   Paced Auditory Serial Addition Test (Gronwall & Sampson, 1974)
   Wisconsin Card Sorting Test[a] (Berg, 1948)
   Categories Test (Halstead, 1947)
   Controlled Word Association Test (Benton, 1973)
Verbal and language function
   WAIS-R: Information, Vocabulary, Similarities, Comprehension[a]
   Controlled Word Association Test[a]
   Boston Naming Test[a] (Kaplan et al., 1983)
   Boston Diagnostic Aphasia Examination, selected subtests (especially Cookie Theft writing
      sample)[b] (Goodglass & Kaplan, 1983)
Motor function
   Finger Tapping[a] (Halstead, 1947)
   Grip Strength[b] (Halstead, 1947)
   Purdue Pegboard[c] (Purdue Research Foundation, 1948)
   WAIS-R Digit Symbol[a]
Visuospatial function
   WAIS-R: Picture Completion, Picture Arrangement, Block Designs, Object Assembly[a]
   Rey–Osterreith Complex Figure (copy)[a] (Rey, 1941)
   Hooper Visual Organization Test[b] (Hooper, 1958)
   Boston Visuospatial Quantitative Battery[a] (Goodglass & Kaplan, 1983)
   Cancellation Test[b] (Weintraub & Mesulam, 1988)
Memory
   WMS or WMS-R (Boston version)[a]
   California Verbal Learning Test[a] (Delis et al., 1987)
   Rey–Osterreith Complex Figure (Recall)[a]
   Delayed Recognition Span Test[c] (Moss et al., 1986)
   Milner Facial Recognition Test (Milner, 1968)
   Tactual Performance Test (Halstead, 1947)
   Peterson Task (Peterson & Peterson, 1959)
   Albert's Famous Faces (Retrograde memory battery)[c] (Albert et al., 1981)

(continued)

TABLE 1. (*Continued*)

Personality/Affect
    Profile of Mood States[c] (McNair et al., 1971)
    Minnesota Multiphasic Personality Inventory—2[c] (Hathaway & McKinley, 1989)
    Nonverbal Analogue Mood Scales (Stern et al., 1997; Diamond & White, unpublished)

---

[a]Core tests used by virtually all process-oriented practitioners.
[b]Tests commonly included in process approach test batteries.
[c]Core test, Boston DVAMC Neuropsychology Service, or common adjunct test in process-oriented batteries.

Woodcock–Johnson tasks (Woodcock & Johnson, 1989, 1990) or the Peabody Picture Vocabulary Test (Dunn & Dunn, 1981). Subtests from the Stanford–Binet (Thorndike, Hagen, & Sattler, 1986) might be applied to a patient who functions at a very low level or needs certain types of nonverbal tasks for linguistic or other reasons. Degraded figures, embedded figures, or a color-matching test might be given under certain circumstances to assess various aspects of visuospatial processing or color detection/naming. Highly specialized tasks assessing the components of anterograde memory or evaluating retrograde memory might be applied. The range of test instruments that can be used is extremely large and is limited mostly by the extent of the clinician's familiarity with test instruments. In some patients, inquiry or testing the patient's limits may result in the clinician's spontaneous or systematic development of tasks.

Once testing is completed, data are scored in a standardized fashion (sometimes with "double scoring" in which the patient's score reflects that earned in a nonstandard administration of a task designed to accommodate special circumstances such as extra time for patients with motor slowing). As noted earlier in this chapter, specialized answer sheets incorporating the process approach to the collection of test data have been designed for many tests and form the basis for scoring tests and summarizing quantitative data (a manual containing these forms is in preparation). At the Boston DVAMC, both quantitative and qualitative data are recorded on patient summary sheets that are divided into functional domains for ease of review and consideration for lesion localization, differential diagnosis, and provision of treatment recommendations. For the purposes of these summary sheets, omnibus tests such a the WAIS-R are summarized by subtest as well as overall scores, so that data can be reviewed most appropriately. With the WAIS-R, for example, the ranges for Full Scale, Verbal, and Performance IQs are recorded in a section aimed at characterizing current and premorbid cognitive abilities (it is recognized here that these abilities may differ significantly in regard to level of performance on standardized tests or they may be very similar). Other sections of the summary sheet are used for subtest scores, however. For example, quantitative and qualitative findings from the Block Design subtest appear in the section summarizing Visuospatial function and Digit Span appears in the section on Attention.

Boston is famous for the length of clinical test reports produced by process practitioners. Although length can vary greatly, generally reports include a section summarizing the referral questions, relevant history and imaging findings, a review of patient's responses to the interview items, a list of tests administered, a results section describing the quantitative and qualitative findings observed in test performance, and a conclusions section. The latter summarizes the clinical questions at the heart of the case. It also provides a succinct description of the pattern of behavioral strengths and weaknesses observed in the patient (including relevant information on qualitative and pathognomonic signs). For many clinicians, this is followed by a statement about the likely cerebral localization of observed dysfunction (if such is noted) and a diagnosis or differential diagnosis of likely neurological and/or psychiatric etiology to which test results may be attributed (if applicable). This is followed by treatment recommendations and recommendations to the patient for use of strengths and special techniques to compensate for any cognitive deficits (if applicable).

NEUROPSYCHOLOGICAL TEST INSTRUMENTS

Although the process-oriented neuropsychological examination generally emphasizes functional domains and various classifications of qualitative findings, we will in this section follow a test-based strategy in describing the application of the process approach. We will first discuss tests developed by process-oriented neuropsychologists and then review the process approach as applied to other psychological and neuropsychological tests.

Tests Developed by Process-Oriented Neuropsychologists

Tests of Naming

The Boston Naming Test (BNT) appeared in two versions: an experimental form with 85 items (Kaplan et al., 1976) and its present 60-item task form (Kaplan et al., 1983). The test, which is used with children 3 years of age and older and with adults, consists of line drawings of objects that the patient is asked to name. If the name is not spontaneously produced within 20 seconds, a semantic cue is provided. A phonemic cue is given when the patient is still unable to name the object. The total score for the test is the number of items correctly named spontaneously plus those named with a semantic cue. Correct responses following a phonemic cue are noted, but these are not included in the "total correct" score on which norms for the BNT are based.

The careful noting of responses as well as response time is essential in interpreting BNT results. Slowed but accurate naming may reflect deficits in the patient's ability to retrieve information from semantic memory efficiently and is common in disorders affecting the basal ganglia (such as Parkinson's disease) and the subcortical white matter (e.g., multiple sclerosis, cerebrovascular disorders).

Response to cuing is also an important clinical indicator. Patients whose performance improves significantly following semantic cues may have visuospatial or visuoperceptual deficits impeding the recognition of the objects depicted in the drawings. Patients who respond well to phonemic cues demonstrate the retention of linguistic information in semantic memory but a deficit in retrieval (as can be seen in subcortical or frontal lobe disorders). Patients who cannot produce object names when provided with phonemic cues may be unfamiliar with the object name (because they never learned it, which can sometimes be ascertained by careful inquiry) or because of a deterioration in semantic memory stores (seen, for example, in AD, certain dementias affecting the frontal lobes, or lesions in cerebral language zones).

Speech characteristics must be noted. The patient may display articulatory groping on the way to producing the target word (in which the sounds of the word are approximated until the word is produced) or semantic groping (in which the patient produces words from the same semantic field as the target word). The former approach suggests a deficit in phoneme production, while the latter raises the issue of a dysfluency in word production. Patients may also produce dysarthric, hypophonic, or stuttered responses, all of which provide clues to the etiology and cerebral localization of language and neuropsychological dysfunction.

Finally, the types of errors noted when the patient produces phonemes or words other than the target are a source of valuable information about the etiology and localization of any observed naming deficits. Phonemic distortions of words (e.g., "beaser" for *beaver*) are referred to as literal or phonemic paraphasias and reflect dysfunction in primary speech zones; they are particularly common in aphasic disorders and the moderate to later stages of AD and can also be seen in patients with language-based learning disabilities. Semantic distortions of speech, in which the patient produces a word substitution for the target name (e.g., "raccoon" for *beaver*), are referred to as verbal or semantic paraphasias; they are also found in patients with dominant hemisphere pathology and are seen in aphasic disorders and the early stages of AD. Neologisms are speech productions that are highly deviant from the target word (e.g., "belatso" for beaver). These are seen in severe aphasic disorders and in advanced AD. (Neologisms or nonsense words that are part of the patient's private vocabulary can be seen in schizophrenics, but this is a different type of neologism than that typically used in language analysis for neuropsychological/aphasia assessments.) Other types of errors seen on the BNT include circumlocutions, in which the patient produces a superordinate word for the target (e.g., "animal" or "mammal" for *beaver*). These indicate retrieval problems and have many etiologies ranging from fatigue to subcortically based retrieval deficits; sometimes they also are seen in the very earliest stages of AD or other primary progressive dementias affecting language, with semantic and literal paraphasias appearing later in the process. Cuing can also elicit other types of language errors, including inaccurate phonemic completions (e.g., "projector" following the "pro" cue for *protractor*) and guesses following semantic cues ("school" for *house*). The sequential naming occurring in the BNT can also give rise to perseverations of prior target names into response to later stimuli ("compass" for *protractor*). Finally, perceptual errors are often seen ("snake" for *pretzel*), suggesting damage in other brain areas (visual cortex, basal ganglia) or primary sensory deficits. (See Goodglass & Kaplan, 1983, for a detailed description of these error types and their interpretation in aphasiology.)

The 60-item BNT has the problem of a low ceiling. Mean score on the test for most adult age groups is about 55 regardless of education. Therefore, it can be very difficult to uncover subtle naming deficits in patients who have superior vocabularies. For this reason, we have developed an ancillary 40-item naming test, the Diamond Naming Test (DNT) (Diamond, Diamond, & White, 1987), using lower frequency names to explore subtle dysnomias in such subjects (items include targets such as *andirons*). It is administered, scored, and qualitatively evaluated in the same manner as the BNT. As a clinical tool, we are finding that it is quite effective. For example, most patients with higher-level vocabularies and no discernible symptoms of language disturbance score 35–40 correct on the DNT. We have seen several patients who earned 58 or 59 on the BNT, but 20–30 on the DNT, clearly demonstrating semantic paraphasic errors when presented with more difficult items.

The Boston Diagnostic Aphasia Examination

The Boston Diagnostic Aphasia Examination (BDAE) (Goodglass & Kaplan, 1976, 1983) was developed in order to allow characterization of specific types of language and language-related deficits. It facilitates exploration of many aspects of linguistic function, including reading (at several levels: letters, sounds, words, phrase, sentences), writing, sound production, naming, body part identification, comprehension, repetition, left–right orientation, finger naming, praxis, simple calculations, and simple visual constructions. Results from the tests permit classification of language dysfunction into severity levels and into subtypes of aphasia. In addition, results may reveal unusual but highly specific and localizable neurobehavioral syndromes (e.g., alexia without agraphia). The BDAE is widely used by speech pathologists, but subtests of the full examination are often used by practitioners of the process approach with patients who have language disorders or who are likely to display specific neurobehavioral syndromes involving language.

Two ancillary tests described in the BDAE manual are especially commonly used by neuropsychologists. One, a primary language test, is the Cookie Theft description task. The stimulus for this task is a picture of events occurring in a kitchen; several events are happening at once. The patient is asked to write a paragraph describing the picture. Responses can be informative at several levels. Motor deficits in writing (overwriting, such as can be seen in occipital pathology; large writing, such as is sometimes observed in cerebellar disorders; micrographia, which is symptomatic of basal ganglia dysfunction) can be well observed, especially since this task requires extensive writing, not just output of single words or a short sentence. Spatial errors can also be seen, including hemispatial inattention (in the patient's perception of events depicted in the stimulus picture, the placement of writing on the page) and problems orienting the writing in space (tendency to go up or downhill, widely disparate placement of words on the page). There are also often psychodynamic cues evident in the subject's interpretation of the events depicted in the drawing. Most importantly, the writing sample allows an analysis of language dysfunction. This can include production of a telegraphic response (which can be seen in patients with agrammatism or dysnomia), omission or misuse of functors, and word distortions of the type described in the section on the BNT (phonemic paraphasics, semantic paraphasics, neologisms, circumlocutions, perseverations of words, letters, or parts of letters). The Cookie Theft stimulus can also be used to elicit spontaneous speech productions if appropriate.

A second group of ancillary tasks associated with the BDAE is the Boston Visuospatial Quantitative Battery (BVSQB). This is a group of tasks analyzing visual constructions (using drawings and replications of designs made of small sticks), map locations, finger location, left–right discrimination of drawings of human and animal body parts, and clock drawings. These tasks were initially designed to uncover parietal lobe dysfunction and were formerly called the Parietal Lobe Battery. They were seen as important in discriminating visuospatial contributions to cerebral dysfunction arising from posterior left and right hemisphere lesions. They continue to constitute an important source of information for process-oriented neuropsychologists on posterior cerebral, subcortical, and cerebellar dysfunction, especially at the qualitative level. The most commonly used tasks in the BVSQB by process practitioners are the drawings, map, and clocks. These tasks are included in the core tasks currently used on the Neuropsychology Service at the Boston DVAMC. They are seen as particularly valuable sources of qualitative information on the likely etiology of visuospatial deficits observed on other neuropsychological tests assessing function in this domain (e.g., WAIS-R Performance tests; WMS-R Visual Memory tasks). In addition, the drawing tasks are often very helpful in patients for whom other tests are inappropriate or impossible because of degree of dementia or other factors. We frequently use them, for example, with patients who do not speak English and have found that the pathognomonic signs of brain pathology observable on these tasks extend to many cultures and language backgrounds. They are also useful for some patients who see drawing as less of a "test" than being timed while constructing a block design or identifying missing parts of pictures.

Stimuli for the drawing task consist of a page that is blank on one side, a line down the middle, and a side containing a drawing at the top of the page. The page is folded in half and the patient is first instructed to draw a specific object on the blank half of the page. After the object has been drawn spontaneously, the patient is presented with the other half of the page and asked to copy the stimulus drawing placed at the top of the page. The usual items used are a clock (draw a picture of a clock, place the numbers on it and draw in hands so that the clock reads "10 after 11"), a daisy, a house (with the front, one side, and the roof showing), an elephant, the Red Cross symbol (without taking the pencil off the page), and a cube (if the patient uses the "trick" for drawing the cube, a second spontaneous drawing is requested). These drawings are so rich in qualitative detail that many pages could be occupied with describing their occurrence and interpretation. Some examples include hemispatial neglect, micro- or macrographia, perseveration of within-drawing elements, perseveration of elements from prior drawings into later drawings ("perseverative contamination," which is quite common, for example, from the clock to the daisy), overdrawing, light drawing, "stimulus pull" to the stimulus example (in which the patient's copy is produced very close to the stimulus example) and stimulus pull in the 10 past 11 clock drawing (in which the patient draws a hand to the number 10), spatial orientation errors (numbers placed in wrong order on the clock, drawings or parts of drawings rotated, drawings going off the page), facing drawings in unusual directions (usually toward the left rather than the right), drawing from right-to-left (left-to-right is more common), omissions of outer outlines or inner details of drawings, disinhibition (e.g., when placing numbers on the clock face, he or she fails to stop at the number 12 but keeps going with higher numbers), inability to represent perspective, writing the name of the object when asked to draw it and considering this production to be a drawing (e.g., writing "daisy" instead of producing a drawing), and writing down the examiner's instructions before producing the drawing.

Other stimuli on this task consist of drawings of clocks. On the upper half of the page, the clocks contain numbers and below each clock is a time written (e.g., 3:00); on the lower half of the page, the clocks are drawn but no numbers appear. The unnumbered clock faces are administered first, followed by the numbered clock faces (the page is folded in half to reveal only one set of the four clock faces at a time). The patient must draw hands on the clock to indicate the written times. Error types include drawing the hands to the wrong numbers (spatial orientation errors), reversing the lengths of the hour and minute hands, placing the arrows so that they point to the center of the clock, neglecting to offset the hour hands when minutes must be indicated (e.g., 9:15, 7:30), drawing multiple arrows (perseveration), and writing in the times on the clock face rather than drawing hands. These error types can indicate dysfunction in the frontal or parietal lobes, and certain error types are common in AD and subcortical disorders (see Freedman et al., 1994, for a detailed description of clock drawing interpretation).

Another BVSQB stimulus is a drawing of a blank map of the United States. The patient must indicate the locations of specified areas. At the Boston DVAMC, we use the following locations: Boston, San Francisco, Texas, Florida, Canada, Mexico, Atlantic Ocean, Pacific Ocean, Mississippi River, and Lake Michigan. This task can provide information on problems with spatial orientation, hemispatial neglect, figure–ground discrimination difficulties, and lack of knowledge about geography (which can sometimes be correlated with errors on the geography questions from the WAIS-R Information subtest).

The Cancellation Test

The Cancellation Test (Weintraub & Mesulam, 1988) is a task assessing spatial attention and planning. These are two types of stimuli presented in two formats. One set of stimuli consists of letters, the other of small visual stimuli. For one format, the stimuli are presented in orderly rows and columns; for the other, the stimuli are scattered across the page. The patient must identify all of the target stimuli in the spatial array for the examiner (one target is chosen for each of the two types of stimulus). The examiner uses a copy of the stimuli to follow the path used by the patient in scanning the stimulus page and identifying the target stimuli. Thus, the examiner can evaluate the patient's approach (haphazard vs. planned) and the tendency to miss stimuli in a specific visual field.

The California Verbal Learning Tests

The California Verbal Learning Tests (CLVT) represent the application of current knowledge about the processing components of memory function to a clinical test. Published forms of the test are available for adults (Delis et al., 1987) and for children (Delis, Kramer, Kaplan, & Ober, 1994), and there is a shorter nine-item form often used for the evaluation of patients with dementia. In all forms, the patient is presented with a list of words that has an internal structure; that is, subgroups of the words can be classified into categories (e.g., spices or clothing). The adult version contains 16 words, the children's version 15 words, and the dementia version 9 words. The patient is presented with the list of words five times; each list presentation is followed by spontaneous immediate recall of the words presented. An interference list of words is then administered once, followed by spontaneous immediate recall of that list. The patient is then asked to recall the initial list spontaneously (short-delayed recall); this is followed by a cued recall, in which the patient is provided with the categories from which the original words were drawn for recall (cued short-delayed recall). After a 20-minute delay, the subject is again asked to spontaneously recall the initial list (long-delayed recall); this is followed by provision of the list categories (cued long-delayed recall). Finally, a list of twice as many words as the original list is given and the subject must indicate whether or not the word was present in the initial list (recognition condition); the foils in the latter condition include words from the interference list as well as other words related to the categories inherent to the structure of the list. At the clinical neuropsychology clinics at the Boston DVAMC and Boston University School of Medicine, we have devised a forced recognition condition in which the subject is presented a page containing twice as many words as on the original list and is asked to choose only a specific number of words (16, 15, or 9, depending on which form of the CVLT is being used) that the patient thinks were on the original list. This allows us a more accurate view of recognition memory, especially in patients who "overendorse" the choices on the orally administered CVLT recognition condition (i.e., indicate more words than were on the initial list).

The CVLT allows the neuropsychologist to examine memory processes in several ways. First, the process of learning can be evaluated by examining the patient's ability to acquire information over the initial five learning trials. Capacity for spontaneous retrieval of information from memory store can also be examined in the patient's performance on recall conditions, especially short and long uncued recall. The effect of providing cuing or structure as an aid in retrieval can also be assessed by evaluating the cued recall conditions. Retention of information over delay or forgetting rates can also be examined by looking at the differences between immediate recall and short-delayed recall and the difference between short-delayed recall and long-delayed recall. This aspect of memory can also be studied by looking at the recognition condition; sometimes recognition is perfect despite impaired recall, suggesting that the problem lies in the realm of retrieval rather than retention. All of these clues are important in localizing the cerebral structures that may subserve impaired memory function. For example, learning problems may reflect frontal, subcortical, or attentional dysfunction and are also seen in alcoholic Korsakoff's disease; retrieval deficits are common in subcortical and frontal disorders; and forgetting (even in the recognition memory condition) is a hallmark of hippocampal dysfunction and is common in AD. Patterns of CVLT deficits have been identified in other disorders as well (see Research section below).

Qualitative aspects of memory performance can also be examined. Susceptibility to interference can be evaluated by comparing first-trial learning on the initial list to the patient's recall for the interference list and by examining intrusion errors. Proactive and retroactive interference can also be evaluated by examining the words recalled by the patient relative to the order in which the list words were presented. The patient's deployment of a strategy (or lack of deploying a strategy) can be assessed by looking at cluster scores, which summarize the patient's use of the internal structure of the word list (categories) as an aid to learning and spontaneous recall of the stimulus words. Perseveration and intrusion errors can also be examined systematically. Many of these qualitative findings suggest an attentional component to memory dysfunction and may suggest primary or secondary frontal lobe dysfunction.

Finally, inconsistent responding can be an important qualitative indicator in evaluating CVLT performance. This can be seen in highly uneven learning from trial to trial in the first five learning trials, recall of totally different words in the five learning trials, extreme differences between long and short recall (with long recall being better), and extreme differences between spontaneous recall and recognition memory. These findings often indicate a problem at the attentional or motivational level and can be seen in patients who are depressed, distracted, exerting less than full effort, or outright malingering. One has to be especially careful in interpreting results when recognition memory is perfect but learning and recall performances are uneven or impaired. One frequently sees such results interpreted as indicating "hippocampal deficit" when this is highly unlikely, especially in disorders such as chronic fatigue syndrome or multiple chemical sensitivity.

The Delayed Recognition Span Test

The Delayed Recognition Span Test (Moss et al., 1986) is a task that also examines subcomponents of memory processing. Based on the delayed nonmatching to a sample paradigm used in cognitive research on monkeys, this test utilizes concrete stimuli and is especially useful for patients who have rather severe cognitive deficits or who are resistant to traditional (usually verbally based) forms of testing.

The stimuli are 14 round plastic disks placed on a board containing five rows and six columns for disk placement. Typically, the disks are plain and contain a word or a color stimulus. In the word and color conditions, the first disk is placed on the board, presented to the patient for 10 seconds, covered, and moved, and a second disk is placed on the board. The patient must indicate the new disk. New disks are successively placed until all 14 are on the board. Because the spatial condition assesses span for spatial orientation, the disks are not moved between trials. Scores consist of span score (number correct to first error) and total correct. For the verbal condition, 15-second incidental spontaneous recall is obtained, followed by 2-minute recall. After the delayed recall, a list of 28 words can be presented with forced-choice responses for 14 words. The verbal and spatial conditions are most commonly used in clinical practice. Verbal stimuli can be easily presented in other languages (we have used Spanish and Russian), and the color condition can be omitted or replaced with other stimuli of interest (e.g., designs, faces). This test has been used extensively both clinically and in research studies in patients with AD, Huntington's disease (HD), and Parkinson's disease (PD). Patients with AD show a characteristic rapid decay in spontaneous recall between the 15-second and 2-minute recall (with poor recognition memory), while patients with PD and HD show poor retrieval on spontaneous recall compared to recognition and also have an interesting tendency to recall different words in the 15-second and 2-minute recall conditions.

Nonverbal Mood Scales

Nonverbal mood scales have been developed by White and Diamond at the Boston VA (Diamond, White, & Moheban, 1990) and Stern (Stern, Arruda, Hooper, Wolfner, & Morey, 1997) for the assessment of mood states using a nonverbal format. For these tasks, a vertical line, 100 mm in length, separates a neutral facial stimulus from a stimulus representing a specific mood state (sad, happy, anxious, angry, etc.). The patient indicates the degree to which the state is currently being experienced on the vertical line. The Boston version uses drawn stimuli that resemble real faces, while the Stern version contains iconic cartoon representations. In the Boston version, a control stimulus in which the patient designates his or her age is included to ascertain that the patient comprehends the task demands. These measures allow us to inquire into the patient's perception of mood state in a nonverbal manner, and are thus usable with patients who are aphasic or dyslexic. Many patients find these self-report measures easier to accept and respond to than the traditional "psychological test" measures. They can also be administered very quickly. Stimuli for these tasks will be included in the upcoming manual containing Boston DVAMC process-oriented stimuli and answer sheets (White, 1996).

Process Applications to Other Psychological Tests

The Wechsler Adult Intelligence Scale—Revised as a Neuropsychological Instrument

The WAIS-R/NI (Kaplan et al., 1991) has appeared as a technique for administering the WAIS-R using a process approach. It provides answer sheets for detailed recording of the steps taken by a patient in responding to WAIS-R stimuli and for scoring patient's responses in a more detailed manner than the standard WAIS-R scoring system. In addition, stimuli for detailed inquiry are provided. For example, the Corsi block task is included so that the examiner can compare verbal and visual attention spans and can get an idea of underlying spatial processing span to be used in interpreting other test data. Also included is a multiple-choice version of the Information task, to be used for inquiry into the word-finding or retrieval deficits that might contribute to a patient's performance on the standard Information test. For each of the subtests, elucidation of the process approach is inherent in the test materials and will not be described in detail here. The recording of responses and scoring systems used in this version of the WAIS-R are somewhat arduous and are probably best applied to research efforts utilizing process methods and concepts. For clinical purposes, the observation of qualitative findings and task strategies is sufficient for interpretative purposes. Most practitioners use a lengthened but less detailed answer sheet to record test item responses verbatim and to record the steps followed by the patient in arriving at a solution to the item.

The Wechsler Memory Scale

The WMS (Wechsler & Stone, 1945) was extensively amended by Boston process clinicians in order to allow a specific analysis of the subcomponents of memory processing that were problematic for individual patients. The Boston version of the test includes cued recall and recognition recall stimuli for Logical Memory, Visual Reproduction, and Paired Associate Learning. In addition, a 20-minute delayed recall was added to the test. Copy and matching conditions were added to the Visual Reproduction task and a reversed presentation of the word pairs was developed for the Paired Associate Learning (PAL) task. Use of the cued, recognition, and copy conditions varies somewhat among Boston practitioners. Some use these conditions after both immediate and delayed recall. Others prefer not to introduce these conditions until after delayed recall (so that forgetting rates can be examined without having to worry about reteaching material between immediate and delayed recall). The reversed PAL condition is generally presented after delayed recall only.

The WMS-R (Wechsler, 1987) was developed with active input from a number of Boston practitioners and contains the delayed recall condition utilized in the Boston version of WMS for many of the tasks. However, it does not include cued recall or recognition conditions for Logical Memory, Visual Reproduction, or Verbal PAL. Likewise, a copy condition was not included for the Visual Reproduction task. Stimuli for these conditions were developed in Boston at the Aphasia Research Center (by Barbara Howarten) and are used locally. We are finding that the WMS-R Visual Reproduction task is easier and less revealing qualitatively than the same task from WMS, and thus we sometimes substitute the latter stimuli when not giving a full WMS-R. In addition, the Visual Span task results are not as stable as the results obtained here using Corsi blocks, and we are interpreting the WMS-R Visual Span findings cautiously (especially differential between forward and backward spans). Here we also typically administer both WAIS-R and WMS-R Digit Spans to patients in order to assess performance and attentional consistency.

The WMS and WMS-R include tasks for assessment of "mental control," a type of attentional task. Because the items are often too simple to pick up real set maintenance problems, auxiliary mental control tasks are often used for limits testing. These generally include reciting the letters of the alphabet containing curves in their printed capital forms, reciting the letters of the alphabet rhyming with the word *tree,* listing the months of the year forward, and providing the months of the year backward.

The Hooper Visual Organization Test

The Hooper Visual Organization Test (HVOT) (Hooper, 1958) is used extensively by process practitioners as a motor-free measure of visuospatial organization that is particularly sensitive to subcortical disorders (especially PD). Special scoring sheets (developed initially to focus on aspects of right hemisphere and frontal lobe function) are used to characterize the types of dysfunction revealed by specific commonly produced erroneous responses. The categories by which error responses are categorized include poor global integration, collate, isolates (divided into right, left, and middle), and parts of isolates (also spatially divided). For each of the 30 HVOT stimuli, four typical responses are listed that fit these categories. These four typical responses plus the correct response can also be given as multiple-choice answers to test limits with patients who are dysnomic or are unable to respond to specific items with any concrete answer.

The Rey–Osterreith Complex Figure

The Rey–Osterreith Complex Figure (ROCF) (Rey, 1941) is so commonly used among Boston process practitioners that it is often viewed as a Boston test. Typically, the figure is presented for copy, followed by immediate recall and a 20-minute delayed recall drawing of the figure. The examiner copies the patient's production of the figure as the patient is drawing it, numbering each line so that the order of construction of figural elements is recorded. Many practitioners have the patient use colored pens to complete the drawing, having the subject change pens frequently, so that the patient's approach can be seen instantaneously, simply by looking at it. (Dr. Tom N. Tombaugh, who recently completed a sabbatical here, innovated a less intrusive approach to the colored pens technique by having the patient use a pencil and having the examiner use colored pens to copy the patient's production.) At the Boston DVAMC, we frequently use an informal recognition condition containing several complex figures as well. Several methods for scoring the test have been devised (Corwin & Bylsma, 1993; Stern et al., 1994; Weber & Holmes, 1985). Stern's method is somewhat more detailed.

A rather complex lore on the meaning of particular aspects of ROCF performance has accumulated and is taught clinically to students specializing in the process approach. This lore has at times found its way into research. Some of the qualitative aspects of ROCF production that have received attention include dramatic size changes (small, large), spatial neglect of figure elements, appreciation of outer gestalt and/or inner gestalt, rotation of the full design or elements, perseveration of elements, overall approach to the drawing (gestalt, detail-oriented, segmented, left-to-right vs. right-to-left), elongation or condensation of the design, fine manual motor dexterity revealed in drawing, dramatic discrepancies between copy and recall productions, and discrepancies between immediate and delayed recall.

Because the ROCF is extremely difficult for patients with advanced or widespread brain damage, we often substitute a simpler form of the figure for these patients. For patients who have recently drawn the ROCF, the Taylor figure (Taylor, 1979) is sometimes substituted, though this figure is an easier one to replicate and remember.

Recurrent Series Writing and Multiple Loops

Recurrent Series and multiple loops (see White, 1992) replications are qualitative tasks drawn from behavioral neurology that are simple to administer and can be completed by patients who are quite impaired. In the recurrent series writing task, the patient is shown a stimulus example of three *mn* pairs (mnmnmn, in cursive) and asked to draw the pattern across the page, first with the preferred hand and then with the nonpreferred hand. This task allows assessment of perseveration, set maintenance and set-switching capacities, and qualitative aspects of graphomotor function. It is harder than the multiple loops tasks, for which the patient is presented with a three-loop pattern ($\substack{333 \\ 333 \\ 333}$) and asked to copy it across the page with the preferred hand and then the nonpreferred hand. Performance on this task can reveal continuous perseveration, stimulus pull (production of the number *3*), spatial rotations, motor problems, and even a remarkable stimulus pull–perseveration combination ($\substack{333 \\ 333 \\ 333}$). These two simple tasks sometimes reveal a surprising degree of frontal lobe dysfunction in patients, though they are sometimes too easy. If so, then other stimuli can be substituted (e.g., $\_\Pi\mathsf{L}\!\diagup\!\diagdown\_$).

Case Report

History

At the time of referral, a 28-year-old female with a college education had carried a diagnosis of probable multiple sclerosis (MS) for 1 year. She had begun experiencing symptoms 2 years prior. These included right eye pain, right arm and leg weakness, dizziness, incontinence, extreme fatigue, and sensitivity to heat. Four exacerbations of symptoms had reportedly occurred in the 2 years since onset, all accompanied by severe symptoms of depression. She was referred for neuropsychological testing in order to determine whether there were cognitive changes suggestive of MS. Magnetic resonance imaging results were pending at the time that she was seen.

Major Findings

Quantitative test results are summarized in Table 2. As can be seen, scores were generally within expectation for the patient's estimated premorbid functioning (average to high average). An exception was her performance on the Santa Ana Formboard Test (a pegboard task), which revealed right-sided weakness, and the Minnesota Multiphasic Personality Inventory (MMPI) profile, which was markedly elevated.

Though quantitative findings were generally as expected, there were some unexpected qualitative findings. Errors in sequencing material were seen at several points in the protocol, particularly on digit spans (worse for backward than forward spans) but also in recalling information from the WMS Logical Memories subtest. She lost set twice on the Wisconsin Card Sorting task (after one 6- and one 7-card sequence) and when doing ancillary mental control testing (reciting the letters of the alphabet that rhyme with *tree*). A perseverative contamination was seen in the Delayed Recall condition of the WMS Visual Reproductions task in which two angled lines with flags (from Fig. A) replaced two straight lines with loops when she drew Fig. C. When copying the Visual Reproduction designs, accuracy was better on the left than the right sides of the drawing. Boston Visuospatial Quantitative Battery productions were notable for a tendency to "close in" to the stimulus example when

TABLE 2. Neuropsychological Test Data: Case Report

1. Attention, executive tasks
   A. WAIS-R Digit Span: ASS = 10 (8F, 6B)
   B. WAIS-R Arithmetic: ASS = 10
   C. WMS Mental Control: no errors/one error on ancillary mental control
   D. Trials A: 75%ile, B:90%ile (no errors)
   E. Wisconsin Card Sorting Test: 6 sorts. 89 trials (loss of set ×2)
2. Motor function
   A. WAIS-R Digit Symbol: ASS = 12
   B. Santa Ana Formboard: R = 18 (expected = 27), L = 23 (expected = 27), both = 35
      (expected = 39)
3. Verbal and language tasks.
   A. WAIS-R Information: ASS = 16
   B. WAIS-R Vocabulary: ASS = 10
   C. WAIS-R Comprehension: ASS = 12
   D. WAIS-R Similarities: ASS = 14
   E. Controlled Word Assn. Test: 55–59%ile (1 perseveration)
   F. Boston Naming Test: 59/60
4. Visuospatial tasks
   A. WAIS-R Picture Completion: ASS = 11
   B. WAIS-R Picture Arrangement: ASS = 11
   C. WAIS-R Block Designs: ASS = 12
   D. WAIS-R Object Assembly: ASS = 11
   E. Boston Visuospatial Quantitative Battery: no errors clocks or map, "closes in" to stimulus
      example, trouble with perspective
5. Memory tests
   A. WMS MQ = 110
   B. Logical Memory, IR = 17 (exact), 27 (including paraphrased), DR = 15, 24
   C. Verbal Paired Associates: IR: 5,3; 6,4; 6,4: DR:6,4
   D. Visual Reproductions, IR = 10; DR = 9

copying and for difficulties in representing three dimensions when drawing a cube and a house. Mood was at times disinhibited and expressed in intense terms. Results suggested problems in the domains of attention, visuospatial function, motor skill, and mood. They were interpreted to be consistent with frontal/subcortical dysfunction with prominent left hemisphere involvement. Magnetic resonance imaging findings (showing white matter lesions in the left corona radiata and right middle cerebral peduncle lesions) were read as consistent with MS, and the patient's clinical course was consistent with this diagnosis.

Discussion

This is an old case but one that clearly demonstrates the utility of examining qualitative detail. The patient's abnormal MMPI and history of depression might have misled the clinician toward the wrong conclusion, particularly given the "normal" scores on cognitive tests. The pathological signs were subtle but consistent and were seen as being diagnostic.

Psychological treatment recommendations focused on monitoring mood and explaining to the patient the relationship between mood change and her disease state. She responded well to this, with a less "catastrophic" response to exacerbation symptoms.

RESEARCH

Because there are few boundaries that limit the application of the process approach's techniques, research is rarely directly self-identified as "process." However, the notion of process is embedded in most neurocognitive research. The following section, therefore, is a review of a select number of studies carried out by some of the principal proponents of the Boston process approach and investigations that best exemplify the application of qualitative analysis to understanding brain–behavior relationships. This section is organized by the cognitive domains typically addressed in neuropsychological research and includes investigations using some of the tests we find to be particularly useful in looking at process variables.

Attention and Executive System

One of the primary purposes of qualitative analysis is to understand the underlying mechanisms that contribute to a particular score on a neuropsychological measure. By analyzing performance on specific tests that ostensibly measure functioning in one cognitive domain, one can often find evidence that scores have been influenced by function and dysfunction in another domain. For instance, Shallice and Evans (1978) analyzed the responses of brain-injured subjects on the WAIS-R. Patients with frontal lobe lesions gave significantly more exaggerated or implausible responses to the Information subtest items relating to number facts than did patients with nonfrontal lesions. By recording and examining such responses, the WAIS-R Information subtest provides not only a measure of general information but also of cognitive estimation skills associated with the executive system.

Performance on the WAIS-R's Digit Span subtest can also be influenced by cognitive processes other than immediate verbal recall. However, examination of such processes is obfuscated by the WAIS-R scoring method of combining the forward and backward span conditions as if the two measured the same cognitive ability (Lezak, 1995). In fact, there is often a large discrepancy between forward and backward spans in normal elderly subjects (Botwinick & Storandt, 1974; Hayslip & Kennelly, 1980) and even more so in brain-damaged populations (Kaplan et al., 1991). Lezak (1995) concluded that, "for neuropsychological purposes, none of the Wechsler scoring systems [for the Digit Span subtest] are useful" (p. 358). The particular processes measured vary greatly. Weinberg, Diller, Gerstman, and Schulman (1972) found that patients with right hemisphere damage performed less well on the digit backward condition than patients with intact right hemispheres. They concluded that the backward span is dependent in part on some form of visualization ability. Rudel and Denckla (1974) also found differences in Digits Forward and Backward in a sample of children with developmental disorders. Specifically, children with right hemisphere damage tended to have impaired performance on Digits Backward, while their Digits Forward performance was generally intact. Visualization ability was again implicated. A factor analytic study by Larrabee and Kane (1986) indicated that backward spans rely on both visual and verbal processes. The forward span, in contrast, is more affected by left hemisphere damage (Black, 1986; Hom & Reitan, 1984).

The Corsi Blocks visual span test (Milner, 1971), a visual analogue to the Digit Span test, has also been shown to be sensitive to various lesions based on patterns of performance. DeRenzi (1983), for example, found that patients with posterior lesions performed worse than patients with anterior lesions. Furthermore, the introduction of a delay between demonstration and response increased the sensitivity to right posterior lesions relative to left posterior lesions. DeRenzi, Faglioni, and Previdi (1977) found that patients with a visual field cut had a shorter forward Corsi span than patients without such defects, independent of lesion side. Corsi Block performance has also been shown to be affected in AD but was not affected by severity of memory deficit (Corkin, 1982), implying that the test is not a "short-term memory" test, as span tests are often interpreted to be. Ruff, Evans, and Marshall (1986) also reported an inverse correlation with Corsi Block span and severity of head injury, such that subjects with moderate head injuries scored approximately 0.5 points below normal controls, and subjects with severe head injuries scored about 1.0 points below normal controls.

One hallmark of executive dysfunction is the presence of perseveration. While the presence of the phenomenon alone is often looked at from a process perspective (e.g., impaired performance on a list learning task may have been due to the presence of a number of perseverative responses as opposed to a failure to respond or recall list items), researchers have described a number of taxonomies that provide further clarification of the cognitive variables involved. Sandson and Albert (1984, 1987) identified three distinct subtypes of perseveration, each presumably controlled by a different mechanism and anatomical locus. Stuck-in-set perseveration is described as an inability to shift from a current set or framework. The perseveration scores from the Wisconsin Card Scoring Test (WCST) (Bert, 1948; Grant & Berg, 1948) best exemplifies this type of perseveration. Recurrent perseveration is the unintentional repetition of a previously emitted response. Within-trial repetitions on generative naming tasks best exemplify this type of perseveration (e.g., Fast . . . Far . . . Forest . . . Fast). According to Sandson and Albert, recurrent perseveration is influenced by a postactivation of memory traces. Their third subtype of perseveration, continuous perseveration, is the continuous and inappropriate repetition of a current behavior without an intervening behavior, such as adding an extra "hump" to a cursive *m*. Sandson and Albert administered a battery of tests to patients with varying lesions and neuropsychological pathology. An examination of the types of perseverative responses led them to conclude that each type was influenced by different anatomical lesions. Recurrent perseveration tended to occur with greater frequency in patients with left hemisphere lesions, stuck-in-set perseveration tended to occur in patients with frontal–subcortical lesions, and continuous perseveration was associated with right hemisphere and sometimes basal ganglia lesions. As a result of Sandson and Albert's work, qualitatively analyzing the influence of perseveration on other neuropsychological test scores improved diagnostic and descriptive clarity.

As noted, the WCST has been associated with executive system function. An increase in perseveration scores has been associated with frontal lobe lesions (Grafman, Jonas, & Salazar, 1990; Janowsky, Shimamura, Kritchevsky, & Squire, 1989; Robinson, Heaton, Lehman, & Stilson, 1980; however, see Mountain & Snow, 1993). Some studies have also found that perseverative errors were associated with left frontal lesions (Grafman et al., 1990; Taylor, 1979) although results have been mixed (e.g., Drewe, 1974; Robinson et al., 1980). Regardless of its localizing qualities, the WCST provides a rich source of data regarding the patient's ability to obtain, test, and shift cognitive sets and to adjust behavior in response to feedback.

An analysis of the ability to interpret proverbs has been investigated as evidence of verbal abstraction ability. A simple yet brief method of assessing this ability can be found by looking at the three proverbs found on the Comprehension subtest of the WAIS-R. The administration of this test at the Boston DVAMC is also frequently supplemented by the administration of additional proverbs as needed. If performance is below expectation, administration of the California Proverbs Test (Delis, Kramer, & Kaplan, 1984) can be used to investigate this ability further. The clinical relevance of proverb interpretation has been investigated by Andree, Hittmair, and Benke (1992), who compared the proverb interpretations of AD patients and normal controls and found both quantitative and qualitative differences between groups. Although recognition testing indicated that AD patients did in fact understand the meanings of proverbs, they were unable to spontaneously provide correct interpretations. They instead made incorrect, incomplete, and circumstantial responses. Interestingly, concrete, or literal, responses were rarely made by these patients.

The Trail Making Test, although typically associated with the Halstead–Reitan Neuropsychological Battery, is another test commonly used in the process-oriented evaluation. While slow performance alone is often indicative of brain damage, the technician is essentially unable to determine whether an impaired score is due to motor slowing, incoordination, visual scanning difficulties, poor motivation, or confusion (Gaudino, Geisler, & Squires, 1995; Lezak, 1995; Newby, Hallenback, & Embretson, 1983). A difference score, Trails B − Trails A, removes some of the variance associated with motor slowing, although Gaudino et al. (1995) observed that Trails B is 56.9 cm longer than Trails A. Thus, mere differences in completion time should be interpreted with caution, particularly in older populations. An analysis of error types, however, can help delineate factors contributing to performance regardless of speed of performance. For instance, errors of impulsivity and perseveration implicate execute system dysfunction, while prolonged delays at one or more points in an otherwise "normal" performance may implicate visual scanning difficulty. As with most graphomotor tests, an analysis of the patient's actual production can also provide evidence of tremor or perseverative overdrawing related to subcortical and executive system dysfunction.

Speech and Language

Application of the Boston process approach to the assessment of speech and language functioning is epitomized by the aphasiology studies of Harold Goodglass. His contributions, using a process approach to assessment, have led to improved diagnosis and description of aphasic syndromes. The Boston Diagnostic Aphasia Examination (Goodglass & Kaplan, 1976, 1983) was developed after years of investigation into the various language impairments seen in aphasia. It is a comprehensive examination using a process approach to language assessment that provides a wealth of data describing precisely where in the language system problems occur. The utility of the BDAE goes beyond the assessment of aphasia, however, and can be used in the assessment of any speech and language disturbance. For example, Appell, Kertesz, and Fisman (1982) and Cummings, Benson, Hill, and Read (1985) have used portions of the BDAE and similar instruments to assess the language disturbance in AD. Appell et al. (1982) found distinct differences in the language impairments of AD and stroke patients with various forms of aphasia, while Cummings et al. (1985) found clear indications of language impairment relative to normal control subjects.

As Goodglass, Kaplan, Weintraub, and Ackerman (1976) acknowledge, simple scores of number correct on a confrontation naming task reveal little in the way of diagnosing the type of aphasia or lesion localization, other than the overall severity of aphasia. These researchers investigated the effects of prior word knowledge on lexical access. Forty-eight line drawings of objects were presented to 42 male patients with unambiguous classification into one of four categories of aphasia: Broca's, Wernicke's, anomic, and conduction. Subjects were asked to name the pictures presented in random order. If the subject was unable to name the item correctly, he was asked to identify the object's initial letter on an alphabet card, to indicate the number of syllables in the word, and to indicate a word association. Finally, the subject responded using a multiple-choice format. Conduction aphasics evidenced superior performance in identifying the initial letter and number of syllables, while the scores of anomic, Wernicke's, and Broca's aphasics were not statistically different from one another. It was concluded that when aphasics are equated by raw scores alone on naming tasks, there are reliable differences in the underlying processes that influence that score.

Tests of confrontation naming are invaluable tools in the process-oriented evaluation because of the clinical utility of analyzing the numerous error types that occur on these tests. For instance, Hodges, Salmon, and Butters (1991) compared the naming performance of AD, HD, and normal control subjects on the Boston Naming Test (Kaplan et al., 1983). Relative to normal controls and HD subjects, AD patients made more semantic associative errors, more semantic supraordinate errors, and more circumlocutions. Perceptual errors tended to increase with disease severity. HD patients, in contrast, made a high number of perceptual errors relative to normal controls. Appell et al. (1982) found a high number of circumlocutory errors and semantic paraphasias but not phonemic paraphasias in their group of AD subjects.

Kohn and Goodglass (1985) administered the 85-item BNT (Kaplan et al., 1976) to groups of Broca's, Wernicke's, anomic, and conduction aphasics. An examination of error types revealed interesting differences. While there were no differences in the number of semantic errors (e.g., "muskrat" for *beaver*) between groups, the number of phonemic paraphasias (e.g., "bran" for *broom*) and circumlocutory responses (e.g., "that sea creature with 8 legs" for *octopus*) were different among the groups. Ignoring the types of errors and relying on scores alone would not have clarified the nature of the naming deficits within aphasic categories. In a similar study, Goodglass, Denes, and Calderon (1974) administered three sets of pictures to aphasic and nonaphasic brain-injured control subjects. One set of pictures was of nonsense figures, one was of phonemically related items (e.g., *tag, bat, cat,* and *bag*), and the last was of unrelated items (e.g., *pipe, bus, clock,* and *hand*). After viewing two, three, or four pictures from each set for several seconds, subjects were to identify those items from a larger array presented after the original stimuli were removed from view. The aphasic subjects made fewer errors when the items were phonemically related than when they were unrelated relative to nonaphasic subjects. Furthermore, aphasic patients exhibited no difference in the number of errors between real and nonsense pictures, whereas nonaphasic subjects almost doubled their scores when matching real pictures relative to nonsense ones. Goodglass et al. (1974) concluded that aphasic subjects do not use verbal mediation in coding pictures of familiar objects in short-term memory. From a process perspective, poor aphasic performance on a visual recognition task may be recorded as globally worse than it actually is if verbal similarity is not taken into account.

Word fluency tasks play an important role in the process-oriented evaluation. Although Bayles, Kaszniak, and Tomoeda (1987) noted that word fluency tasks can also be thought of as a measure of semantic memory, the task will be discussed here because of its greater face validity as a naming and therefore language task. Performance on word list generation tasks is typically impaired in most aphasias, but poor performance is also related to a number of other disorders and lends itself to qualitative analysis. Lezak (1995) describes several strategies used on the task that can be investigated as evidence of efficient verbal search strategies. These including phonological similarity (sun, son, sunken) and variations of a theme (e.g., shoe, sandal, sock). Frontal lesions in general depress fluency scores, with left frontal lesions resulting in the lowest scores overall (Miceli, Caltagirone, Gainotti, Masullo, & Silveri, 1981; Perret, 1974). When words generated to a specific letter of the alphabet are compared to words generated to a specific semantic category, several researchers (Butters, Granholm, Salmon, Grant, & Wolfe, 1987; Monsch, Bondi, Butters, Salmon, Katzman, & Thal, 1992; Weingartner et al., 1981; Zec et al., 1990) found that semantic word fluency was more impaired than phonemic word fluency in AD patients, and that specific error types tended to separate AD patients from normals and from patient's diagnosed with other dementias such as HD and Korsakoff's disease. Randolph, Braun, Goldberg, and Chase (1993) also found that providing cues during the 60-second blocks of semantic word list generation trials greatly improved the scores of PD and HD patients but not AD patients.

Gardner, Strub, and Albert (1975) described a patient with global aphasia, who after 11 years had recovered major language functioning and remained unable to understand numerical terms or perform numerical operations when presented aurally but not when presented in any other modality. Furthermore, other tests of abstract thinking were performed well within the patient's estimated level of premorbid functioning. Using a behavioral neurology approach to assess the apparent dissociation between this patient's oral and written numerical abilities, a number of specific tests were administered. The patient, J. O., exhibited varying levels of impairment when matching aurally presented numbers to written numbers, when reading written numbers aloud, and when writing numbers to dictation. The ability to solve arithmetic problems was largely intact in the written sphere and numerical comprehension was generally intact when assessed in written, tactile, and visual modalities, but not in the auditory modality. Interestingly, J. O. also exhibited difficulty answering questions relating to time-sequencing (e.g., "Has it been tomorrow yet?") but not any other dimension such as size (e.g., "Which is taller, a giraffe or a rabbit?"). Written performance on time-series questions, in contrast, was more successful. Numerous other tests were administered that effectively subdivided the facets of speech–language comprehension, numerical reasoning, audition, and so forth into component parts in order to identify the precise point at which the process broke down. As a result, Gardner and colleagues concluded that J. O. was unable to perform logical operations when the task was presented in the auditory modality alone. All other rival hypotheses were ruled out based on their process-oriented approach. As the authors conclude, if their patient had been tested only in the auditory modality, a strikingly different conclusion would have been drawn regarding J. O.'s facility in performing mental operations than was in fact the case.

Yamadori and Albert (1973) described a patient who, after a left hemisphere depressed skull fracture, displayed a word–category aphasia. What was interesting about this patient was that his everyday speech and language abilities, according to the authors, were grossly intact. Aside from a degree of circumstantiality and emptiness, he displayed no deficit in fluency, prosody, or amount of spontaneous speech. Language comprehension, again in everyday speech, appeared unremarkable. Only when asked to identify objects by their description or to name specific objects did a rather striking deficit appear. For instance, when asked to point to a chair, he stood up, looked around the room, sat back down, spelling to himself "c-h-a-i-r, c-h-a-i-r." He then remarked, "I'll have to double check that later." A rather profound difficulty in understanding body parts was also observed. Although other mild language deficits were also described (e.g., impaired story comprehension for long stories), this inability to understand the meaning of words in certain specific categories, in conjunction with anomia, was rather unique. Yamadori and Albert (1973) concluded by postulating a stepwise series of neuropsychological processes, one of which involves activating or accessing categorical associations. They argued (in a manner consistent with the general theme of this section) that without closely investigating the entire language process, the distinction between word sound perception and word meaning comprehension may have been overlooked.

Visuospatial Functioning

The qualitative analysis of drawings can provide insight into visuospatial functioning in various population groups. Several researchers (Brantjes & Bouma, 1991; Moore & Wyke, 1984; Ober, Jagust, Koss, Delis, & Friedland, 1991; Rouleau, Salmon, Butters, Kennedy, & McGuire, 1992) have identified qualitative anomalies in the drawings of AD patients. The omission of essential elements of object drawings was a common finding. Brantjes and Bouma (1991) and Rouleau et al. (1992) attributed omissions to a loss of semantic knowledge about objects. That is, AD patients were unable to invoke semantic representations of the to-be-drawn object in order to successfully draw it. Moore and Wyke (1984) reported that attention deficits may also contribute to some of the omission errors found in drawings. Brantjes and Bouma (1991) also found that similar amounts of extra information contained in drawings was seen in both AD patients and controls, though the type of information differed. AD patients tended to confabulate (adding irrelevant or free-associated material that may or may not be recognizable) aspects of drawings, while normals added stereotypes (adding more details than are necessary but are nonetheless correct associations). Evidence of object simplification or impoverishment, continuous perseveration, and recurrent perseveration were all seen in AD patients to a greater extent than normal controls.

Clock drawings have been a hallmark of the process approach and are included in the Boston Visuospatial Quantitative Battery described earlier in this chapter (also known as Parietal Lobe Battery) (Goodglass & Kaplan, 1983). The quality of clock drawings have been found to remain relatively stable with advancing age up into the eighth decade (Albert, Wolfe, & Lafleche, 1990), so significant deviations from generally good representations should raise suspicion of impairment. Although the drawing of clocks was originally used to assess unilateral neglect in patients with right hemisphere dysfunction (Battersby, Bender, Pollack, & Kahn, 1956), performance can be affected by a variety of neurological disorders. As noted above, Rouleau et al. (1992) found qualitative distinctions between the clock drawings of demented patients (AD and HD) and normal controls. Furthermore, differences between the two patient groups were found in patients in the early stages of illness. The differences included the size of the clock face, graphic difficulty (e.g., inability to draw a reasonably symmetrical circle), stimulus boundedness (e.g., drawing clock hands to the 10 and 11 when asked to set them to "10 past 11"), conceptual impairment, spatial–planning deficits, and perseveration. In general, AD patients tended to draw larger clocks, made more conceptual errors, perseverated more, and had more stimulus-bound responses than HD patients or normals.

The Rey–Osterreith Complex Figure (Osterrieth, 1944; Rey, 1941) lends itself exceptionally well to the analysis of process variables involved in visual construction. The manner in which the subject approaches the task is particularly useful. Osterrieth (cited in Lezak, 1995) identified seven procedural approaches to the figure; 83% of his normal adults began with either the large central rectangle or with a detail attached to the rectangle and then completed the rectangle, filling in details last. Binder (1982) obtained three scores involving the degree to which elements were drawn as a complete unit, as fragmented details, and those that were omitted. Patients with left hemisphere strokes tended to draw the figure in a more fragmented fashion, while right hemisphere patients omitted more details. Right hemisphere patients also made a greater number of configurational errors, indicating difficulty in processing the gestalt aspects of the figure. Recently, Stern et al. (1994) devised a qualitative scoring system for the ROCF. This system includes 16 dimensions for scoring, including aspects of fragmentation, planning, organization, presence and accuracy of features, placement, size distortions, perseveration, confabulation, rotation, neatness, symmetry, and immediate and delayed retention. Stern and colleagues scored the copy and immediate and delayed recall ROCF drawings of 60 patients with various neurological disorders and normal controls. Results indicated generally high kappa values for 11 of the 16 scores, with fair reliability for two other scores. Scores for confabulation and neatness were more variable. Although somewhat time consuming, the system is comprehensive in its coverage of variables important in determining the underlying mechanisms contributing to performance on the task. Such analyses are important, because using the more traditional scoring systems (e.g., Osterrieth, 1944) can result in similar composite scores despite qualitatively different performances.

Performance on various WAIS-R subtests has also be enlightening from a process perspective. Picture Arrangement performance can be affected by a passive approach that results in very few cards being arranged. For instance, if cards are presented in the order "1-2-3-4-5," a passive approach may result in only moving one card ("2-3-4-5-1"). McFie (1975; cited in Kaplan et al., 1991) reported that patients with damage in the right frontal lobe tend to use such a passive approach. As noted earlier, application of the process approach to this subtest frequently entails having the patient tell the story for each production in a testing of limits exercise at the subtest's conclusion. Story variants may reflect difficulty with specific details while getting the overall gist of the intended story, or a correct arrangement may have been achieved without really understanding the point or humor inherent in the story. These differences may be associated with left hemisphere dysfunction in the former case (Delis, Kiefner, & Fridlund, 1988; Delis, Robertson, & Efron, 1986) and right hemisphere dysfunction in the latter (Gardner, Brownell, Wapner, & Michelow, 1983).

That the right hemisphere is involved in the processing of gestalt aspects of stimuli while the left hemisphere has greater specificity for processing details has received considerable support in the literature. Delis and colleagues (1986, 1988) have consistently found that patients with left hemisphere damage have greater difficulty in processing local aspects of stimuli. However, the global–local dissociation is not exclusively related to the right hemisphere. Kramer, Kaplan, Blusewicz, and Preston (1991) observed that a group of alcoholic patients who made configurational errors on Block Design also made errors in matching figures based on global relative to local similarity. Their alcoholic subjects had no known right hemisphere impairment. Similarly, Filoteo et al. (1994) found that PD patients made a greater number of errors in a divided attention task relative to normal controls, regardless of the hierarchical level of stimuli. In other words, errors at both the global and local levels were made in patients with bilateral basal ganglia dysfunction. Different subgroups of AD patients have also been found to differ in their processing of global and local stimuli, which can be identified by a qualitative analysis of neuropsychological test data (Delis et al., 1992; Massman, Delis, Filoteo et al., 1993).

The Block Design and Object Assembly subtests of the WAIS-R are also useful for looking at process variables. Performance can be hindered or enhanced in a variety of ways. As noted above, right hemisphere lesions can result in a failure to appreciate the outer configuration or gestalt of the figure, while left hemisphere lesions impair effective processing of specific details. Commissurotomized patients using their left hand (right hemisphere) were able to appreciate and represent the correct square configuration of Block Design items but frequently misaligned specific details. Patients using their right hand (left hemisphere), in contrast, frequently broke the square configuration of the designs (Kaplan, 1988; Kaplan, Palmer, Weinstein, Baker, & Weintraub, 1981). Researchers (Akshoomoff, Delis, & Kiefner, 1989; Kaplan et al., 1981) have also found that the broken configuration on the Block Design subtest was the single best indicator of right hemisphere damage when compared to both normal controls and patients with left hemisphere damage. Akshoomoff et al. (1989) arrived at a rough cutoff of greater than 25% broken configurations to suggest at least right hemisphere and possible bilateral damage. Kramer et al. (1990) assessed the ability of groups of alcoholic patients to rate which of two hierarchically constructed figures best matched a target figure. Subjects who demonstrated an increased frequency of broken configurations on the Block Design subtest were less likely to select the figure that most resembled the target at the global level. This finding was interpreted as evidence that broken configurations in the WAIS-R Block Design subtest are indicative of an impaired ability to process information at the global or gestalt level, even in populations without specific right hemisphere damage.

The manner in which patients construct their Block Designs is also of interest from a process perspective. Akshoomoff et al. (1989) noted that although right-handed subjects tended to construct their block designs beginning on the left side of the figure, left-handed patients did so more consistently. Their interpretation was that left-handed subjects demonstrated a perceptual bias toward the left side of space. Right-handers, in contrast, do not show such a consistent bias (Kaplan et al., 1991). Although the meaning behind such biases is unclear, significant deviations from this pattern may suggest brain pathology.

Analysis of patient performance during the Object Assembly subtest is similar to that used on Block Design. Specifically, Kaplan et al. (1991) describe three approaches to the puzzles originally reported by Wechsler (1944) (see also Matarazzo, 1972). These three approaches include an immediate reaction to the entire puzzle and the interrelationships among the pieces, the rapid identification of the figure with difficulty identifying the relationships among pieces, and the use of a trial-and-error approach based on a failure to identify the gestalt aspects of the figure. The distinction between these types reflect the global–local hierarchical processing biases, with a blend of the two (i.e., the first strategy described) being the most efficient.

Memory Function

Although the majority of Boston process procedures involve adapting existing tests to better allow the analysis of qualitative findings, a number of tests have been developed exclusively on the basis of process variables. Perhaps the most well known and most widely researched is the California Verbal Learning Test (Delis et al., 1987). As described in the Tests section, this is a 16-item list-learning task that allows the analysis of multiple variables that contribute to successful and unsuccessful learning. The results of factor analytic studies with neurological and normal populations were generally similar, supporting the theoretical framework of the test (Lezak, 1995). Studies involving the CVLT have demonstrated unique patterns of performance among populations of head-injured patients (Crosson, Novack, Treneery, & Craig, 1988, 1989), left temporal lobe epileptics (Hermann, Wyler, Richey, & Rea, 1987), depression (Massman, Delis,

Butters, Dupont, & Gillin, 1992), and various dementing illnesses (Delis et al., 1991; Kramer, Levin, Brandt, & Delis, 1989; Massman, Delis, Butters, Levin, & Salmon, 1990).

Because of the rich data generated by the CVLT, its ability to distinguish various forms of memory impairment found to exist in different dementias is promising. Massman, Delis, and Butters (1993), for example, found different degrees and sources of serial position effects among AD and HD patients relative to each other and to normal controls. They concluded, based on their qualitative analysis of list learning and recognition performance, that the impaired primacy effects seen in both patient groups were attributable to different processes and not solely to a deficit in long-term storage as such a memory pattern is often interpreted.

Rey's Auditory Verbal Learning Test (AVLT) has also been shown to assist in the differential diagnosis of various patient groups. The AVLT is a 15-item list of unrelated nouns that, like the CVLT, is presented over five learning trials and again after the presentation of an interference list. Delayed recall is also frequently employed. Gainotti and Marra (1994) found significant differences in the pattern of AVLT learning and recall between AD patients and depressive pseudodementia patients. In addition to impaired learning and retention relative to pseudodementia patients, AD patients exhibited a high rate of intrusion errors (the "recall" of extralist items). However, only recognition scores reliably distinguished individual patients. This was due primarily to the AD patients' positive response bias relative to the depressive patients' more conservative approach. AD patients had a high number of false-positive errors, while the depressed patients had a high number of misses.

Some patient groups exhibit forgetting on memory tests using a delayed recall procedure. One qualitative variable that has been investigated is the speed with which similar amounts of information are forgotten and the extent to which group differences exist on this variable. Moss et al. (1986) assessed the rate of forgetting in groups of normal controls, AD patients, alcoholic Korsakoff's patients, and HD patients using the Delayed Recognition Span Test (DRST) (described earlier). Although there were no differences among patient groups in their recognition span for nonverbal stimuli, HD patients showed a longer span than the other groups when verbal stimuli were used. Substantial differences emerged during the delayed recall condition, however. Although all three patient groups were impaired on the 15-second delayed recall condition, only the AD patients showed a dramatic decrease in recall on the 2-minute delay condition, demonstrating their rapid rate of forgetting relative to other memory-impaired patient groups. Moss and Albert (1988), using the DRST, reported that patients with frontal lobe dementia also have better delayed recall scores than AD patients even when patient groups were equated for overall level of dementia severity. As later research has revealed, it is the rate of forgetting and not necessarily the amount of forgetting that distinguishes the memory impairment of AD patients

(Hart, Kwentus, Harkins, & Taylor, 1988). As Albert and Moss (1992) conclude, assessing the rate of forgetting using relatively brief delays provides maximum discrimination between AD and other patient groups. Delays longer than 10 minutes, they argue, make it more difficult to distinguish different populations of patients with memory impairment.

The assessment of retrograde amnesia has also been investigated from a process perspective. Albert et al. (1979) developed a test consisting of various personalities during specific decades going back to the 1920s. Relative to normal controls, Albert and co-workers found that Korsakoff's patients showed a steep temporal gradient in their ability to identify the names of the personalities, with names from the distant past recalled to a greater extent than those from more recent decades. Use of Albert's Famous Faces and similar tests has been fruitful in identifying the remote memory capacity of patients with HD (Albert, Butters, & Brandt, 1981), PD (Freedman, Rivoira, Butters, Sax, & Feldman, 1984), MS (Beatty, Goodkin, Monson, Beatty, & Hertsgaard, 1988), and AD (Beatty, Salmon, Butters, Heindel, & Granholm, 1988). Qualitative differences between patient groups have been found, even when overall test scores may be similar. Beatty, Salmon et al. (1988), for instance, found that AD patients demonstrated a slight but significant temporal gradient and overall depressed scores, whereas HD patients showed an equal loss across decades.

FUTURE DIRECTIONS

The field of behavioral neuroscience continues to expand. In particular, knowledge about the brain–behavior relationships subserving the completion of simple processing tasks is becoming more detailed. Functional imaging techniques used with normal as well as brain-damaged patients are beginning to provide rich sources of information on neural system contributions to the completion of cognitive tasks. These sources of scientific data will greatly enrich the array of information available to the process practitioner and will almost certainly affect the task elements and tests used to evaluate the functional sequelae of brain damage in the future. In particular, the use of computer-assisted testing is likely to be quite important in sampling behavioral processing in a highly detailed, precise, and consistent manner. One attempt has been made by process-oriented practitioners to develop computerized testing (Microcog: Powell et al., 1993). In collaboration with Richard Letz, White and colleagues are combining new techniques available for use with the computer (drawing pads, touch screens, voice recording) with process-oriented tasks and validating these techniques in patients with specific types of brain damage (Letz & Baker, 1988; White, Diamond, Krengel, Lindem & Feldman, 1997). In this work, the computer is seen as an instrument that will assist the clinician in gathering cognitive data. Given all of these trends, future work will certainly involve novel tasks, new equipment, innovative imaging-related validation methods, and surprising new ideas about cognitive processing and neural systems.

REFERENCES

Akshoomoff, N. A., Delis, D. C., & Kiefner, M. G. (1989). Block constructions of chronic alcoholic and unilateral brain-damaged patients: A test of the right hemisphere vulnerability hypothesis of alcoholism. *Archives of Clinical Neuropsychology, 4,* 275–281.

Albert, M. L., Feldman, R. G., & Willis, A. L. (1974). The subcortical dementia of progressive supranuclear palsy. *Journal of Neurology, Neurosurgery, and Psychiatry, 37,* 121–130.

Albert, M. S., Butters, N., & Brandt, J. (1981). Patterns of remote memory in amnesic and demented patients. *Archives of Neurology, 38,* 495–500.

Albert, M. S., Butters, N., & Levin, J. (1979). Temporal gradients in the retrograde amnesia of patients with alcoholic Korsakoff's disease. *Archives of Neurology, 36,* 211–216.

Albert, M. S., & Moss, M. B. (1988). *Geriatric neuropsychology.* New York: Guilford Press.

Albert, M. S., & Moss, M. B. (1992). The assessment of memory disorders in patients with Alzheimer's disease. In L. R. Squire & N. Butters (Eds.), *Neuropsychology of memory* (2nd ed., pp. 211–219). New York: Guilford Press.

Albert, M. S., Wolfe, J., & Lafleche, G. (1990). Differences in abstraction ability with age. *Psychology and Aging, 5,* 94–100.

Andree, B., Hittmair, M., & Benke, T. H. (1992). Recognition and explanation of proverbs in Alzheimer's disease. *Journal of Clinical and Experimental Neuropsychology, 14,* 372.

Appell, J., Kertesz, A., & Fisman, M. (1982). A study of language functioning in Alzheimer's patients. *Brain and Language, 17,* 73–91.

Battersby, W. S., Bender, M. B., Pollack, M., & Kahn, R. L. (1956). Unilateral "spatial agnosia" ("inattention") in patients with cerebral lesions. *Brain, 79,* 68–93.

Bayles, K. A., Kaszniak, A. W., & Tomoeda, C. K. (1987). *Communication and cognition in normal aging and dementia.* Boston: College Hill Little, Brown & Company.

Beatty, W. W., Goodkin, D. E., Monson, N., Beatty, P. A., & Hertsgaard, D. (1988). Anterograde and retrograde amnesia in patients with chronic progressive multiple sclerosis. *Archives of Neurology, 45,* 611–619.

Beatty, W. W., Salmon, D. P., Butters, N., Heindel, W. C., & Granholm, E. L. (1988). Retrograde amnesia in patients with Alzheimer's disease. *Neurobiology of Aging, 9,* 181–186.

Benton, A. L. (1973). The measurement of aphasic disorder. In A. C. Belasquez (Ed.), *Aspectos patologicos del lingage.* Centro Neuropsicologico.

Berg, E. A. (1948). A simple objective technique for measuring flexibility in thinking using a card sorting method. *Journal of General Psychology, 39,* 15–22.

Binder, L. M. (1982). Constructional strategies on Complex Figure drawings after unilateral brain damage. *Journal of Clinical Neuropsychology, 4,* 51–58.

Black, F. W. (1986). Digit repetition in brain-damaged adults: Clinical and theoretical implications. *Journal of Clinical Psychology, 42,* 770–782.

Botwinick, J., & Storandt, M. (1974). *Memory related functions and age.* Springfield, IL: Thomas.

Brantjes, M., & Bouma, A. (1991). Qualitative analysis of the drawings of Alzheimer's patients. *The Clinical Neuropsychologist, 1,* 41–52.

Butters, N., Granholm, E., Salmon, D. P., Grant, I., & Wolfe, J. (1987). Episodic and semantic memory: A comparison of amnestic and dementia patients. *Journal of Clinical and Experimental Neuropsychology, 9,* 479–597.

Corkin, S. (1982). Some relationships between global amnesias and the memory impairment in Alzheimer's disease. In S. Corkin, K. L. Davis, J. H. Growdon, & E. Usdin (Eds.), *Alzheimer's disease: A report of progress* (pp. 149–164). New York: Raven Press.

Corwin, J., & Bylsma, F. W. (1993). Translation: Psychological examination of traumatic encephalopathy and the Complex Figure Copy Test. *The Clinical Neuropsychologist, 7,* 3–21.

Crosson, B., Novack, T. A., Trenerry, M. R., & Craig, P. L. (1988). California Verbal Learning Test (CVLT) performance in severely head-injured and neurologically normal adult males. *Journal of Clinical and Experimental Neuropsychology, 10,* 754–768.

Crosson, B., Novack, T. A., Trenerry, M. R., & Craig, P. L. (1989). Differentiation of verbal memory deficits in blunt head injury using the recognition trial of the California Verbal Learning Test: An exploratory study. *The Clinical Neuropsychologist, 3,* 29–44.

Cummings, J. L., Benson, D. F., Hill, M., & Read, S. (1985). Aphasia in dementia of the Alzheimer type. *Neurology, 35,* 394–397.

Delis, D. C., Kiefner, M., & Fridlund, A. J. (1988). Visuospatial dysfunction following unilateral brain damage: Dissociations in hierarchical and hemispatial analysis. *Journal of Clinical and Experimental Neuropsychology, 10,* 421–431.

Delis, D. C., Kramer, J. H., & Kaplan, E. (1984). *The California Proverbs Test.* Boston: Boston Neuropsychological Foundation.

Delis, D. C., Kramer, J. H., Kaplan, E., & Ober, B. A. (1987). *The California Verbal Learning Test— Research Edition.* San Antonio, TX: The Psychological Corporation.

Delis, D. C., Kramer, J. H., Kaplan, E., & Ober, B. A. (1994). *The California Verbal Learning Test— Children.* San Antonio, TS: The Psychological Corporation.

Delis, D. C., Massman, P. J., Butters, N., Salmon, D. P., Shear, P. K., Demadura, T., & Filoteo, J. V. (1992). Spatial cognition in Alzheimer's disease: Subtypes of global–local impairment. *Journal of Clinical and Experimental Neuropsychology, 14,* 463–477.

Delis, D. C., Robertson, L. C., & Efron, R. (1986). Hemispheric specialization of memory for visual hierarchical organization. *Neuropsychologia, 24,* 205–214.

DeRenzi, E. (1983). *Disorders of space exploration and cognition.* Chichester, England: Wiley.

DeRenzi, E., Faglioni, P., & Previdi, P. (1977). Spatial memory and hemispheric locus of control. *Cortex, 13,* 424–433.

Diamond, R., Diamond, J., & White, R. F. (1987). *The Diamond Naming Test.*

Diamond, R., White, R. F., & Moheban, C. (1990). *Nonverbal Analogue Profile of Mood States.* Unpublished test.

Drewe, E. A. (1974). The effect of type and area of brain lesions on Wisconsin Card Sorting Test performance. *Cortex, 10,* 159–170.

Dunn, L. M., & Dunn, L. M. (1981). *Peabody Picture Vocabulary Test—Revised manual.* Circle Pines, MN: American Guidance Service.

Filoteo, J. B., Delis, D. C., Demadura, T. L., Salmon, D. P., Roman, M. J., & Shults, C. W. (1994). Abnormally rapid disengagement of covert attention to global and local stimulus levels may underlie the visuoperceptual impairment in Parkinson's disease. *Neuropsychology, 8,* 210–217.

Folstein, M. F., Folstein, S., & McHugh, P. R. (1975). Mini-mental state: A practical method for grading the cognitive state of patients for the clinician. *Journal of Psychiatric Research, 12,* 189–198.

Freedman, M., Leach, L., Kaplan, E., Winocur, G., Shulman, K. I., & Delis, D. C. (1994). *Clock drawing: A neuropsychological analysis.* New York: Oxford University Press.

Freedman, M., Rivoira, P., Butters, N., Sax, D. S., & Feldman, R. (1984). Retrograde amnesia in Parkinson's disease. *Canadian Journal of the Neurological Sciences, 11,* 297–301.

Gainotti, G., & Marra, C. (1994). Some aspects of memory disorders clearly distinguish dementia of the Alzheimer's type from depressive pseudo-dementia. *Journal of Clinical and Experimental Neuropsychology, 16,* 65–78.

Gardner, H., Brownell, H. H., Wapner, W., & Michelow, D. (1983). Missing the point: The role of the right hemisphere in the processing of complex linguistic materials. In E. Perecman (Ed.), *Cognitive processing in the right hemisphere* (pp. 169–191). New York: Academic Press.

Gardner, H., Strub, R., & Albert, M. L. (1975). A unimodal deficit in operational thinking. *Brain and Language, 2,* 333–344.

Gaudino, E. A., Geisler, M. W., & Squires, N. K. (1995). Construct validity in the Trail Making Test: What makes part B harder? *Journal of Clinical and Experimental Neuropsychology, 17,* 529–535.

Goodglass, H., Denes, G., & Calderon, M. (1974). The absence of covert verbal mediation in aphasia. *Cortex, 10,* 264–269.

Goodglass, H., & Kaplan, E. (1976). *The assessment of aphasia and related disorders.* Philadelphia: Lea & Febiger.

Goodglass, H., & Kaplan, E. (1983). *The assessment of aphasia and related disorders* (2nd ed.). Philadelphia: Lea & Febiger.

Goodglass, H., Kaplan, E., Weintraub, S., & Ackerman, N. (1976). The "tip-of-the-tongue" phenomenon in aphasia. *Cortex, 12,* 145–153.

Grafman, J., Jonas B., & Salazar, A. (1990). Wisconsin Card Sorting Test performances based on location and size of neuroanatomical lesion in Vietnam veterans with penetrating head injury. *Perceptual and Motor Skills, 71,* 1120–1122.

Grant, D. A. & Berg, E. A. (1948). A behavioral analysis of the degree of reinforcement and ease of shifting to new responses in a Weigl-type card sorting problem. *Journal of Experimental Psychology, 38,* 404–411.

Gronwall, D. M. A., & Sampson, H. (1974). *The psychological effects of concussion.* Auckland, NZ: The Auckland University Press.

Halstead, W. C. (1947). *Brain and intelligence.* Chicago: University of Chicago Press.

Hart, R. P., Kwentus, J. A., Harkins, S. W., & Taylor, J. R. (1988). Rate of forgetting in mild Alzheimer's-type dementia. *Brain and Cognition, 7,* 31–38.

Hathaway, S. R., & McKinley, J. C. (1989). *Minnesota Multiphasic Personality Inventory—2.* Minneapolis: University of Minnesota.

Hayslip, B., & Kennelly, K. J. (1980, August). *Short-term memory and crystallized-fluid intelligence in adulthood.* Paper presented at the 88th annual convention of the American Psychological Association, Montreal, Canada.

Hermann, B. P., Wyler, A. R., Richey, E. T., & Rea, J. M (1987). Memory function and verbal learning ability in patients with complex partial seizures of temporal lobe origin. *Epilepsia, 28,* 547–554.

Hodges, J. R., Salmon, D. P., & Butters, N. (1991). The nature of the naming deficit in Alzheimer's and Huntington's disease. *Brain, 114,* 1547–1558.

Hom, J., & Reitan, R. M. (1984). Neuropsychological correlates of rapidly vs. slowly growing intrinsic cerebral neoplasms. *Journal of Clinical and Experimental Neuropsychology, 6,* 309–324.

Hooper, H. E. (1958). *The Hooper Visual Organization Test Manual.* Los Angeles: Western Psychological Services.

Janowsky, J. S., Shimamura, A. P., Kritchevksy, M., & Squire, L. R. (1989). Cognitive impairment following frontal lobe damage and its relevance to human amnesia. *Behavioral Neuroscience, 103,* 548–560.

Kaplan, E. (1988). A process approach to neuropsychological assessment. In T. Boll & B. K. Bryant (Eds.), *Clinical neuropsychology and brain function: Research, measurement, and practice.* Washington, DC: American Psychological Association.

Kaplan, E., Fein, D., Morris, R., & Delis, D. C. (1991). *WAIS-R as a neuropsychological instrument.* San Antonio, TX: The Psychological Corporation.

Kaplan, E., Goodglass, H., & Weintraub, S. (1976). *The Boston Naming Test.* Philadelphia: Lea & Febiger.

Kaplan, E., Goodglass, H., & Weintraub, S. (1983). *The Boston Naming Test* (2nd ed.). Philadelphia: Lea & Febiger.

Kaplan, E., Palmer, E. P., Weinstein, C., Baker, E., & Weintraub, S. (1981, July). *Block design: A brain–behavior based analysis.* Paper presented at the meeting of the International Neuropsychological Society, Bergen, Norway.

Kohn, S., & Goodglass, H. (1985). Picture naming in aphasia. *Brain and Language, 24,* 266–283.

Kramer, J. G., Levin, B. E., Brandt, J., & Delis, D. C. (1989). Differentiation of Alzheimer's, Huntington's, and Parkinson's disease patients on the basis of verbal learning characteristics. *Neuropsychology, 3,* 111–120.

Kramer, J. H., Kaplan, E., Blusewicz, M. J., & Preston, K. A. (1991). Visual hierarchical analysis of Block Design configural errors. *Journal of Clinical and Experimental Neuropsychology, 13,* 455–465.

Larrabee, G. J., & Kane, R. L. (1986). Reversed digit repetition involves visual and verbal processes. *International Journal of Neuroscience, 30,* 11–15.

Letz, R., & Baker, E. Z. (1988). *Neurobehavioral Evaluation System: User's manual.* Winchester, MA: Neurobehavioral Systems.

Lezak, M. D. (1995). *Neuropsychological assessment* (3rd ed.). New York: Oxford University Press.

Luria, A. R. (1982). *Higher cortical functions in man* (2nd ed.). New York: Basic Books.

MacGinitie, W. H. (1978). *Gates–MacGinitie Reading Test* (2nd ed.). Chicago: The Riverside Publishing Company.

Massman, P. J., Delis, D. C., & Butters, N. (1993). Does impaired primacy recall equal impaired long-term storage? Serial position effects in Huntington's disease and Alzheimer's disease. *Developmental Neuropsychology, 9,* 1–15.

Massman, P. J., Delis, D. C., Butters, N., Dupont, R., & Gillin, J. C. (1992). The subcortical dysfunction hypothesis of memory deficits in depression: Neuropsychological validation in a subgroup of patients. *Journal of Clinical and Experimental Neuropsychology, 14,* 687–706.

Massman, P. J., Delis, D. C., Butters, N., Levin, B. E., & Salmon, D. P. (1990). Are all subcortical dementias alike? Verbal learning and memory in Parkinson's and Huntington's disease patients. *Journal of Clinical and Experimental Neuropsychology, 12,* 729–744.

Massman, P. J., Delis, D. C., Filoteo, J. V., Butters, N., Salmon, D. P., & Demadura, T. L. (1993). Mechanisms of spatial impairment in Alzheimer's disease subgroups: Differential breakdown of directed attention to global–local stimuli. Neuropsychology, 7, 172–181.

Matarazzo, J. D. (1972). *Wechsler's measurement and appraisal of adult intelligence* (5th ed.) New York: Oxford University Press.

McFie, J. (1975). *Assessment of organic intellectual impairment.* London: Academic Press.

McNair, D. M., Lorr, M., & Droppleman, L. F. (1971). *Profile of Mood States.* San Diego: Educational and Industrial Testing Service.

Miceli, G., Caltagirone, C., Gainotti, G., Masullo, C., & Silveri, M. C. (1981). Neuropsychological correlates of localized cerebral lesions in nonaphasic brain-damaged patients. *Journal of Clinical Neuropsychology, 3,* 53–63.

Milberg, W. P., Hebben, N., & Kaplan, E. (1986). The Boston process approach to neuropsychological assessment. In I. Grant & K. M. Adams (Eds.), *Neuropsychological assessment of neuropsychiatric disorders* (pp. 65–86). New York: Oxford University Press.

Milner, B. (1968). Visual recognition and recall after right temporal lobe excision in man. *Neuropsychologia, 6,* 191–209.

Milner, B. (1971). Interhemispheric differences in the localization of psychological processes in man. *British Medical Bulletin, 27,* 272–277.

Monsch, A. U., Bondi, M. W., Butters, N., Salmon, D. P., Katzman, R., & Thal, L. J. (1992). Comparisons of verbal fluency tasks in the detection of dementia of the Alzheimer's type. *Archives of Neurology, 49,* 1253–1258.

Moore, V., & Wyke, M. A. (1984). Drawing disability in patients with senile dementia. *Psychological Medicine, 14,* 97–105.

Moss, M. B., & Albert, M. S. (1988). Alzheimer's disease and other dementing disorders. In M. S. Albert & M. B. Moss (Eds.), *Geriatric neuropsychology* (pp. 293–304). New York: Guilford Press.

Moss, M. B., Albert, M. S., Butters, N., & Payne, M. (1986). Differential patterns of memory loss among patients with Alzheimer's disease, Huntington's disease, and alcoholic Korsakoff's syndrome. *Archives of Neurology, 43,* 239–246.

Mountain, M. A., & Snow, W. G. (1993). Wisconsin Card Sorting Test as a measure of frontal pathology: A review. *The Clinical Neuropsychologist, 7,* 108–118.

Nelson, H. E. (1982). *The National Adult Reading Test (NART): Test manual.* Windsor, Berks, England: NFER, Nelson.

Newby, R. F., Hallenback, C. E., & Embretson, S. (1983). Confirmatory factor analysis of four general neuropsychological models with a modified Halstead–Reitan Battery. *Journal of Clinical Neuropsychology, 5,* 115–133.

Ober, B. A., Jagust, W. J., Koss, E., Delis, D. C., & Friedland, R. P. (1991). Visuoconstructive performance and regional cerebral glucose metabolism in Alzheimer's disease. *Journal of Clinical and Experimental Neuropsychology, 13,* 752–772.

Osterrieth, P. A. (1944). Le test de copie d'une figure complexe. *Archives de Psychologie, 30,* 206–356. [In Corwin, J., & Bylsma, F. W. (1993). Psychological examination of traumatic encephalopathy and the Complex Figure Copy Test. *The Clinical Neuropsychologist, 7,* 3–21].

Perret, E. (1974). The left frontal lobe of man and the suppression of habitual responses in verbal categorical behavior. *Neuropsychologia, 12.* 323–330.

Peterson, L. R. & Peterson, M. J. (1959). Short-term retention of individual verbal items. *Journal of Experimental Psychology, 58,* 193–198.

Powell, D. H., Kaplan, E. G., Whitla, D., Weintraub, S., Catlin, R., & Funkenstein, H. H. (1993). *Microcog: Assessment of cognitive functions.* San Antonio, TX: The Psychological Corporation.

Purdue Research Foundation. (1948). *Examiner's manual for the Purdue Pegboard.* Chicago: Science Research Associates.

Randolph, C., Braun, A. R., Goldberg, T. E., & Chase, T. N. (1993). Semantic fluency in Alzheimer's, Parkinson's, and Huntington's disease: Dissociation of storage and retrieval failures. *Neuropsychology, 7,* 82–88.

Raven, J. C. (1958). *Standard Progressive Matrices.* London: HK Lewis.

Raven, J. C. (1962). *Coloured Progressive Matrices.* London: HK Lewis.

Rey, A. (1941). L'examen psychologique dans les cas d'encephalopathie traumatique. *Archives de Psychologie, 28,* 286–340.

Robinson, A. L., Heaton, R. K., Lehman, R. A. W., & Stilson, D. W. (1980). The utility of the Wisconsin Card Sorting Test in detecting and localizing frontal lobe lesions. *Journal of Consulting and Clinical Psychology, 48,* 605–614.

Rosvold, H., Mirsky, A., Sarason, I., Bronsome, E., & Beck, L. (1956). A continuous performance test of brain damage. *Journal of Consulting and Clinical Psychology, 20,* 343–350.

Rouleau, I., Salmon, D. P., Butters, N., Kennedy, C., & McGuire, K. (1992). Quantitative and qualitative analyses of clock drawings in Alzheimer's and Huntington's disease. *Brain and Cognition, 18,* 70–87.

Rudel, R. G., & Denckla, M. B. (1974). Relation of forward and backward digit repetition to neurological impairment in children with learning disability. *Neuropsychologia, 12,* 109–118.

Ruff, R. M., Evans, R., & Marshall, L. F. (1986). Impaired verbal and figural fluency after head injury. *Archives of Clinical Neuropsychology, 1,* 87–101.

Sandson, J., & Albert, M. L. (1984). Varieties of perseveration. *Neuropsychologia, 22,* 715–732.

Sandson, J., & Albert, M. L. (1987). Perseveration in behavioral neurology. *Neurology, 37,* 1736–1741.

Shallice, T., & Evans, M. E. (1978). The involvement of the frontal lobes in cognitive estimation. *Cortex, 14,* 294–303.

Stern, R. A., Arruda, J. E., Hooper, C. R., Wolfner, G. D., & Morey, C. E. (1997). Visual Analogue Mood Scales to measure internal mood state in neurologically impaired patients: Description and initial validity evidence. *Aphasiology, 11,* 59–71.

Stern, R. A., Singer, E. A., Duke, L. M., Singer, N. G., Morey, C. E., Daughtrey, E. W., & Kaplan, E. (1994). The Boston qualitative scoring system for the Rey–Osterrieth Complex Figure: Description and interrater reliability. *The Clinical Neuropsychologist, 8,* 309–322.

Taylor, L. B. (1979). Psychological assessment of neurosurgical patients. In T. Rasmussen & R. Marino (Eds.), *Functional neurosurgery* (165–180). New York: Raven Press.

Thorndike, R. L., Hagen, E. P., & Sattler, J. M. (1986). *The Stanford Binet Intelligence Scale* (4th ed.). Chicago: The Riverside Publishing Company.

Weber, W. P., & Holmes, J. M. (1985). Assessing children's copy productions of the Rey–Osterrieth Complex Figure. *Journal of Clinical and Experimental Neuropsychology, 7,* 264–280.

Wechsler, D. (1946). *The Wechsler–Bellevue Intelligence Scale (W-B).* New York: The Psychological Corporation.

Wechsler, D. (1955). *The Wechsler Adult Intelligence Scale (WAIS) manual.* New York: The Psychological Corporation.

Wechsler, D. (1981). *Wechsler Adult Intelligence Scale—Revised (WAIS-R) manual.* New York: The Psychological Corporation.

Wechsler, D. (1987). *Wechsler Memory Scale—Revised.* San Antonio, TX: The Psychological Corporation.

Wechsler, D., & Stone, C. (1945). The Wechsler Memory Scale. *Journal of Psychology, 19,* 87–95.

Weinberg, J., Diller, L., Gerstman, L., & Schulman, P. (1972). Digit span in right and left hemiplegics. *Journal of Clinical Psychology, 28,* 361.

Weingartner, H., Kaye, W., Smallberg, S. A., Ebert, M. H., Gillin, J. C., & Sitaram, B. (1981). Memory failures in progressive idiopathic dementia. *Journal of Abnormal Psychology, 90,* 187–196.

Weintraub, S., & Mesulam, M. M. (1988). Visual hemispatial inattention: Stimulus parameters and exploratory strategies. *Journal of Neurology, Neurosurgery, and Psychiatry, 51,* 1481–1488.

Werner, H. (1937). Process and achievement: A basic problem of education and developmental psychology. *Harvard Education Review, 7,* 353–368.

White, R. F. (Ed.). (1992). *Clinical syndromes in neuropsychology.* Amsterdam: Elsevier.

White, R. F., Diamond, R., Krengel, M., Lindem, K., & Feldman, R. G. (in press). Validation of the NES in patients with neurologic disorders. *Neurotoxicology and Teratology.*

White, R. F., Nyenhuis, D. S., & Sax, D. S. (1992). Multiple sclerosis. In R. F. White (Ed.), *Clinical syndromes in neuropsychology* (pp. 177–212). Amsterdam: Elsevier.

Wilkinson, G. S. (1993). *The Wide Range Achievement Test 3.* Wilmington, DE: Jastak Associates.

Wolfe, N., Linn, R., Babikian, V., Knoefel, J., & Albert, M. L. (1990). Frontal systems impairment following multiple lacunar infarcts. *Archives of Neurology, 47,* 129–132.

Woodcock, R. W., & Johnson, M. B. (1989, 1990). *Woodcock–Johnson Psycho-Educational Battery—Revised.* Allen, TX: DLM Teaching Resources.

Yamadori, A., & Albert, M. L. (1973). Word category aphasia. *Cortex, 9,* 112–125.

Zec, R. F., Andrise, A. B., Vicari, S., Feldman, E., Belman, J., Landreth, E., & Markwell, S. (1990). A comparison of phonemic and semantic word fluency in Alzheimer patients and elderly controls. *Journal of Clinical and Experimental Neuropsychology, 12,* 18.

7

What, Where, and Why

What Cognitive Psychology Can Contribute to Clinical Assessment

MARCIE WALLACE RITTER AND LISA MORROW

Cognitive psychology is the science of discovering the mechanisms by which the brain processes the outside world. By examining behavior, cognitive psychologists attempt to infer the existence of systems in the brain that work together to analyze conditions external and internal to the animal (usually humans) and to decide what actions should be produced. Cognitive psychology evolved as a reaction to behaviorism, which was popular in the mid-1900s. Behaviorism said that the mind was an impenetrable black box and science could only study the inputs and the resulting outputs and should not make assumptions about the operations that connect the two. In contrast, cognitive psychology's main goal is to understand the transformations that occur between the input the organism receives and the output or behavior the organism produces. The types of behaviors (and underlying systems) that cognitive psychologists study include: learning, memory, attention, visual perception, reasoning, and language perception (reading and hearing) and production (writing and speaking). Cognitive psychology seeks to understand how the brain translates the pattern of photons hitting the retina (in seeing) or the pattern of sound waves hitting the eardrum (in hearing) into meaningful units. These meaningful units must be interpreted so the organism knows how to respond to its environment immediately and how it might be stored for later reference. To accomplish these goals, the brain comprises a conglomeration of multiple subsystems that have specialized duties. Cognitive psychology studies what goes in and

MARCIE WALLACE RITTER • Department of Psychology, Carnegie-Mellon University, Pittsburgh, Pennsylvania 15213   LISA MORROW • Western Psychiatric Institute and Clinic, Pittsburgh, Pennsylvania 15213 what comes out in order to try and understand the organization of these subsystems and how they work together in order to produce a unified cognitive experience. The related field of cognitive neuropsychology has similar goals and accomplishes them by the study of how these subsystems work and how they fail when brain damage occurs. By studying the types and co-occurrences of failure, its goal is to learn how the various systems work together or independently of one another. Posner and Rafal (1987) explain a cognitive system as being

> ... similar to what is known in physiology as an organ system—a set of component functions performed in pursuit of a common goal by several specialized organs. . . . Similarly, a cognitive system is a set of mental operations performed in pursuit of common processing goals that are carried out by a common neural system. (pp. 186–187)

The goal of cognitive psychology and cognitive neuropsychology is to discover those component functions that define the various systems.

The question we address in this chapter is, "What can cognitive psychology contribute to clinical neuropsychology and patient assessment?" The short and easy answer is that cognitive psychology provides a structural framework for understanding cognition and a method for answering new questions, such as, "What is the nature and scope of this particular patient's cognitive deficits?" A better understanding of the underlying mental architecture allows for a better understanding of the specificity and generalizability of deficits incurred due to brain damage. This in turn allows for better and more efficient rehabilitation strategies. The more that is known about a deficit, the better the treatment can be tailored to address the specific problem.

In this chapter we will briefly present a history of cognitive psychology in order to give some context to the current purpose and future goals. We will also provide examples of current research on various visual deficits, attentional deficits, and information processing deficits in brain-damaged populations that have been derived from the cognitive psychology literature.

Mandler (1985) traces the origins of cognitive psychology to a mid-twentieth century revolution in thought. Previously, the field of psychology and philosophy of mind had been troubled by the lack of a physiological seat for thought, specifically consciousness. Dualism—the belief that mind and body were separate entities—was the prevailing view. The lack of a place to locate the occurrence of mental processes caused behaviorists to abandon the search for the processes that intervened between the stimulus and response. They instead chose to assume a direct link between stimulus and response. In contrast, cognitive psychology—also known as the information-processing approach—is the study of all that intervenes between the stimulus and the response. Cognitive neuropsychology is the study of how these intervening processes are grounded in the nervous system. According to Reed (1982), the seeds of cognitive psychology had been sown by some, including William James (1890) and F. C. Bartlett (1932), before Watson's (1924) book, *Behaviorism,* spawned its own field, but cognitive psychology did not come into its own until the late 1950s. One of the pioneers of cognitive psychology was George Miller (1956), who published the paper that defined normal short-term memory capacity as "seven plus or minus two items." Miller's work is the basis of the digit span assessment of short-term memory.

VISUAL COGNITION

At first glance, vision might seem more like a perceptual process than a cognitive one. Extensive research has shown, however, that there is a great deal of computation and interpretation that occurs between the time the visual signal hits the brain and when an appropriate response can be formed. Someone who becomes blind as a result of some problem with their eyes might be much less incapacitated than someone whose eyes are still capable of transmitting signals to their brain, but whose brain can no longer process those signals in meaningful ways (e.g., visual agnosia[1]). An individual who has lost vision because of an eye problem can still remember and imagine what things look like. Some adults who have damage to the visual parts of their brains are incapable of generating a mental picture of the ways things look (cf, Farah, Hammond, Mehta, & Ratcliff, 1989). Those who have lost their ability to pay attention to one side (spatial neglect) are often more hindered than those who are blind in one visual hemifield (homonymous hemianopia). Those with the hemifield blindness can compensate by turning their head or eyes toward the affected side. Those with the attentional defect do not realize they are missing anything and need constant reminding to attend to the affected side.

There are many different visual problems that can occur following brain lesions, and cognitive psychology can help to differentiate the contributions of the various subsystems that work together to make visual cognition possible. We will examine some of the classic experiments that have been done in the field of vision to enumerate the subsystems. First, we will begin with a short overview of the visual system and then explain the experiments that contributed some of the major findings.

Light hitting the eye is focused on the retina by the lens. At the retina, it is transduced into signals that can be carried by the optic nerve into the brain. On its way to the cortex of the brain, the optic nerve divides and crosses sides so that information coming from the left visual field travels to the right hemisphere and vice versa. The signal passes through subcortical structures and then enters the cortex. The first cortical area the signal enters is the occipital lobe, the primary visual cortex. In the occipital lobe, the signal is analyzed in many different ways, but the various analyses share a common feature: They work on a raw version of the signal, which has the information arranged in the same manner in which it was organized

---

[1]See Farah (1990) for a complete review of the agnosia literature.

on the retina. Areas that were contiguous in the representation on the retina are contiguous in the first representations in the occipital lobe. This type of representation is known as an analogue representation. While an analogue organization might seem natural because it matches our subjective experience of the world, it is not the way most brain systems, even many of those dealing with visual representation, are set up.

"Where" and "What" in the Visual System

At the level of the occipital lobe, there are already multiple representations of the visual scene. As the signals move through the primary visual cortex and into more abstract levels of processing, an interesting dichotomy emerges. The visual processing system splits into a dorsal (upper) and ventral (lower) stream. The dorsal stream leaves the occipital lobe and enters the parietal lobe. The ventral stream goes into the temporal lobe. This split represents more than a physical division; it also represents a division in labor. The dorsal (parietal lobe) stream is specialized for encoding locations and spatial relations, whereas the ventral (temporal lobe) system is specialized for encoding object appearance and identity. The shorthand names for these streams are the "where" and "what" systems, respectively (cf, Kolb & Wishaw, 1990).

Mishkin, Ungerleider, and Macko (1983) demonstrated that the dorsal and ventral visual pathways in the brain coded separate information. Bilateral lesions of the dorsal, occipitoparietal pathway in monkeys caused them to have difficulty in making discriminations based on spatial location but not object identity. Bilateral lesions of the ventral, occipitotemporal pathway resulted in the opposite deficit. The experiment involved two tasks. One task tested the monkeys' ability to determine the spatial location of an object and the other determined the monkeys' ability to recognize a previously seen object. Both tasks allow the monkeys to open one of two covered food wells in a table. If the monkeys open the correct well, they are allowed to retrieve the piece of food inside. The incorrect well is empty. The spatial task rewarded monkeys for choosing the food well located closer to the one object on the table. In order to perform this task, the monkeys need to determine the relative distances between the objects and the two food wells and choose the shorter of the two. There were two steps in the identity discrimination task. In step one, the monkey is shown an object in the center of the table. The table is hidden from the monkey's view and the object the monkey was just shown is placed near one well and a novel object is placed near the other. In step two, the monkey is rewarded for picking the well closer to the new object. In order to perform this task, the monkey must be able to identify the first object and discriminate it from the novel object it is paired with in step two. The monkeys are trained until they can perform the task correctly and then one of the two lesions is made and the monkeys are tested again.

There are also many studies that show a dissociation between what and where. Levine, Warach, and Farah (1985) describe two patients with imagery disorders. The first patient had bilateral lesions, primarily in the temporal lobe, but with some extension into the occipital lobe on the left and into the frontal lobe on the right. He had no difficulty on spatial tasks, such as reaching for objects, copying simple geometric diagrams, and navigating around the city. He did have, however, great difficulty in recognizing or forming a mental image of people and animals. The second patient had bilateral parieto-occipital lesions, larger on the left than the right. He had difficulty determining which of two objects was closer, copying even the simplest figures, and finding his way around even his own house. He was able to identify objects, people, and animals once he was able to find the picture in his visual field. Both patients had imagery deficits that were very similar to their perceptual deficits. The similarity between deficits is quite common, but there are some notable exceptions, such as Behrmann, Moscovitch, and Winocur (1994). Their patient, C. K., had perceptual deficits that were more severe than his equivalent imagery deficits.

The behavioral differences found following the dorsal and ventral lesions are a good example of a double dissociation. Cognitive neuropsychologists find double dissociations in lesion–deficit pairs helpful in understanding the organization of the brain.[2] Mishkin et al. (1983) found that a dorsal lesion produced a spatial localization deficit without producing an identity discrimination deficit. Likewise, a ventral lesion produces an identity discrimination deficit without also producing a spatial deficit. This double dissociation suggests that identity and spatial location are processed separately in the brain.

Imagery in Visual Cognition

Cognitive psychology has done much to advance our understanding of how information is represented in the brain. This, in turn, has helped neuropsychologists to better understand many disorders of visual cognition. Kosslyn, Ball, and Reiser (1978) showed that mental images are represented in an analogue manner in the brain. Critics of this view, such as Pylyshyn (1973) claimed that visual information is represented propositionally, the same way in which language is represented, and has no special format. He argued that if visual things were represented visually in the brain, then it would be necessary to invoke a homunculus to look at the representations. Another way of saying this is that a computer can store the image of a line in two different forms; the first is bit map or topographic where each pixel in the image is represented in memory as either "on" or "off." So, to set the pixels using the digit 1 to signify on and 0 to signify off for a 4×3 pixel square bordered by 1 pixel of blank space, one could say:

[2]See Shallice (1988) for a discussion of when it is and is not appropriate to conclude that the dissociations indicate separate processors.

row 1 = 0 0 0 0 0 0
row 2 = 0 1 1 1 1 0
row 3 = 0 1 1 1 1 0
row 4 = 0 1 1 1 1 0
row 5 = 0 0 0 0 0 0

In the above representation, it is possible to actually see the square being represented. However, the information could also be represented in the computer as:

square (2, 2) to (4, 5)

Someone with minor knowledge of programming could figure out that the hypothetical programming language was instructing the computer to draw a square from the pixel second from the top and second from the left, to the pixel 4 down and 5 to the right. The identity and location of the square are given in a form of language. The computer is capable of storing the information in either form, but in the first example the square is only apparent if it is looked at. If someone were to read the code to you, "row one equals zero, one, one, one, one, zero. Row two equals zero, one . . . ," it would not be obvious that the person was reading the instructions for drawing a square. However, the word "square" is in the second example, so you would figure it out if it were read to you. Pylyshyn's point is that there is no one in your head to look at the 1's and 0's and see the square, so the information must be stored in propositional form.

A classic experiment that supported the idea that mental images do have actual size and shape and not just descriptions was performed by Kosslyn et al. (1978). They presented subjects with a drawing of an island containing a number of landmarks (e.g., tree, lake, well). The subjects were asked to memorize the layout of the island and its landmarks. Once the memorization was complete, the map was removed and subjects were required to use their mental image of the map to perform the following tasks. The subjects were asked to focus on a particular landmark (e.g., the tree), and once they had it in focus, the experimenter named another landmark (e.g., the lake) to which the subjects were supposed to move their gaze. The time it took the subject to scan the mental image from the first landmark to the second was measured. If the configuration of the island was stored propositionally by the subjects (for example, "the well is on the western edge of the island, one inch from the most southern point, and half an inch northwest of the well"), it should take no longer to change the focus of attention from one landmark to another as a function of the distance between the landmarks. If, however, the representation does actually have spatial extent, then there should be a difference in the amount of time it takes to look from one to another. Moving one's gaze from one object to a far away object takes longer than moving it to a nearby object. This is the result they obtained. The further the two landmarks were from each other, the longer people took to move their attention from one to the other.

Kosslyn and Shinn (1994) assert that the fact that visual imagery uses visual rather than language-based representations is not as paradoxical if one considers that the brain is already designed to handle such representations—in the visual perceptual system. When we look at the world, our brains need to take the information received from the eyes (essentially a bit map representation) and translate that into meaning. When we see a square, the eyes do not send back word that they have seen a square; they send back signals that are similar to the pattern of 1's and 0's mentioned in the earlier computer analogy. The brain must take that information and assign the meaning, "square." Thus, the brain must have processors capable of representing the information received from the eyes and processing it to obtain meaning. If these systems are already available for perception, why should not the brain also take advantage of them for representing visual images generated inside the head. If this is the case, then people who have visual problems caused by damage to the parts of the brain that process visual input should also have similar deficits in their ability to form visual images.

Mental Representations

If visual images are truly visual and if we do have analogue representations of the outside world within our minds, Pylyshyn (1973) might ask, Onto what screen are they projected? Farah, Soso, and Dasheiff (1992) performed an elegant experiment to demonstrate that there is a mental movie screen. They were able to measure the size of the "screen" onto which the mind's eye projects its images before and after an operation that would drastically alter a young woman's visual perceptual fields. The woman, whose intractable epilepsy was found to have its focus in the occipital lobe, agreed to participate in the study before and after her occipital lobectomy. She was asked to close her eyes and imagine an object. Twelve objects were tested, ranging in size from a banana to a car. After she had the picture clearly in mind, she was asked to imagine moving closer to the item until the item filled her field of vision. When the items filled her vision, she was asked to estimate how far in front of her the item would be to produce this view. Her answers were compared to those of college students. Before her operation, her estimates were similar to those of the students. Following the operation to remove her entire right occipital lobe, her estimates of the distance at which the items would fill her mind's eye were approximately twice that of her preoperative estimates. This suggests that the screen that the postoperative image is filling is only half the size of the preoperative one. The removal of her occipital lobe effectively removed half of the screen on which her mind's eye could display images. The experimenters were careful to avoid the suggestion that she should imagine what she was capable of seeing, as she had a left homonymous hemianopia as a result of her surgery. They made it clear that they were interested in seeing how her mind worked when she imagined the images and not what she was capable of seeing when she opened her eyes.

Mental Representation and Neglect

People with visual neglect fail to notice or attend to stimuli on the contrale-sional side. As neglect has become better understood, it has become apparent that what is neglected is the person's mental representation of space rather than the actual space. Bisiach, Luzzatti, and Perani (1979) and Ogden (1985) showed neglect patients pairs of abstract shapes and asked them to make same–different judgments about them. In order to make sure that all parts of the figure were equally well attended, the subjects viewed the items as they moved past a narrow slit in a screen covering the stimuli. This procedure ensured that the subject paid equal attention to the left and right side of the object because the entire object was viewed in the center of the visual field. Despite this restriction, subjects still made more errors in detecting differences on the left sides of the figures than the right. Thus, even though the patients saw the entire figure, they still neglected the left side of the mental representation they constructed.

Bisiach and Luzzatti (1978) also tested the ability of subjects to use mental representations that were formed before their lesions. They asked two subjects with left neglect to imagine standing at one end of a familiar plaza in Milan facing the other end and to describe the view. Both subjects described a number of buildings that were on their right in the particular point of view, but described very few from the left side of that point of view. The subjects were then asked to describe the plaza from the opposite end. They now named many of the buildings they failed to mention in the first description and they did not mention many that they had mentioned in the first view. Note that the items on the right that the subjects mentioned in the first point of view are the same ones ignored because they are on the left in the second point of view, and vice versa. They interpreted these findings as supporting the hypothesis that the deficit in neglect is one of representing the left side of space.

Morrow (1987) replicated Bisiach and Luzzatti's (1978) findings with a similar task. She had subjects—neglectors and nonlesioned controls—imagine a map of the United States and name as many states as possible. Subjects with neglect displayed a very high East Coast to West Coast ratio in their naming. The normal controls did not show an equivalent asymmetry in their naming. Morrow ruled out differences in travel experience and geographic knowledge as explanations for the differences in performance between the two groups of subjects. In fact, she cites one particular case of a subject with neglect, who after failing to name almost any states west of the Mississippi, said that he had traveled to California, Colorado, and Texas. He had not named any of those states during the imagery task.

Bisiach, Capitani, Luzzatti, and Perani (1981) used the plaza description task with a large group of subjects: nonlesioned controls; two groups of right-hemisphere-lesioned patients with no neglect, one group who did and one group who did not have a hemianopia; and a group of right-hemisphere-lesioned patients who had both neglect and a hemianopia. In addition to the free report condition used in Bisiach and Luzzatti (1978), they included a cued report condition. After subjects had performed the free report task, they were asked to name the buildings on the right side of the first perspective and then the left side of the first perspective and then the left and right sides of the second perspective. They found that the only group that was significantly different from the others on the free report task was the group with visual neglect. They reported many fewer buildings on the left side of each view than the right. On the cued report task, the people with neglect did not show significantly different performances on the right and left sides. The authors interpreted this as evidence for the hypothesis that neglect is a deficit of representation of the left; but an alternative explanation is that neglect causes an inability to spontaneously attend to the left side of the representation, which can be overcome when the subjects are specifically instructed to attend to the left. Other studies (e.g., Riddoch & Humphreys, 1983) have shown that cuing patients with neglect to attend to the left can improve their performance.

ATTENTION AND COGNITION

The Components of Visual Attention

Posner and his colleagues have done a great deal of research to elucidate the mechanisms of the visual attention system. The combination of experiments employing both college students and people with brain lesions exemplifies the cognitive neuropsychological approach to understanding the mechanisms of the human brain. We will discuss many of the studies performed by Posner and his colleagues to understand the attention mechanisms of the brain.

Posner and Rafal (1987) divide attentional processes into two main subgroups: phasic arousal and selective orienting. We will concentrate on the selective orienting aspect in this chapter. Why would selection and orienting be important? Selection is important because it reduces the amount of information the brain must process at a time (cf, LaBerge, 1990). When an animal is searching for a mate, the color of the sky is rarely relevant, and therefore it would be a waste of cognitive resources to be analyzing it. Orienting is important because it is often necessary to have some way for important information outside the realm of what is currently selected to be interrupted. Searching for a mate suddenly becomes less important when motion in the animal's peripheral vision makes the animal aware of a predator. It is important that the animal interrupt the mate seeking and orient its attention to the predator's approach, so as to avoid being caught.

The work of Posner and his colleagues dissects how the brain's attentional-orienting system works. The basic experimental paradigm used by Posner and his colleagues is quite simple. Three boxes are outlined on a computer screen. The first box is in the horizontal and vertical center of the screen, the second is to its left, and the third is to the right of the center box. In some experiments, the center box is replaced with a plus sign, "+." All the paradigms measure the time it takes the subject to respond to a stimulus appearing on the computer screen. There is a complex theory behind the use and interpretation of reaction time measures,[3] but we will explain only what is necessary for the purpose of this discussion. The basic theory is that the reaction time is a reflection of the amount of processing necessary to process the stimulus and to formulate and execute a response. For example, it takes much less time to push a single button as soon as something appears on the computer screen than to push one of two buttons in response to looking at a string of five letters presented on the computer screen and determining whether or not they form an English word. In the latter case, the brain must first identify the letters and decide whether they form a word and then decide which of the two buttons (yes or no) to push to indicate the appropriate response. In the former case, the brain only has to notice a change and then send a message to the finger to push the button.

Posner's experiments involve the simpler case. Subjects simply have to push a button as soon as they see an asterisk appear in one of the boxes visible on the computer screen. Even in a task this simple, there are still many things the brain must do in order to respond to the stimulus. By making slight changes in the task, we can add or delete steps we hypothesize the brain must complete in order to perform the task. We test these hypotheses by examining the reaction times of subjects. If we hypothesize that task A takes one less step or process than task B, an otherwise similar task, then we would predict there should also be less time taken to perform task A. If the reaction time is shorter for the simpler task, there is support for the hypothesis.

Posner's basic task requires subjects to push a button as quickly as possible if they see an asterisk appear in one of the boxes on the computer screen. He hypothesized that giving subjects a hint about where the asterisk would appear would improve their performance. He brightened one of the outside boxes before the presentation of each asterisk. He predicted that if the asterisk appeared in the brightened box, the subjects would be able to respond faster (have a shorter reaction time) than if they were misled and the asterisk appeared in the opposite box. The cue was predictive of the asterisk's location on 70 to 80% of trials, so there was motivation for the subjects to use the information provided by the cue. His reasoning for this prediction is that, when the box brightened, subjects would move their attention to the cued box. If the asterisk did not appear in the expected location, the subjects would need to move their attention to the other box to see if the asterisk was there before they could respond. Moving their attention to the other box takes time, and therefore the subjects' reaction times will be longer.

Posner and his colleagues (Posner & Cohen, 1984; Posner, 1988) have defined two different ways that attention can be moved: overtly and covertly. Overt movements are obvious to the observer because they involve eye movements. The

[3]For original theory, see Sternberg (1969a). For critique, see McClelland (1979).

subjects move their eyes to the new location to which they wish to attend. The other type of attentional shift is covert. This term is used because there is no physical sign that can be observed. It is possible to move one's attention separate from one's eyes. A concrete example of when this could happen outside the laboratory is when an innocent person in an action movie is cornered by the villain holding a gun. The person's eyes are obviously fixed on the gun. If the victim detects movement in the room behind the villain, he can covertly move his attention to see what's there. His eyes will remain fixed on the gun because he does not want to alert the villain of the hero creeping across the room to disable the villain.

Posner, Walker, Friedrich, and Rafal (1984) examined the performance of patients with parietal lesions on their task. The patients were selected for having a lesion in the pariental lobe. Some had mild visual neglect, some had none. Patients whose neglect was too strong were unable to do the task, because they would be unable to notice the cue (box brightening) or the target (asterisk) when it appeared on the contralesional (impaired) side. Approximately half of the patients had right parietal lesions, the rest had left parietal lesions. They also tested three patients with frontal lobe lesions and four patients who had temporal lobectomies as neurological controls. If the patients had a hemianopia, the boxes were arranged so they were entirely within the subjects' field of view. In the first experiment, only the right or left box was used for cue and target presentation, but not the center box. The left-parietal-lesioned subjects showed faster reaction times than the right-parietal-lesioned subjects, but the overall pattern of performance was similar for both groups. When the cue correctly predicted the side on which the asterisk would appear (valid trials), the parietal patients responded quickly, regardless of the side on which the target appeared. There is a small effect of target side, so the subjects are slightly slower to detect a validly cued contralesional target as compared to a validly cue ipsilesional target, but the effect is very small. The more interesting finding is that the parietal patients are impaired when the cue appears on the ipsilesional side and the target appears on the contralesional side. When the subjects are led to believe that the asterisk will appear in their good field but it actually appears in their bad field, it takes them much longer to respond than when they are misled in the other direction. The authors call this the extinctionlike reaction time pattern because it occurs only when the subject's attention is engaged on the ipsilateral side and the subject needs to respond to a stimulus on the contralesional side. If the subject's attention is engaged ipsilaterally and the subject needs to respond to an ipsilesional target, the response is fastest. If the subject's attention is incorrectly engaged on the contralesional side but the target appears on the ipsilesional side, there is little or no delay over the ipsilesional cue/ipsilesional target condition. If the subject's attention is engaged contralesionally and the subject needs to respond to a contralesional target, there is only a very slight delay. However, when the subject's attention is incorrectly summoned to the ipsilesional side and the target appears on the contralesional side, there is a tremendous increase in reaction time.

Posner et al. (1984) interpret this reaction time pattern as a deficit of the disengage mechanism. They propose that there are three components to selective attention: disengage, move, and engage. In order to move attention to a new location, one must first disengage it from its current location, move it, and then engage it at the new location. Posner, Walker, Friedrich, and Rafal (1987) tested whether the deficit in parietal patients applied only to switching attention from the ipsilesional visual hemifield to the contralesional hemifield, or whether it applied to any movement in a contralesional direction. They found that the effect prevailed any time attention needed to be disengaged for movement in a contralesional direction, even if the movement was between two locations in the ipsilesional hemifield. The deficit arises only when their attention is first engaged at any location but needs to be disengaged in order to be moved in the contralesional direction. Morrow and Ratcliff (1988) repeated Posner's attention-switching task with both right- and left-hemisphere-lesioned patients. Like the findings of Posner et al. (1987), they found that patients with right hemisphere lesions were impaired when required to disengage attention to the contralateral side. However, unlike Posner et al. (1987), they did not find that patients with left hemisphere damage had a deficit in disengaging attention. Morover, Morrow and Ratcliff (1988) found that the extent of clinical neglect (as measured by standardized tests) was related to the magnitude of the disengage deficit.

Posner and his colleagues (for summary, see Posner, 1988) have identified other patient groups as having move and engage deficits. Patients with supranuclear palsy due to midbrain lesions have difficulty voluntarily moving their eyes vertically. They also seem to have difficulty moving their attention even when eye movements are not permitted. As mentioned above, normal subjects and parietal patients benefit from a cue that predicts where the target will appear. Patients with supranuclear palsy can benefit from the valid cue when the attentional movement is horizontal, but not at short delays when it is in the vertical direction. The cue needs to come on well before the target for the benefit to emerge in vertical movements. Patients with thalamic lesions have been shown to have short reaction times for targets appearing in the ipsilesional field, but longer reaction times for targets appearing in the contralesional field, both for validly and invalidly cued trials (Rafal & Posner, 1987). The reaction times in the contralesional field are both longer than in the ipsilesional field, but the invalid trials have the longest reaction times of all. These patients seem to have difficulty engaging attention in the contralesional field; thus, the reaction times are longest. In sum, specific localized lesions can cause problems in either the engage, move, or disengage part of the attentional system.

The Distribution of Attention in Neglect

Ladavas and her colleagues (Ladavas, DelPesce, & Provinciali, 1989; Ladavas, Petronio, & Umilta, 1990) tested two hypotheses about the nature of the deficit in visual neglect. They compare a hypothesis that explains left neglect[4] as a deficit of attending to the left in combination with normal attention on the right (Heilman, Bowers, Coslett, Whelan, & Watson, 1985; Heilman, Bowers, Valenstein, & Watson, 1987) to the hypothesis that neglect is caused by a disruption in the right–left balance of attention causing a bias to attend to the rightmost position (Kinsbourne, 1977, 1987). The theory by Heilman et al. (1985, 1987) is that neglect is a unilateral arousal/orienting deficit. People with left neglect have a deficit of arousal of the right hemisphere, and the lack of arousal causes them to fail to process information coming in from the left and organize a response to it. In contrast, Kinsbourne's (1977, 1987) theory is an opponent process theory. He proposes that the left and right hemispheres each have an attentional bias. The left hemisphere directs attention to the right and the right hemisphere to the left. In a normally functioning brain, these two biases balance each other and we can direct our attention where we want. Following damage, the lesioned hemisphere is no longer able to temper the bias of the intact hemisphere, so the intact hemisphere biases attention in the ipsilesional direction. This produces a gradient of attention such that attention is predisposed to orient to the most ipsilesional item of interest.

The hypothesis that attention is preferentially allocated to the most ipsilesional item predicts that people with visual neglect will perform better when asked to respond to an ipsilesional peripheral target than to one located more centrally located in the visual field. Normal subjects show preference for the centrally located target, because it is closer to the fovea (the center of the visual field). Ladavas et al. (1989) demonstrated that people with left visual neglect are faster at processing the more ipsilesional stimulus of a pair even if the more contralesional stimulus is closer to the fovea.

Ladavas et al. (1990) extended this finding by demonstrating that the ipsilesional stimulus is processed not only more rapidly than the more contralesionally situated one, but also more rapidly than a control group. This is significant because most theories of neglect state that the lesion damages the person's ability to pay attention to the contralesional side but leaves the person's ability to pay attention to the ipsilesional side normal. The opponent process theory says that the lesion that produces neglect damages the component of the attentional-orienting system that directs attention in the contralesional direction. However, the lesion leaves the opponent process (directing attention in the ipsilesional direction) untouched and unchallenged. Because the ipsilesional orienting system is uncontested, the patient's attentional resources are more concentrated in the ipsilesional periphery than they would be in a normal, balanced system. This allows focused attention to be stronger in the ipsilesional field than it would be normally. So the opponent process theory predicts that attention to the right in people with left neglect would

---

[4]The deficit of left neglect following right hemisphere damage is more common than the deficit of right neglect following left hemisphere damage (cf, Weintraub & Mesulam, 1987). Thus, many studies of neglect focus on left neglect.

be stronger than in those without neglect. Other theories would simply predict weaker attention to the left without an increase in ability above normal on the right.

To test this hypothesis, Ladavas et al. (1990) compared the reaction times of patients with left visual neglect to a control group of other patients with right hemisphere damage who did not show any signs of neglect. Nonneglecting patients with right hemisphere lesions were used as controls, because lesions to the right hemisphere have been shown to cause a slowing of reaction times (Howes & Boller, 1975). In order to directly compare reaction times for targets on the ipsilesional (right) side, comparable base rate reaction times are necessary. Subjects were instructed to push a button whenever a target was detected and to do nothing if a distracter item appeared instead. The items could appear in one of two boxes on a computer screen. Both boxes were located to the right (ipsilesional) side of a central fixation point. The control patients were faster at responding when the target appeared in the box located closer to the fixation point than to targets appearing in the more ipsilesional location. This is the same pattern shown by people with no history of neurological problems. It is easier to detect the target closer to the fixation point, because acuity is better in that region of the visual field. In contrast, the patients with neglect responded faster to the targets when they appeared in the box farther to the right (and farther from fixation). This suggests that they were attending to the right side of the screen more strongly than to the center. The experimenters monitored eye position and made sure that the subject's eyes were on the fixation point before initiating each trial, so it was not the case that the patients with neglect were preferentially fixating on the ipsilesional box. Ladavas concluded that the preference shown by the neglect patients for the more ipsilesional box supports Kinsbourne's theory that neglect is not simply a deficit of attention to the left, but a bias of attention to the right. Attention is strongest in the ipsilesional periphery and declines through the center of the visual field to be the weakest in the contralesional periphery.

SERIAL VERSUS PARALLEL PROCESSING

The length of time it takes a subject to respond to a stimulus contains a great deal of information about the type of processing that takes place inside our heads to perform a particular task. Sternberg's (1969b) memory search experiment was one of the first investigations of serial versus parallel processing. He gave subjects a list of digits to remember. Once the set was memorized, he presented subjects with a probe digit and they had to decide whether the digit was in their memorized set or not. He found that the subjects' reaction time increased linearly with the number of items in the memorized set. If they had simultaneously compared all the memorized digits to the target, reaction time would not be affected by the number of items memorized. The linear increase in reaction time suggests that the subjects are making a comparison between the probe and each member of the set until the target (if present) is identified.[5] When the time to respond is graphed against the number of items in the memory set, a linear function is obtained. The slope of the function indicates the time to check each item, and the intercept reflects the time to perceive the probe and execute the response. Thus, making a change in the procedure that results in an increased intercept indicates that the time to perceive or form a response to the stimulus has increased, whereas a change that increased the slope of the line indicates that time to compare individual items to the probe has increased.

Nebes, Brady, and Reynolds (1992) performed an elegant study based on the Sternberg model of parallel versus serial processing to compare depressed patients with patients with Alzheimer's disease. Elderly patients with depression often resemble those with Alzheimer's disease and both groups show increased reaction time on cognitive tasks. Nebes and his coauthors were interested in testing the hypothesis that people with Alzheimer's disease have increased reaction times due to a slowing of cognitive processing in contrast to people with depression, who show slowing only in initiating and executing the motor task required for processing. The study looked at the ability to differentiate the time needed to initiate a response from the time needed to make a probe–list item comparison using a Sternberg procedure. As we noted above, the Sternberg task separates the cognitive (comparison) part of the process from the motor component (response execution). Previous studies using Sternberg's (1975) procedure (Hart & Kwentus, 1987; Hilbert, Niederehe, & Kahn, 1976) cited by Nebes et al., 1992 had already shown that depressed elderly patients show an increased intercept but not slope relative to normal elderly adults. In the current study, the task was modified to remove the memory component that was extremely difficult for the Alzheimer's patients. Their task required subjects to determine the number of items (1–4) in a brief (300 msec) visual array. They noted that Anders, Fozard, and Lillyquist (1972) had found that normal aging increases the intercept more than the slope.

The current study compared four groups: Alzheimer's patients, depressed elderly patients, normal elderly, and normal young. Nebes et al. (1992) predicted that all the elderly populations would show a higher intercept than the normal young subjects, but the Alzheimer's patients should show an increased slope relative to the other populations. Overall, the Alzheimer's patients were slower than all other groups. The elderly normal and depressed subjects were slower than the normal young subjects. The Alzheimer's group showed a significantly greater slope than the three other groups, but none of the other groups differed from each other. The intercept of the Alzheimer's patient data also did not differ from the other two elderly groups.

The prediction that the Alzheimer's patient data would differ from the two other elderly groups on slope but not intercept was upheld. The previous finding that normal elderly subjects are slower than (or have an increased intercept

---

[5]This is slightly oversimplified, but sufficient for understanding the next experiment.

relative to) normal young was replicated. However, the previous finding that depressed elderly have an increased intercept relative to normal elderly was not replicated. The authors explain that the disparity between the findings could be a result of differences in patient selection criteria or the constraints imposed by the current study's use of a voice key response system. In any case, the critical difference between the two patient populations—that Alzheimer's patients show an increased slope relative to normal elderly people and depressed elderly do not—was obtained. The authors hope that the finding that Alzheimer's patients have slowed cognitive processing but depressed elderly do not may have some clinical use, although further testing and a simpler form are needed before it can be widely used.

SUMMARY

In this chapter we have reviewed a number of studies that have focused on the assessment of visual cognition, attention, and serial versus parallel processing as applied to clinical populations of brain-damaged patients. The findings of Farah, Posner, Ladavas, Nebes, and other researchers have shown, quite elegantly, how the application of experiments developed in the cognitive psychology laboratory can help to identify specific underlying operations that are disrupted by focal brain lesions. Not only do these studies confirm the existence of cortical and subcortical areas that are specialized for cognitive operations, they also help to confirm, or disconfirm, underlying theories of mental processing. Moreover, the findings have far-reaching implications for rehabilitation. That is, once specific operations have been identified with certain disorders, e.g., patients with neglect have a bias to attend to the ipsilateral side and have difficulty disengaging attention, rehabilitation measures can be focused on those operations. The application of methods in cognitive psychology to the study of clinical populations are valuable and represent a technique that will, over time, set the standard for providing the most sensitive means of evaluating cognitive deficits in brain-lesioned patients.

REFERENCES

Anders, T. R., Fozard, J. L., & Lillyquist, T. D. (1972). Effects of age upon retrieval from short-term memory. *Developmental Psychology, 6*, 214–217.

Bartlett, F. C. (1932). *Remembering: A study in experimental and social psychology.* New York: Macmillan.

Behrmann, M., Moscovitch, M., & Winocur, G. (1994). Intact visual imagery and impaired visual perception in a patient with visual agnosia. *Journal of Experimental Psychology: Human Perception and Performance, 20*(5), 1068–1087.

Bisiach, E., Capitani, E., Luzzatti, C., & Perani, D. (1981). Brain and conscious representation of outside reality. *Neuropsychologia, 19*, 543–551.

Bisiach, E., & Luzzatti, C. (1978). Unilateral neglect of representational space. *Cortex, 14,* 129–133.

Bisiach, E., Luzzatti, C., & Perani, D. (1979). Unilateral neglect, representational schema and consciousness. *Brain, 102,* 609–618.

Farah, M. F. (1990). *Visual agnosia: Disorders of object recognition and what they tell us about normal vision.* Cambridge, MA: MIT Press.

Farah, M. J., Hammond, K. H., Mehta, Z., & Ratcliff, G. (1989). Category-specificity and modality-specificity in semantic memory. *Neuropsychologia, 27,* 193–200.

Farah, M. J., Soso, M. J., & Dasheiff, R. M. (1992). The visual angle of the mind's eye before and after unilateral occipital lobectomy. *Journal of Experimental Psychology: Human Perception and Performance, 18,* 241–246.

Hart, R. P., & Kwentus, J. A. (1987). Psychomotor slowing and subcortical-type dysfunction in depression. *Journal of Neurology, Neurosurgery and Psychiatry, 50,* 1263–1266.

Heilman, K. M., Bowers, D., Coslett, H. B., Whelan, H., & Watson, R. T. (1985). Directional hypokinesia. *Neurology, 35,* 855–859.

Heilman, K. M., Bowers, D., Valenstein, E., & Watson, R. T. (1987). Hemispace and hemispatial neglect. In M. Jeannerod (Ed.), *Neurophysiological and neuropsychological aspects of spatial neglect* (pp. 115–150). Amsterdam: North-Holland.

Hilbert, T. N. M., Niederehe, G., & Kahn, R. L. (1976). Accuracy and speed of memory in depressed and organic aged. *Educational Gerontology, 1,* 131–146.

Howes, D., & Boller, F. (1975). Simple reaction time: Evidence for focal impairment from lesions of the right hemisphere. *Brain, 98,* 317–332.

James, W. (1890). *Principles of psychology.* New York: Holt.

Kinsbourne, M. (1977). Hemineglect and hemispheric rivalry. In E. A. Weinstein & R. P. Friedland (Eds.), *Advances in neurology* (pp. 41–49). New York: Raven Press.

Kinsbourne, M. (1987). Mechanisms of unilateral neglect. In M. Jeannerod (Ed.), *Neurophysiological and neuropsychological aspects of spatial neglect* (pp. 69–86). New York: Elsevier.

Kolb, B., & Wishaw, I. Q. (1990). *Fundamentals of human neuropsychology* (3rd ed.). New York: Freeman.

Kosslyn, S. M., Ball, T. M., & Reiser, B. J. (1978). Visual images preserve metric spatial information: Evidence from studies of image scanning. *Journal of Experimental Psychology: Human Perception and Performance, 4,* 47–60.

Kosslyn, S. M., & Shinn, L. M. (1994). Visual mental images in the brain: Current issues. In M. J. Farah & G. Ratcliff (Eds.), *The neuropsychology of high-level vision: Collected tutorial essays* (pp. 269–296). Hillsdale, NJ: Lawrence Erlbaum.

LaBerge, D. (1990). Thalamic and cortical mechanisms of attention suggested by recent positron tomographic experiments. *Journal of Cognitive Neuroscience, 2*(4), 358–372.

Ladavas, E., DelPesce, M., & Provinciali, L. (1989). Unilateral attentional deficits and hemispheric asymmetries in the control of visual attention. *Neuropsychologia, 27,* 353–366.

Ladavas, E., Petronio, A., & Umilta, C. (1990). The deployment of visual attention in the intact field of hemineglect patients. *Cortex, 26,* 307–317.

Levine, D. N., Warach, J., & Farah, M. J. (1985). Two visual systems in mental imagery: Dissociation of "what" and "where" in imagery disorders due to bilateral posterior cerebral lesions. *Neurology, 35,* 1010–1018.

Mandler, G. (1985). *Cognitive psychology: An essay in cognitive science.* Hillsdale, NJ: Erlbaum.

McClelland, J. L. (1979). On the time relations of mental processes: An examination of systems of processes in cascade. *Psychological Review, 86,* 287–324.

Miller, G. A. (1956). The magical number seven, plus or minus two: Some limits on our capacity for processing information. *Psychological Review, 63,* 81–97.

Mishkin, M., Ungerleider, L. G., & Macko, K. A. (1983). Object vision and spatial vision: Two cortical pathways. *Trends in Neurosciences, 6,* 414–417.

Morrow, L. A. (1987). Cerebral lesions and internal spatial representations. In P. Ellen & C. Thinus-Blac (Eds.), *Cognitive processes and spatial orientation in animal and man:* Vol. II. *Neurophysiology and developmental aspects* (pp. 156–164). Boston: Martinus Nijhoff.

Morrow, L., & Ratcliff, G. (1988). The disengagement of covert attention and the neglect syndrome. *Psychobiology, 16,* 261–269.

Nebes, R. D., Brady, C. B., & Reynolds, C. F. (1992). Cognitive slowing in Alzheimer's disease and geriatric depression. *Journal of Gerontology: Psychological Sciences, 47*(5), 331–336.

Ogden, J. A. (1985). Contralesional neglect of constructed visual images in right and left brain-damaged patients. *Neuropsychologia, 23*(2), 273–277.

Posner, M. I. (1988). Structures and functions of selective attention. In T. Boll & B. Bryant (Eds.), *Clinical Neuropsychology and brain function: Research measurement and practice* (pp. 171–202). Washington, DC: American Psychological Association.

Posner, M. I., & Cohen, Y. (1984). Components of visual orienting. In H. Bouma & D. Bowhuis (Eds.), *Attention and performance* (pp. 531–556). Hillsdale, NJ: Erlbaum.

Posner, M. I., & Rafal, R. D. (1987). Cognitive theories of attention and the rehabilitation of attentional deficits. In M. Meier, A. Benton, & L. Diller (Eds.), *Neuropsychological rehabilitation* (pp. 182–201). New York: Guilford Press.

Posner, M. I., Walker, J. A., Friedrich, F. J., & Rafal, R. D. (1984). Effects of parietal lobe injury on covert orienting of visual attention. *Journal of Neuroscience, 4*(7), 1863–1874.

Posner, M. I., Walker, J. A., Friedrich, F. A., & Rafal, R. D. (1987). How do the parietal lobes direct covert attention? *Neuropsychologia, 25,* 135–145.

Pylyshyn, Z. W. (1973). What the mind's eye tells the mind's brain: A critique of mental imagery. *Psychological Bulletin, 80,* 1–24.

Rafal, R. D., & Posner, M. I. (1987). Deficits in visual spatial attention following thalamic lesions. *Proceedings of the National Academy, 84,* 7349–7353.

Reed, S. K. (1982). *Cognition: Theory and applications.* Monterey, CA: Brooks/Cole.

Riddoch, M. J., & Humphreys, G. W. (1983). The effect of cueing on unilateral neglect. *Neuropsychologia, 21,* 589–599.

Shallice, T. (1988). *From neuropsychology to mental structure.* New York: Cambridge University Press.

Sternberg, S. (1969a). The discovery of processing stages: Extensions of Donders' method. *Acta Psychologica, 30,* 276–315.

Sternberg, S. (1969b). Memory scanning: Mental processes revealed by reaction-time experiments. *American Scientist, 57,* 421–457.

Sternberg, S. (1975). Memory scanning: New findings and current controversies. *Quarterly Journal of Experimental Psychology [A], 27,* 1–32.

Watson, J. B. (1924). *Behaviorism.* New York: Norton.

Weintraub, S., & Mesulam, M. M. (1987). Right cerebral dominance in spatial attention. *Archives of Neurology, 44,* 621–625.

8

Recent Advances in Neuropsychological Assessment of Children

MARK A. WILLIAMS AND THOMAS J. BOLL

INTRODUCTION

Neuropsychological assessment of children has expanded substantially in recent years, with a broadening of goals, assessment approaches, and populations served. Knowledge acquired from various disciplines including developmental and cognitive psychology, clinical neurosciences, and child psychiatry is increasingly being incorporated into child neuropsychological assessment models. An attempt is made in this chapter to highlight recent trends in child neuropsychological assessment. A broad presentation of the major domains, issues, and developments is presented. Our goal is to provide clinically useful information and multiple citations to point the reader to sources where more detailed consideration of each issue is provided.

Historical Perspective: Changing Goals

Tramontana and Hooper (1988) discussed four stages of development in clinical child neuropsychology. They referred to the first stage as the "single-test" stage. This approach emphasized the use of single measures, such as the Bender Visual Motor Gestalt Test (Bender, 1938) for the assessment of "organicity." This approach was popular between the mid-1940s through the 1960s. It was based on the belief that single tests could be used to identify brain damage, regardless of the location or pathological process involved. The second stage of development has been called the "test battery/lesion specification" stage. Beginning in the 1960s,

MARK A. WILLIAMS and THOMAS J. BOLL • Department of Surgery, Division of Neurological Surgery, Section of Neuropsychology, University of Alabama at Birmingham, Birmingham, Alabama 35294-4551.

researchers demonstrated that selected batteries of tests had substantially better discriminant validity than single tests for correctly identifying brain-damaged children (e.g., Ernhart, Graham, Eichman, Marshall, & Thurston, 1963; Reed, Reitan, and Klove, 1965). During this time, the original Halstead Neuropsychological Test Battery, already expanded for clinical use with adults by Reitan, was modified for use with children and adolescents (Boll, 1974; Reitan, 1974). The Halstead–Reitan batteries quickly became the most commonly used formal neuropsychological assessment batteries for children and adolescents.

In the mid-1970s, there was a shift in focus from emphasizing detection of brain injury with neuropsychological tests to emphasizing the use of neuropsychological tests to comprehensively evaluate functionally important cognitive and behavioral sequelae of brain damage. This has been called the "functional profile stage" (Tramontana & Hooper, 1988). While many of the same assessment instruments continued to be used, increased interest was directed toward examining the utility of neuropsychological tests for predicting functional capacities in the real world (ecological validity). At the same time, attempts to link neuropsychological assessment results to rehabilitation planning and deficit management grew. Also, traditional neuropsychological assessment measures began to be applied to a broader category of children to include not just those with documented acquired brain damage, but also to those with cognitive deficits believed to stem from developmentally based brain dysfunction (e.g., specific learning disorders) or from a history of poorly documented neurological insults such as prenatal brain damage.

Rourke (1992) has elaborated on a more recent stage of development in clinical child neuropsychology, which he calls the "dynamic phase." This approach continues to emphasize the ecological validity of neuropsychological assessment. In addition, however, influences from empirical and theoretical work in cognitive and developmental psychology have become more apparent in both the design of assessment instruments and in the interpretation of test performance. With this stage has come an increased use of narrow-band tests reflecting the influence of component models from cognitive psychology (e.g., specific components of attention, language, and memory). By assessing specific cognitive processes according to the various elemental components believed to make up the more complex cognitive processes (e.g., reading or memory abilities), more specific treatment recommendations can potentially be offered. The dynamic phase continues to exert the dominant influence in clinical child neuropsychology. Currently, in most situations, the emphasis is not on diagnosing brain impairment, but on providing a comprehensive functional assessment of the child from a "biopsychosocial" framework from which inferences can be drawn for purposes of treatment and management.

Broadening the Referral Base

At least three factors can be related to the growth of child neuropsychological assessment services. The first factor is passage of the Education for All Handicapped Children Act in 1976 (Public Law 94-142, Federal Register, 1976). This legislation required all states to provide adequate educational services to all handicapped children. As a result, an increased need for neuropsychological assessment was created to assist in diagnosis, description of functional capacities, psychological intervention, and educational planning for children with neurodevelopmentally based and acquired brain damage (Tramontana & Hooper, 1988).

Advances in medical technology are a second factor responsible for the growth of clinical child neuropsychology. Improved survival rates from a broad range of previously fatal medical conditions have increased the number of infants and children who survive neurologically related conditions. Unfortunately, many of these children are left with substantial cognitive and/or behavioral deficits. Examples include increased survival rates of very low birth weight babies and increased survival rates from traumatic brain injury, intracranial tumors, and cancers (Hynd, 1988).

An increase in the use of neuropsychological tests in medical research represents a third area of growth. Clinical medicine has become more concerned with considering "quality of life" issues in treatment outcome studies as opposed to purely physical measures of morbidity. Neuropsychological assessment provides a quantitative measure of cognitive and behavioral capacities that can be included under the umbrella of quality of life assessment and adds much to treatment outcome studies dealing with disorders affecting the brain. In addition, the emerging area sometimes referred to as "medical neuropsychology" has gained impetus. A sizable empirical knowledge base has developed demonstrating that medical disorders primarily affecting nonbrain organ systems can, under certain conditions, have neuropsychological sequelae. Examples include the research relating cardiac, renal, pulmonary, and immune disorders to neuropsychological deficits (e.g., Tarter, Van Theil, & Edwards, 1988). In response to these data, clinical neuropsychological services have broadened to include assessment of general medical populations (e.g., Williams et al., 1995).

MULTIDISCIPLINARY INFLUENCES ON CHILD NEUROPSYCHOLOGICAL ASSESSMENT

Neurodevelopmental Psychology

Research in neurodevelopment has provided evidence that models of functional organization of the adult brain do not apply evenly to children (Slomka & Tarter, 1993). Early attempts to relate locus and lesion type to specific cognitive deficits in children produced substantial variation in outcomes. It became clear that inferences about brain-lesion–deficit relationships in adults could not be generalized to children.

In children, the age of onset of brain damage is of primary importance to understanding lesion–deficit relationships. The maturational stage of brain development, the environmental demands placed on children at different stages of development, and the nature of the brain lesion interact in a complex fashion, leading to neuropsychological outcome. Children with a history of documented brain damage with only minimal or no neuropsychological deficits on age-referenced neuropsychological tests during one stage of development many nevertheless show neuropsychological deficits on follow-up testing during a subsequent developmental stage (Rudel, 1978).

With improved understanding of the relationship between brain maturation, overt indications of development, and brain damage has come an increased emphasis on the need to develop measures capable of assessing aspects of normal cognitive development at different age-referenced points in development. Limitations in current assessment tools are easily discovered. For example, despite the general agreement that memory functions are of primary importance in academic performance, memory tests specifically designed for children of different ages based on current models of memory development have been slow to develop. The downward extension of adult memory tests applied to children has provided limited utility and can be misleading when clinicians assume that a "general memory ability" factor exists in children (Boyd, 1988). For example, using a large group of 5-year-olds, Stevenson, Parker, and Wilkinson (1975, cited in Boyd, 1988) found a median correlation of only .14 among 11 memory tasks. Among a sample of 8- and 9-year-olds, Kail (1975, cited in Boyd, 1988) found a median correlation of only .18 among eight memory tests. Based on their review of the literature, Kail and Hagen (1982) proposed that the concept of a "general memory ability" factor in children is inadequate. With increased age, normally developing children will show more consistency in their performance across different types of memory tasks due apparently to the increased use of specific memory strategies that occurs with development.

Knowledge gained from developmental psychology is also in an ongoing process of influencing the assessment of other cognitive domains such as language (e.g., Crary, Voeller, & Haak, 1988), attentional processes (e.g., Barkley, 1988), and executive functions (e.g., Pennington, 1991). These advances provide increased ability to usefully quantify specific cognitive strengths and weaknesses across developmental levels. In addition, the increased incorporation of models from developmental psychology promises to better inform child neuropsychologists about the outcome of brain injury and provide an improved bases from which to develop remediation and management strategies.

Cognitive Psychology

Cognitive psychology has influenced child neuropsychological assessment in recent years. With increased efforts in cognitive psychology to understand the basic building blocks of complex cognitive processes, such as attention, memory, language, and academic skills development, have come efforts to evaluate cognitive abilities in a more elemental or component-oriented fashion. This has resulted in the development and inclusion of more narrow-band tests designed to evaluate the specific putatively disrupted processes that underlie deficits at the more complex level of functioning (e.g., on tests of reading, memory, math, etc.). Neuropsychological assessment guided by cognitive neuropsychological models lends itself easily toward theory-driven remediation programs. However, much work is needed to determine whether or not a focus on narrow-band assessment and theory-driven rehabilitation programs leads to improved neuropsychological outcome compared to the use of more traditional broadband assessment and more empirically driven remediation and management programs.

Pediatric Neurology and Neurodiagnostics

Recent advances in neurodiagnostics, which include magnetic resonance imaging, single photon emission computed tomography, and video-electroencephalography monitoring, have influenced child neuropsychology (Bigler, 1988). With the rapidly developing ability to obtain sensitive structural and physiological examination of the brain has come a decreased need for the use of neuropsychological assessment for the purpose of diagnosing and localizing brain damage. However, the use of neuropsychological assessment for determining the functional capacities of children has not been supplanted by advances in neurodiagnostics.

Correlation of data obtained from neuropsychological and neurodiagnostic techniques has advanced our understanding of brain–behavior relationships in both acquired central nervous system (CNS) damage and developmentally based neurological dysfunction (e.g., traumatic brain injury, learning disorders, and attention deficit hyperactivity disorder). Clinically, knowledge of the child's neurodiagnostic and neurological examination results can assist the clinician in selecting a battery of tests, interpreting test results, predicting the course of recovery, and in treatment planning.

Child Psychopathology

Recent research in child psychopathology has demonstrated, using many of the newer neurodiagnostic techniques now available, that many of the disorders of childhood previously only presumed to result in large part from dysfunctional brain systems are in fact in many cases correlated with abnormal neurodiagnostic findings. In like fashion, application of neuropsychological tests to various child psychiatric groups has resulted in the finding of interesting relationships. For example, neuropsychological approaches to the description of different types of specific learning disorders has become commonplace. In addition, several of the *Diagnostic and Statistical Manual of Mental Disorders,* 4th edition (DSM-IV) (American Psychiatric Association, 1994) childhood behavior disorders (e.g., conduct disorder, attention deficit hyperactivity disorder) have a high prevalence of comorbidity with learning problems, making the use of neuropsychological assessment among child psychiatric groups commonly indicated.

APPROACHES TO NEUROPSYCHOLOGICAL ASSESSMENT OF CHILDREN

Various approaches to the neuropsychological assessment of children are currently in use. Selection of approach is determined by the primary purpose for the examination, assets and limitations of the setting, and the theoretical bias of the neuropsychologist.

Fixed Battery Approaches

The Halstead–Reitan Batteries for Children

Reitan and his colleagues developed two neuropsychological test batteries for children. The Halstead–Reitan Neuropsychological Battery is used for children between the ages of 9 and 14 (Boll, 1974) and the Reitan–Indiana Neuropsychological Test Battery is designed for children between 5 and 8 years of age (Reitan, 1969, 1974). Both batteries include several of the tests from the Halstead–Reitan Neuropsychological Battery for adults, modified for use with children. The Reitan–Indiana battery includes several subtests that were newly devised for use with young children, and therefore does not resemble the adult battery as closely as the Halstead–Reitan Neuropsychological Battery for 9- to 14-year-olds. Interestingly, however, many of the subtests developed specifically for use with the 5- to 8-year-olds (e.g., Marching test, Target test, etc.) have been shown to be the least useful clinically (Boll, 1981). Table 1 provides an overview of the subtests that comprise both batteries. In addition, a standardized intelligence test (e.g., age-appropriate Wechsler IQ test) and a standardized achievement test are also administered.

The Reitan batteries have been widely used. They offer the advantage of being supported by a larger research database than any other formal neuropsychological test battery, with much of the research focused on examining its ability to discriminate between children with documented brain damage and controls (Slomka & Tarter, 1993). The Reitan batteries have been found to have adequate validity in discriminating between brain-damaged, learning disabled (LD), and normal children (e.g., Reitan & Boll, 1973; for review, see Hynd, 1988). Rourke and co-workers (Rourke & Finlayson, 1978; Rourke & Gates, 1981) have applied multivariate statistical procedures to the performance of LD children on the Reitan batteries, resulting in identification of subtypes of learning disabilities. For example, the early work that led to the distinction between "verbal" and "nonverbal" learning disabilities emerged from multivariate analyses of Reitan batteries. These studies found that children with different neuropsychological profiles tended to have predictable strengths and weaknesses on standardized academic achievement tests (Hynd, 1988).

TABLE 1. Halstead–Reitan Neuropsychological Test Batteries for Children and Adolescents[a]

Subtest	Primary abilities assessed	Ages 9–14	Ages 5–8
Category Test	Abstract reasoning and concept formation	X	X
Tactual Performance Test	Tactile form discrimination, manual dexterity, spatial memory, problem solving	X	X
Finger Tapping Test	Right/left-sided manual speed	X	X
Aphasia Screening Test	Basic reading, spelling, math, articulation, naming, right–left confusion, copy abilities	X	X
Grip Strength Test	Right/left-sided grip strength	X	X
Lateral Dominance	Right/left-sided preference	X	X
Sensory-Perceptual Examination	Tactile, auditory, and visual sensory recognition, perception, and localization (minor differences in administration for two age groups)	X	X
Tactile Finger Localization Test	Perceive and localize sensory stimulation	X	X
Fingertip Number/Symbol Writing Test	Perceive written numbers (or symbols) on finger tips (graphesthesia) (X's and O's are the symbols used for the 5–8 age group)	X	X
Tactile Form Recognition Test	Intact tactile recognition (stereognosis)	X	X
Seashore Rhythm Test	Sustained auditory attention; match rhythmic sequences	X	
Speech Sounds Perception Test	Sustained attention, auditory perception, auditory–visual integration	X	
Trail Making Test	Cognitive set shifting, sequencing, psychomotor speed	X	
Color Form Test	Cognitive flexibility, sequential reasoning		X
Progressive Figures Test	Visual–spatial reasoning, cognitive flexibility, sequential reasoning		X
Matching Pictures Test	Ability to categorize		X
Target Test	Pattern perception, ability to copy		X
Individual Performance Test	Visual perception, visual–motor integration		X
Marching Test	Visual–motor integration, coordination		X

[a]Table adapted from Hynd (1988), with permission.

A major limitation of the Reitan neuropsychological batteries for children includes the fact that language and memory processes are not explicitly examined. Many clinicians continue to use the Reitan neuropsychological batteries for children, but include additional tests in an attempt to more fully evaluate language and memory functions.

The Luria–Nebraska Neuropsychological Battery—Children's Revision

The Luria–Nebraska Neuropsychological Battery—Children's Revision (LNNB-CR) (Golden, 1981) was developed for use with children ages 8 to 12.

When developing the LNNB-CR, Golden (1981) noted the importance of systematically considering maturational variables. It is difficult to appreciate, however, that this has actually been accomplished. Instead, the LNNB-CR appears primarily to be a downsized version of the adult LNNB, including similar tests that have been modified to be easier (Hynd, 1988). The LNNB-CR includes 149 "procedures" that constitute 11 scales. The scales are multifactorial and should not be considered as measures of specific skills. Table 2 presents a descriptive overview of LNNB-CR.

Several studies have addressed the discriminant validity of the LNNB-CR by comparing the performance of brain-damaged children and non-brain-damaged children (e.g., Carr, 1983; Gustavson et al., 1984; Wilkening, Golden, MacInnes, Plaisted, & Hermann, 1981). Golden (1988) reviewed these studies and reported that on the average, an 86% correct classification rate was obtained.

Concurrent validity of the LNNB-CR has been established by comparing childrens' performance on the LNNB-CR and the Halstead–Reitan battery for children (Tramontana, Sherrets, & Wolf, 1983). Tramontana et al. (1983) reported that the 11 scales from the LNNB-CR were significantly correlated with scaled scores obtained from the Halstead–Reitan battery for children, with coefficients ranging from .54 to .80. Within a group of brain-injured children, Berg et al. (1984) reported a 91% rate of agreement between the LNNB-CR and Halstead–Reitan in classifying the children as brain damaged.

The discriminant validity of the LNNB-CR has also been examined among LD children. Geary and Gilger (1984) compared a group of LD children to age- and Full Scale IQ-matched controls on the LNNB-CR. The LNNB-CR correctly

TABLE 2. Luria–Nebraska Neuropsychological Battery—Children's Revision[a]

Scales	Primary abilities assessed
Motor Skills	Motor speed, coordination, ability to imitate motor movements
Rhythm	Perceive and repeat rhythmic patterns, sing a song from memory
Tactile	Finger localization, arm localization, 2-point discrimination, movement discrimination, shape discrimination, stereognosis
Visual	Visual recognition, visual discrimination
Receptive Speech	Follow simple commands, comprehend verbal directions, decode phonemes
Expressive Language	Ability to read and repeat words and simple sentences, names objects from description, use automated speech
Writing	Analyze letter sequences, spell, write from dictation
Reading	Letter and word recognition, sentence and paragraph reading, nonsense syllable reading
Arithmetic	Simple arithmetic abilities, number writing and number recognition
Memory	Verbal and nonverbal memory
Intelligence	Vocabulary development, verbal reasoning, picture comprehension, social reasoning, deductive reasoning

[a]Table adapted from Hynd (1988), with permission.

classified all of the LD children, with only two false positives being found within the normal control group. However, less impressive results have been reported from other discriminant validity studies (e.g., Snow & Hynd, 1985a; Snow, Hynd, & Hartlage, 1984). While the LNNB-CR has shown substantial success in discriminating reading and spelling LD children from normal controls, its ability to discriminate math LD children from normals and from reading and spelling disabled children has been poor (Nolan, Hammeke, & Barkley, 1983). These findings have been explained by the LNNB-CR's relatively weak sampling of visual–spatial processes, which have been proposed as typically deficient among math LD children (Rourke & Finlayson, 1978).

It should also be noted that most of the performance variability on the LNNB-CR is explained by variability in general cognitive ability. For example, Tramontana et al. (1983) examined the relationship between LNNB-CR and the Wechsler Intelligence Scale for Children—Revised (WISC-R) among a sample of child and adolescent psychiatric patients. They found significant correlations between the WISC-R Full Scale IQ and each of the 11 LNNB-CR scales (ranging from .38 to −.63). Also, Snow and Hynd (1985b) conducted a factor analysis across the 11 scales and reported a three-factor solution, with the first factor reflecting "Language–General Intelligence." As a result, in clinical evaluation of children with suspected acquired brain damage, the influence of premorbid IQ on LNNB-CR must be considered and performance expectations adjusted.

Flexible Battery Approach

The "flexible" or sometimes called "eclectic" approach to child neuropsychological assessment also emphasizes the use of standardized test procedures to quantify aspects of cognitive and behavioral functioning. In addition, however, the eclectic approach encourages flexibility in test selection in an attempt to make the evaluation of each child more specific to the referral question and primary deficits suspected. This approach begins with a core battery of measures designed to assess a broad domain of cognitive functions. Based on the child's performance on the core battery, additional tests are added to supplement the evaluation providing a comprehensive and individualized assessment. Fletcher and colleagues (e.g., Fletcher, 1988; Fletcher & Taylor, 1984; Taylor & Fletcher, 1990) have discussed a flexible approach to neuropsychological assessment that not only encourages flexibility in cognitive test selection, but also emphasizes the importance of comprehensive assessment of psychosocial, environmental, and biological functioning. In order to accomplish this, the neuropsychologist must have expertise with a broad array of tests, models of higher cognitive functioning, clinical assessment, and developmental psychopathology.

The use of flexible batteries is currently common practice and will likely continue to be a dominant approach to child neuropsychological assessment. As new and improved tests become available and research examining the validity of various measures evolves, the flexible approach will allow for continued modification of assessment batteries. Unfortunately, all too often clinicians begin including newly available tests into their batteries before adequate validation studies are performed. This substitution of face validity for scientific validity is responsible for substantial amounts of misuse of psychometric tests. A second concern about the flexible approach is that it may lead to a "pathology search," selecting additional tests in areas of deficiency but inadvertently not providing adequate coverage of areas of strength. This becomes quite relevant in an educational or rehabilitation setting. For example, attempts at remediating areas of deficit may result in limited, if any, true gains. However, teaching skills aimed at the child's areas of strength represents a promising strategy.

Process Approach

The process approach to neuropsychological assessment is an extension of the flexible approach. It provides both nomothetic and extensive idiographic information. The evaluation begins with the use of standardized tests to allow for norm-referenced quantification of areas of strength and weakness. After identifying areas of deficiency, efforts are made to understand the specific processing deficits responsible for the poor quantitative performance. A hypothesis-testing process is followed, which requires the examiner to "test limits" and break down tests into their presumed component parts. An attempt is made to determine the specific elemental deficits that are present and believed to be responsible for poor performance on the standardized tests. The term "satellite tests" is sometimes used to describe the specific procedures performed by the examiner to test specific hypotheses regarding the component skill deficits that account for poor performance on the standardized tests.

An advantage of the process approach is that to the extent that a better understanding of the patient's processing deficits and remaining abilities can be obtained from this approach, the more detailed and potentially useful remediation and management recommendations can be made. However, as mentioned above, if this pathology search results in an inadequate evaluation of areas of strength, then informed management attempts are substantially decreased.

RECENT TRENDS IN TEST DEVELOPMENT

Comprehensive neuropsychological evaluation of children involves assessing each of the following domains: global intelligence, academic achievement, language, visual–spatial, somatosensory, motor, attention, memory, learning, and problem solving. In addition, psychosocial and environmental factors should be adequately considered. Previous authors have provided an overview of commonly used tests (e.g., Taylor & Fletcher, 1990). What follows is a selective descriptive review of cognitive tests that have become available more recently, as well as those that have been in use for quite some time but continue to be commonly used.

Intelligence Tests

Wechsler Intelligence Scale for Children—3rd Edition

The Wechsler Intelligence Scale for Children—3rd edition (WISC-III) has been available since 1991 (Wechsler, 1991). It retains the basic design of the previous editions with inclusion of three composite scores [Verbal IQ (VIQ), Performance IQ (PIQ), and Full Scale IQ (FSIQ)]. Although the major goal of the revision was to obtain contemporary norms, other changes have also occurred. First, a new supplementary subtest called Symbol Search was added. This subtest can either be substituted for the Coding subtests in computing the PIQ or used to supplement the PIQ. Factor analysis of the WISC-III subtests reveals the same three factors as found from previous editions (Verbal Comprehension Factor, Perceptual Organization Factor, Freedom from Distractibility Factor), but with an additional factor emerging called Processing Speed, which is made up of the Coding and Symbol Search subtests. Longitudinal consistency is obtained by retaining all of the subtests from previous editions. However, the specific content of the items making up each subtest has been modified in an attempt to make items more reliable and up to date. The WISC-III also delivers substantial improvements in the physical design of the test materials, making them more esthetically interesting. Revised administration and scoring procedures are provided in a fashion that makes the use of the WISC-III substantially easier for the examiner.

Additional changes found in the WISC-III include an attempt to further minimize gender, ethnic, and regional bias. Also, certain subtests were redesigned to further reduce the outcome of obtaining a "bottomed out" or "topped out" performance. To accomplish this goal, additional items were added to several of the subtests, allowing for more downward and upward extension. Taken together, the WISC-III provides the advantages of more contemporary norms and improved test materials, while maintaining the essential theoretical structure of previous versions, making the use of the WISC-III an easy and appropriate switch for the clinician (Wechsler, 1991).

Stanford–Binet Intelligence Scale—4th Edition

The Stanford–Binet Intelligence Scale—4th Edition (SB4) (Thorndike, Hagen, & Sattler, 1986) was released in 1986 as a revision of the Stanford–Binet Intelligence Scale—Form LM (SB-LM) edition. The SB4 is appropriate for ages 2 through adult. The format includes both features common to the SB-LM as well as several new features. For example, the SB4 includes 15 subtests that are clustered into four theoretically derived "area" scores: Verbal Reasoning, Quantitative Reasoning, Abstract/Visual Reasoning, and Short-Term Memory. The SB4 continues to use a "composite" or general ability score that is a global index of intelligence. By inclusion of the four area scores in the SB4, potentially useful additional information is obtained regarding the pattern of cognitive strengths and weaknesses.

The SB4 test materials are significantly improved over the SB-LM. Changes include more straightforward directions to the examinee and the use of easels that provide convenient access for the examiner to most of the decision and scoring rules. By using specific rules for determining "entry levels" into each subtest, examinees are exposed only to the range of difficulty appropriate to them. In addition, the familiar use of basal and ceiling rules continue to be used.

The scaling of individual subtests comprising the SB4 is unusual. Specifically, the subtests scaling system establishes the mean at 50 and the standard deviation at 8. Fortunately, the four area scores and the composite score use the more familiar Stanford–Binet metric (mean = 100, SD = 16). In addition, a table is provided in the SB4 manual that allows the examiner to convert each of the subtests scores to the more familiar Wechsler Metric (mean = 100, SD = 15).

A primary disadvantage of the SB4 relative to the SB-LM is that there is a higher "floor effect," making it no longer possible to obtain scores in the Moderate Retardation range until the child reaches the age of 5. The SB-LM is capable of obtaining scores consistent with moderate mental retardation as early as 3½ years of age. At the high end of the ability continuum, the SB4 offers improved discrimination between examinees relative to the SB-LM, making this a better measure for assessing gifted adults, but improvement is not appreciated for children (Glutting & Kaplan, 1990).

Achievement Tests

Measures of academic achievement are an integral part of the comprehensive neuropsychological evaluation of the child. Numerous academic achievement tests have been developed, all of which share the inclusion of at least a measure of reading and mathematics abilities. A common use of these measures is to look for significant discrepancies between achievement test performance and IQ test scores, since this is a commonly used procedure for defining specific learning disorders.

Wide Range Achievement Test—3rd Edition

The Wide Range Achievement Test—3rd edition (WRAT-3) was released in 1993 (Wilkinson, 1993). It includes a few changes in format while retaining the basic goal of providing an age- and grade-referenced test of reading (word recognition), spelling, and mathematics. The WRAT-3 includes normative data covering a broad age range (5–74) for two separate record forms, allowing for improved test validity when repeat testing is performed. The alternate form reliability coefficients for the total sample across reading, spelling, and arithmetic are .98, .98, and .98, respectively (Wilkinson, 1993).

Discriminant validity is of primary importance when a test is used to assist in diagnosis. The discriminant validity of the WRAT-3 has been examined and it has produced respectable results. For example, Wilkinson (1993) reports a study in which children enrolled in special education programs were compared to children from the normative sample matched on the basis of age, gender, and race. Discriminant analysis resulted in the following correct group classification rates: 85% for students assigned to gifted programs, 72% for learning disabled, 83% for educably mentally handicapped, and 56% for normal children.

The WRAT-3 continues to serve its purpose as a relatively brief measure of basic academic achievement. After identifying performance deficits in the basic areas of reading, spelling, and mathematics, more narrow-band tests can be given in an attempt to more fully understand the nature of the deficiency.

Wechsler Individual Achievement Test

The Wechsler Individual Achievement Test (WIAT) was released in 1992 (Wechsler, 1992). It was designed to assess academic achievement in children ranging in age from 5 yeas to 19 years, 11 months. The WIAT consists of eight subtests including basic reading, mathematics reasoning, spelling, reading comprehension, numerical operations, listening comprehension, oral expression, and written expression. The first three subtests can be used as a screening battery. The subsequent subtests can be administered to more extensively examine performance deficits found on the screening tests. A major advantage of the WIAT is that is was co-normed with the series of Wechsler Intelligence tests [Wechsler Preschool and Primary Scale of Intelligence—Revised (WPPSI-R), WISC-III, and Wechsler Adult Intelligence Scale—Revised (WAIS-R)]. This provides improved psychometric grounding for examination of significant discrepancies between performance on the IQ tests and tests of achievement. A second advantage is that the WIAT subtests were devised to assess all of the areas of learning disabilities described in the Education for All Handicapped Children Act (Public Law 94-142; Federal Register, 1976).

The WIAT has good reliability and validity. For example, split-half reliability coefficients for the subtests have been reported as ranging between .81 to .92. Test–retest reliability of the subtests averaged across all grades ranges from .76 to .94. Construct validity of the WIAT, as determined by examining its relationship to other academic achievement tests, has been reported to be at acceptable levels. For example, the WIAT basic reading, numerical operations, and spelling subtests were found to correlate .84, .77, and .84 with the WRAT-R reading, arithmetic, and spelling subtests, respectively.

The Woodcock–Johnson Psycho-Educational Battery—Revised

The Woodcock–Johnson Psycho-Educational Battery—Revised (WJ-R) (Woodcock & Johnson, 1989) was released in 1989 with several additions and modifications compared to the 1977 version. The WJ-R includes two major components: The Woodcock–Johnson Test of Academic Achievement (WJ-R/ACH) and the Woodcock–Johnson Test of Cognitive Ability (WJ-R/COG). Within each of the two components exists a standard battery of tests and a supplementary battery of tests. This gives the examiner the option of administering either a relatively brief or an extended battery of tests. The WJ-R/ACH offers the advantage of alternate forms (form A or B). WJ-R/COG is designed as a measure of cognitive ability as opposed to academic achievement, and therefore is not reviewed here. Fortunately, the WJ-R/ACH can be used separately from the WJ-R/COG.

The WJ-R/ACH standard battery consists of nine tests and the supplemental battery consists of an additional nine tests. The examiner is encouraged to selectively use subtests, depending on assessment needs. Collectively, the standard and supplemental batteries assess abilities in four areas: reading, mathematics, written language, and knowledge.

Normative data for the WJ-R/ACH was obtained from over 6000 subjects, including preschoolers (ages 2–5), school-aged children (grades K–12), a college sample, and an adult nonschool sample ranging from 14 to 90+ years of age. Alternate forms reliability coefficients for the 18 subtests ranges from .76 to .93. The manual reports respectable levels of construct validity of the WJ-R achievement categories with other achievement tests across the different age groups. For example, among a group of 9-year-olds, the concurrent validity coefficients between WJ-R Reading, Math, and Language Domains and the WRAT-R Reading, Math, and Spelling Domains were .83, .63, and .69, respectively.

Language Testing

Deficits in language functions are commonly found among children with learning disorders and documented brain damage. Trends in the assessment of language abilities have included attempts to relate knowledge obtained in research on language development to clinical neuropsychological assessment (Crary et al., 1988). As of this writing, the authors are not aware of the existence of a complete battery of language tests derived from a comprehensive model of neurolinguistic development. However, the Psycholinguistic Assessment of Language (PAL) battery is currently in development by David Caplan and Daniel Bub and may soon be available to clinicians (Caplan, 1995). At present, attempts can be made to combine currently existing tests into a comprehensive assessment of language functions for children of various ages (Crary et al., 1988).

Crary et al. (1988) have presented a developmental neurolinguistic assessment model. This framework is discussed here as an example of how component models of cognitive constructs taken from research in basic developmental and cognitive psychology can be used in a clinical context. This approach holds promise for improving syndrome identification by using assessment procedures linked to experimentally derived models of cognitive functions.

Crary et al. (1988) assert that language development follows an invariant path evolving through three general stages. The first stage is called the *prelinguistic stage* and represents prelanguage development corresponding to the time period from birth to approximately 12 months of age. During this stage, the normal infant learns to communicate needs through the use of basic movements and nonspecific vocalizations. For example, the infant may change the pitch of his voice in a meaningful and predictable fashion, with the function of communicating excitement or displeasure. Prelinguistic assessment is carried out through parent interview and direct observation to ascertain the range of prelinguistic communication behaviors elicited by the infant. Readiness scales typically include communication scales that can be used to indicate the infant's communication development relative to available normative data. These scales include the Receptive–Expressive Emergent Language Scale (Bzoch & League, 1971) and the Denver Developmental Screening Test (Frankenburg, Dodds, Fandel, Kazuk, & Cohrs, 1975).

The second stage of neurolinguistic development is called the *lexical expansion stage* (Crary et al., 1988). This stage involves growth in the semantic (meaning) and phonological (organization and production of sounds) aspects of language. Evidence of growth in the semantic system is seen as children begin to be more discriminating in their use of terms, suggesting that word meaning is associated with an increasingly complex number of organizational features. For example, a child early in the lexical expansion stage may use the word "doggie" to label any four-legged animal. As the semantic system develops, the child begins to use "doggie" more discriminantly, requiring more than just the presence of four legs. Phonological development involves the acquisition of abilities to discriminate and produce various language sounds and to accurately connect different sounds to a specific meaning. Prosody is a paralinguistic component of communication in which speech is varied in pitch, stress on specific sounds, and rhythm to express differential meaning. Substantial expansion in prosodic aspects of language is seen during the lexical expansion stage. For example, Menyuk and Bernholts (1969) found that the use of prosodic variation to discriminate between statements and questions or to indicate emphasis was common among 18- to 20-month-old children.

Standardized batteries of language development of children in the lexical expansion stage (12 to 24 months) have not been developed. Readiness scales such as the Receptive–Expressive Emergent Language Scale (Bzoch & League, 1971) and the Denver Developmental Screening Test (Frankenburg et al., 1975) are useful for assessing performance level in receptive and expressive functions. These measures, however, do not provide adequate evaluation of semantic knowledge, phonological development, pragmatic functions (e.g., requesting, commenting, directing, etc.), or prosodic recognition and production. Development of formal assessment batteries of these functions is needed.

The third stage of neurolinguistic development is called the *grammatical expansion stage,* which corresponds in the normal child between 2 to 4+ years of age (Crary et al., 1988). During this stage, there is a rapid increase in word use, increased verbal and phonological complexity, and an increased use of multiword productions with increased syntactic complexity. Toward the end of this stage, the basic phonological system should be almost fully developed. Once the child reaches the grammatical expansion stage, multiple components of the language system can be categorized for assessment, and various formal tests are available for use. Crary et al. (1988) review several available tests, only a few of which are selected below for discussion.

Comprehension of spoken language is of obvious importance to learning and primary to any examination of language processes. The Test for Auditory Comprehension of Language—Revised (Carrow, 1985) assesses comprehension of words from various classes, understanding of grammar, and ability to comprehend complex sentences.

Expressive language functions are assessed by using standardized phonological measures such as the Templin–Darley Tests of Articulation (Templin & Darley, 1969). Appropriate use of grammar and syntax can be assessed with tests such as the Grammatic Completion subtest of the Test of Language Development (Hammill & Newcomer, 1982), and the Northwestern Syntax Screening Test (Lee, 1971).

Repetition and naming are commonly measured as part of comprehensive language testing. Crary et al. (1988) have questioned the utility of these procedures in characterizing developmentally based language deficits. However, for older children with suspected acquired language deficits, these procedures, particularly tests of confrontational naming, are of substantial use because of their sensitivity to brain dysfunction (Dennis, 1992).

Pragmatic language functions and prosody are typically poorly assessed. Recently, however, increased attention has been focused on the importance of these aspects of linguistic functioning. A series of checklists has been developed by Wiig (Wiig, 1982a, b; Wiig & Bray, 1983) to assist in the evaluation of pragmatic language functions in children 3 years of age or older. Assessment of prosodic functions requires consideration of both abilities to produce a range of prosodic variation in a meaningful fashion, as well as ability to comprehend prosodic aspects of communications received.

Assessment of language functions, as is true for other functions, is never performed within a vacuum separate from consideration of integrative functions, such as motor ability, memory, sustained concentration, and motivation. Motor speech abilities may be assessed by asking children to perform speech diadochokinetic tasks, with reference to normative data to ascertain performance expectation levels (e.g., Fletcher, 1978; Riley & Riley, 1985). Impaired attending and memory can also obviously impair performance on a multitude of formal tests, including language tests.

Visual–Spatial and Constructional Testing

Tests of visual–spatial skills are best accomplished by tasks requiring little or no fine or gross motor activity, memory, or complex problem-solving abilities. Tests of constructional abilities are more integrative, requiring coordination of both fine-motor manual skills and visuoperceptual skills.

Basic ability to correctly perceive the angular relationship of various lines making up an object is presumed to be an elemental requirement for intact complex visual–perceptual processing. Judgment of Line Orientation (JLO) (Benton, Hamsher, Varney, & Spreen, 1993) is a commonly used measure to assess this ability. While JLO has been found to be reliable among children of 7–14 years of age (Lindgren & Benton, 1980), validity data with children need to be obtained.

Constructional tasks combine visuoperceptive processes and graphomotor processes. The Developmental Test of Visual–Motor Integration (VMI) (Beery & Buktenica, 1989) is a copying task that has been in use for a number of years. A restandardization was undertaken for the 1989 edition, and the long-form is appropriate for use with children age 3–18. The VMI has acceptable reliability (e.g., .63 after 7 months, .92 after 2 weeks) (Ryckman & Rentfrow, 1971), but the predictive validity of the VMI has been assessed with mixed results. Gates (1984) found that VMI scores obtained in kindergarten significantly predicted school achievement in grade 5. Other studies, however, have found that the VMI is not a reliable predictor of later school achievement (Duffy, Ritter, & Fedner, 1976).

Somatosensory and Motor Testing

The Reitan–Klove Sensory Perceptual Examination was originally developed for use with adults but has been downsized for use with children. Two forms exist, for children 9–15 and children 5–8 years. The measures include assessment of finger localization, stereognosis, graphesthesia, and sensory extinction. These procedures are particularly germane to neuropsychological assessment because of their sensitivity to brain damage. The presence of sensory and motor deficits has been related to learning difficulties among brain-damaged children (Fletcher & Satz, 1980; Rourke & Orr, 1977). These tests may also be of importance in subtyping LD children (Fisk & Rourke, 1979).

Manual motor testing is standardly included in neuropsychological assessment because of its significance with regard to lateralization of cortical dysfunction. Measures of grip strength, finger tapping speed, and a pegboard test have been standard for several years and continue to hold their value as potential indicators of cortical damage. It is most useful to include all three measures in a comprehensive assessment battery because significant bimanual performance discrepancies on any one of these measures occurs with unacceptable frequency in the normal population to be used diagnostically. However, findings of the same lateralized pattern of bimanual performance differences across all three of these motor tests is quite rare in the normal population and is strongly suggestive of neuropathology (Thompson, Heaton, Mathews & Grant, 1987).

Tests of Attention

Attention is perhaps the most difficult cognitive construct to compartmentalize and quantify. At least minimally sufficient attentional capacities must be present before higher cognitive abilities can be validly assessed. Performance on a number of tasks labeled as measuring memory, problem solving, constructional skills, and so on are at times limited by deficiencies in underlying attentional processes. Specific measures of "attention" by necessity should require very limited amounts of other skills such as language, memory, constructional skills, problem solving, or motor responding. In addition, integrity of attentional processes can be inferred by examining performance on multiple tasks involving both redundancy and uniqueness with regards to the cognitive skills and attentional resources required. This can lead to hypotheses about the extent to which a primary attentional deficit may be present versus primary deficiencies in other cognitive functions.

Current conceptualizations view attention as a multidimensional construct. There is substantial agreement in the literature that the following five components of attention can be usefully conceived: alertness, selective attention, sustained attention, span of apprehension, and hemi-inattention (Barkley, 1988). In addition, numerous authors discuss the construct of "supervisory attentional control" as an important component of the attentional system (e.g., van Zomeren & Brouwer, 1994). While these components are obviously not independent (Klee & Garfinkel, 1983), they are also not identical, and research has demonstrated the usefulness of considering them separately.

Alertness or arousal refers to the general responsivity of the child to the surrounding environment. Deficient alertness is apparent on observation and brief mental status examination. Poor alertness or arousal is indicated by a generalized and substantial deficiency in responsivity to the environment and precludes valid examinations of higher cognitive processes.

Selective attention refers to the ability to focus one's attention on a specified task without being unduly disrupted by distracting stimuli. Inattentiveness and distractibility are terms expressing deficits in selective attention (Barkley, 1988). Sustained attention or vigilance refers to the ability to direct one's attention toward a specified task for a relatively extended period of time.

A number of psychometric tests of selective and sustained attention have been devised. Computer-based reaction time tests have become popular for assessing aspects of selective and sustained attention. In simple reaction time tests, the primary measure is the average reaction time across a number of trials in which the child presses or releases a key in response to the presentation of a target stimulus on a screen. Variability of reaction time is also commonly examined. Commission errors (responding at incorrect times) are considered signs of impulsivity and omission errors (failure to respond within time limits following stimulus presentation) are considered a sign of inattentiveness.

Continuous performance tasks (CPTs) are commonly considered a better measure of vigilance or sustained attention than are simple reaction time tests. CPTs are devised such that the child is continuously presented with an array of stimuli (usually visual), and instructed to respond (e.g., lever press) only when a specified goal is met (e.g., respond to the letter X only when it follows the letter A). For CPTs, errors of omission and commission are the primary performance measures, reflective of inattentiveness and impulsivity.

Similar non-computer-based tasks of selective and sustained attention are available. The Underlining Test (Rourke & Gates, 1980) is a cancellation task consisting of 14 subtests that differ in terms of specific stimulus objects used (e.g., numbers, geometric shapes, letters, etc.). Each of the subtests requires the child to scan rows of stimuli as quickly as possible and to underline the ones that match the predetermined stimulus at the top of the page. As with CPTs, errors of omission and commission can be obtained. Other tests involving a primary component of attention include the Children's Embedded Figures Test (CEFT) (Witken, Oltman, Raskin, & Karp, 1971), the mazes subtest from the WISC-R, and the Matching Familiar Figures Task (MFST) (Kagan, Rosman, Day, Albert, & Phillips, 1964).

Hemi-inattention, or neglect, refers to the phenomena of deficient selective attention to half of a sensory field. While uncommon in adults, it is believed to be even less common in children. When seen in children, it occurs during the acute stages of neurological disruption and disappears within a few hours. Neglect is almost always seen as a result of damage to the posterior region of the right hemisphere. Visual neglect can be assessed by asking the child to copy simple drawings. Children with neglect will fail to copy the left half of the drawing. A visual field cut (homonymous hemianopsia) must be ruled out before neglect can be concluded (Barkley, 1988).

Span of apprehension refers to the amount of information to which one can simultaneously attend. Experimental procedures designed to assess span of apprehension involve use of a tachistoscope to briefly present (e.g., 100 msec) matrices of stimuli arranged in various arrays. The number of stimuli accurately scanned during the brief exposure is the span of apprehension (Barkley, 1988). This test has been shown to discriminate children with attention deficit disorder from normal children (Denton & McIntyre, 1978). While this procedure is promising, in its current form it is impractical due to the required tachistoscope. With advances is use of computerized testing, these procedures will likely become easily obtainable to the clinician in the near future.

Supervisory attentional control is discussed by Shallice (1982, 1988) as being a dimension of the attention construct. Supervisory attentional control is the system proposed as being responsible for regulating the tasks of focusing, dividing, switching, and sustaining attention. This construct is considered by many as being part of the executive functions construct and is associated strongly with integrity of the frontal lobes. The Tower of London test has been developed as a measure of supervisory attentional control (Shallice, 1982). This planning test is modeled after the Tower of Hanoi. It includes three vertical pegs of different lengths and three colored beads. The object is to move the beads from one peg to another, arrange them in a specified order, and correctly complete the task in a minimal number of moves.

Tests of Memory and Learning

Memory assessment in children has been relatively neglected in the past. For example, the Halstead–Reitan Neuropsychological Battery for children is lacking in explicitly labeled tests of memory. While the Luria–Nebraska Neuropyschological Battery for Children includes a memory scale, its coverage of the memory construct is quite limited and inadequate. Several individual tests of learning and memory originally designed for adults have been modified for use with children. These include the Rey Auditory–Verbal Learning Test (Crawford, Stewart, & Moore, 1989), the Selective Reminding Test (Buschke, 1974; Clodfelter, Dickson, Newton-Wilkes, & Johnson, 1987; Morgan, 1982), the Rey–Osterrieth Complex Figure Test (Kolb & Whishaw, 1985), and Logical Memory, Visual Reproduction, and Associate Learning subtests from the Wechsler Memory Scale (Curry, Logue, & Butler, 1986; Halperin, Healey, Zeitchik, Ludman, & Weinstein, 1989). However, only recently have batteries of memory tests become available that were developed specifically for children. Four memory batteries now available for children are the Wide Range Assessment of Memory and Learning (WRAML) (Sheslow & Adams, 1990), the California Verbal Learning Test for Children (CVLT-C) (Delis, Kramer, Kaplan, & Ober, 1994), the Children's Memory Scale (CMS) (Wechsler, 1995), and the Test of Memory and Learning (TOMAL) (Reynolds & Bigler, 1994).

The WRAML is a standardized memory assessment battery that provides normative data from a large group of children 5 through 17 years of age. Table 3 describes the nine subtests included in the WRAML. The WRAML offers the benefits of allowing for the examination of various aspects of memory that have been identified as potentially important in previous research. These include discriminating between verbal and visual stimulus modalities, separating episodic from semantic memory, use of list-learning subtests that allows for assessment of strategy use and learning curve, and the opportunity to examine immediate, delayed, and recognition memory.

As we mentioned earlier, researchers have found that children's performance across different tests of learning and memory tends to be variable. As a result, use of only one or two brief memory tasks is likely to produce misleading and inadequate characterization of a child's learning and memory abilities. For example, the mean correlation between subtests making up the WRAML is only $r = .24$ for the normative sample of children 8 and younger. For the 9 and older group, the mean correlation between WRAML subtests is not much better ($r = .29$). As a result, we recommend that several memory tests be administered prior to drawing conclusions about a child's memory functions.

TABLE 3. Wide Range Assessment of Memory and Learning

Scales and subtests	Description

Verbal memory scale

Number/Letter Memory. This subtest is a modification of the "digit span test." A random sequence of numbers and letters ranging in unit length from 2 to 10 are presented and the child is asked to recite the number/letter sequence. This approach prevents clustering of units allowing for assessment of strategy free short-term recall. Discontinuation criteria are applied.

Sentence Memory. This is a sentence repetition subtest. The child is to repeat a series of meaningful sentences, which gradually increase in length. Discontinuation criteria are applied.

Story Memory. This is a test of memory for narrative information. Two brief stories are read to the child and the child is asked to recall as much of each story as he can.

Visual memory scale

Finger Windows. This is a test of memory for spatial sequences. A series of trials are presented in which the examiner points to stimulus "windows" on a page in a specific order, which is then to be reproduced from memory by the child. The sequence gradually becomes longer. Discontinuation criteria are applied.

Design Memory. This is a test of memory for geometrical designs. After a brief stimulus presentation and delay, the child is asked to draw the designs from memory. To factor in the influence of perceptual–motor skills in the reproduction, a series of seven designs are copied prior to beginning this subtest. If constructional difficulties are made on the copy of any of the designs, these can be used to modify the scoring of the reproduction of the designs made from memory.

Picture Memory. This is a test of visual memory for a meaningful scene. Four pictures are presented one at a time. After briefly viewing each picture, another scene is presented on which several changes and additions have been made. The child is asked to mark an "X" through each change noted.

Learning scale

Verbal Learning. This is a test of learning ability for a list of unrelated words. Four presentation and immediate recall trials are given.

Visual Learning. This is a test of visual learning. Four presentation and immediate recall trials are given for the child to display learning of the particular position in which various designs have been placed on a board.

Sound Symbol. This is a paired-associate learning task. Four presentation and immediate recall trials are given in which the child's ability to recall the correct sound and symbol pairs is tested.

Delayed recall

Optional delayed recall trials can be given for Verbal Learning, Visual Learning, Sound Symbol, and Story Memory.

Types of memory that are not typically assessed but may be of relevance with regard to treatment include incidental memory, procedural memory, and metamemory. Incidental learning is information that is automatically acquired through experience without imposed (self or other) attempts to remember. Procedural memory refers to the learning of a complex series of motor behaviors needed to accomplish a task such as putting together a complex puzzle or learning to play a musical instrument. Finally, metamemory refers to a child's knowledge of memory and learning rules. For example, knowing that it is more difficult to recall information verbatim than in a paraphrased fashion is helpful to a child as he attempts to encode information for subsequent recall. This is a clearly important area because of its potential relevance to treatment. Along these lines, Kreutzer, Leonard, and Flavell (1975) have developed a metamemory interview that may be helpful in assessing a child's knowledge of mnemonic principles and strategy use.

Tests of Problem Solving

Problem-solving tasks are complex and may require the effective use of a multitude of component skills including motor, visual–spatial, attention, memory, and language functions. Due to the complexity of problem-solving tests, deficient performance does not lend itself easily toward interpretation with regard to the underlying deficit in component skills. Nevertheless, assessment of problem-solving abilities is of much relevance to understanding the functional capacities of the child. Other constructs typically included under the umbrella of problem solving include metacognition (e.g., Brown, 1975), executive functions (e.g., Kistner & Torgesen, 1987), and abstract reasoning (e.g., Richman & Lindgren, 1981).

Numerous tests have already been mentioned that fall under the umbrella of problem solving. For example, the WISC-III includes the Block Design and Similarity subtests. The Halstead–Retain Neuropsychological Battery for Children includes the Category Test and the Tactual Performance Test. The Woodcock–Johnson Psycho-Educational Battery includes several subtests of problem-solving abilities.

Recently developed or revised independent tests of problem solving include the Wisconsin Card Sorting Test (WCST) (Chelune & Thompson, 1987) and the Children's Category Test (CCT) (Boll, 1993). The revised WCST manual includes normative data on a large sample ranging in age from 6.5 to 89 years. The CCT was co-normed with the California Verbal Learning Test for Children (CVLT-C). Two levels are available: Level 1 (color) for ages 5 through 8, and Level 2 (numbers) for ages 9 through 16. Normative data are provided based on a national sample stratified across age, gender, race, region, and parent education level. The CCT can be administered individually or used during the 20-minute delayed recall section of the CVLT-C.

ASSESSMENT OF PSYCHOSOCIAL, BEHAVIORAL, AND ENVIRONMENTAL FACTORS

Evaluation of psychosocial, behavioral, and environmental factors is of no less importance in clinical child neuropsychology than it is in general clinical child psychological assessment. Variables such as motivation, impulsivity, and anxiety/

depression are important to consider with respect to performance on neuropsychological tests and the influence they have in contributing to maladaptive behavior in the natural environment. Understanding the broader social context is also necessary. Specifically, "Who makes up the primary family unit?" "How stable is the family unit?" "What is the nature of the power structure?" "What modes of discipline are used?" "What are the family strengths and limitations with regards to their ability to contribute to and carry out treatment procedures?" Information about nonfamilial environment such as school, church, and broader community involvement is useful for some types of evaluative issues and diagnostic questions.

Obtaining information from multiple sources using different data collection methods is common practice in child psychological assessment. Assessment modalities include self-report scales; behavior rating scales completed by parents and/or other informed persons; structured interview of the child, parents, and/or teachers; and direct behavioral observation. Each of these methods has advantages and disadvantages, with the most informative picture being derived from integrating information from the various measures. For example, self-report measures have the potential advantage of obtaining information about the child's covert experiences (thoughts and feelings). Unfortunately, children many times fail to accurately represent their functioning on self-report scales. This may be due to a number of reasons, including developmental limitations with regards to self-monitoring of behavior, poor reading abilities, or a noncooperative attitude (e.g., Lachar, 1990).

Structured diagnostic interviews provide the advantage of being able to follow an organized list of questions that cover the major domains of maladaptive behavior. There are several structured interviews that have been developed for use with children. Most of them provide questions written in language easy to understand for young children and are structured such that minimal verbal responding is required to endorse symptoms. Like self-report scales, however, structured interviews are prone to being invalidated by a child's attitude toward the task, whether it be that of denial or overendorsement. Also, most investigators agree that it is difficult to obtain reliable self-report information from preschool aged children because of their immature level of conceptual development (e.g., Stone & LeManek, 1990).

Behavior rating scales, completed by parents or other informed party (e.g., teacher), are the most commonly used assessment modality with children. These escape the biases and limitations of self-report scales but introduce limitations of their own. The primary advantage of behavior checklists is that information about the child's behavioral functioning across a broad range of behaviors can be ascertained. Also, narrow-band behavior rating scales can be used to assess for characteristics of specific syndromes such as attention deficit hyperactivity disorder. The validity of behavior rating scales are anchored to the accuracy with which the person completing the form responds. Parents own psychological difficulties can influence their perception and report of their child's behavioral difficulties (Forehand & Brody, 1985). Also, parents' retrospective reports of the child's problem behaviors may show poor stability over time (Hetherington & Martin, 1979).

Direct behavioral observation, while appearing to be the most objective form of assessment, suffers from impracticality and problems with interrater reliability and reactivity on the part of the observers (Foster & Cone, 1986). Table 4 provides a list of commonly used assessment tools to include structured interviews, behavior rating scales, self-report scales, and behavioral observation systems.

NEUROPSYCHOLOGICAL CORRELATES OF SELECTED SYNDROMES

Below we provide a review of neuropsychological findings associated with three diagnostic groups commonly referred to child neuropsychologists: traumatic brain injury, learning disability, and attention deficit hyperactivity disorder.

TABLE 4. Standardized Interviews, Broad-Band Rating Scales, and Self-Report Inventories

---

Standardized interviews

    Diagnostic Interview for Children and Adolescents (DICA) (Herjanic & Campbell, 1977; Herjanic & Reich, 1982)
    Diagnostic Interview Schedule for Children (DISC) (Costello, Edelbrock, Kalas, Kessler, & Klaric, 1984)
    Children's Assessment Schedule (CAS) (Hodges, McKnew, Cytryn, Stern, & Klein, 1982)
    Kiddie SADS (K-SADS) (Chambers et al., 1985; Puig-Antich & Chambers, 1978)
    Interview Schedule for Children (ISC) (Kovacs, 1982)
    Semistructured Clinical Interview for Children (SCIC) (McConaughy & Achenbach, 1990)

Broad-band rating scales

    Child Behavior Checklist (CBC) (Achenbach & Edelbrock, 1983)
    Conners Parent Symptom Questionnaire—Revised (CPSQ-R) (Goyette, Conners, & Ulrich, 1978)
    Conners Teacher Rating Scale—Revised (CTRS-R) (Goyette et al., 1978)
    Personality Inventory for Children (PIC) (Lachar, 1982)
    Revised Behavior Problem Checklist (BPC-R) (Quay & Peterson, 1983)
    Yale Children's Inventory (YCI) (Shaywitz, Schnell, Shaywitz, & Towle, 1986)
    Behavior Rating Profile (BRP) (Brown & Hammill, 1983)
    Direct Observation Form (DOF) (Achenbach, 1986; McConaughy & Achenbach, 1988)

Self report inventories

    Personality Inventory for Youth (PIY) (Lachar & Gruber, 1994)
    Child Behavior Checklist—Youth Self Report (CBC-YSR) (Achenbach, 1991)
    Minnesota Multiphasic Personality Inventory/Adolescent (MMPI-A) (Butcher et al., 1992)
    Revised Children's Manifest Anxiety Scale (RCMAS) (Reyolds & Richmond, 1985)
    Reynolds Adolescent Depression Inventory (RADI) (Reynolds, 1986)
    Child Self Report Questionnaire (SRQ) (Beitchman & Corradini, 1988)
    Children's Depression Inventory (CDI) (Kovacs, 1985)

Traumatic Brain Injury

Traumatic brain injury (TBI) is the most common cause of death in children and adolescents (Fenichel, 1988). Among survivors, the factors that determine the extent of deficit to cognitive functions include the severity of the injury, the presence of secondary complications, and the age of onset.

The Glasgow Coma Scale (GCS) (Teasdale & Jennett, 1974) is a commonly used TBI severity classification system. A score ranging from 3 to 15 is assigned based on the child's ability to open his eyes, respond verbally, and follow simple motor commands following head injury. Because of the verbal demands of the GCS, this rating scale is inappropriate for infants and very young children. Modifications of the GCS for preverbal children are available (e.g., Levin, Aldrich, & Saydjari, 1992). A head injury resulting in a GCS greater than 12 is classified as a mild head injury, GCS of 9 to 12 is classified as moderate head injury, and GCS of 8 or lower is classified as a severe head injury. As with adults, the GCS has been found to be useful in predicting the probability of lasting neurocognitive deficits in children. For example, in a study of the outcome from traumatic brain injury among a pediatric population hospitalized in San Diego County (Kraus, Rock, & Hemyari, 1990), it was found that the GCS was useful in staging extent of recovery.

Secondary complications to TBI can occur, increasing the severity of neuro-psychological sequelae. Secondary complications include intracranial hemorrhage, edema, and increased intracranial pressure. Age-related differences in the pathophysiological process of TBI have been described. For example, Shapiro and Smith (1993) reported that diffuse cerebral swelling is a more frequent complication among children than adults. On the other hand, the infant brain is at less risk for contusion secondary to striking the inward-facing surface of the skull, which is smoother in infants. The epidemiology of TBI is different in infants and young children relative to adults. Older children and adults are most likely to experience head injury in the context of motor vehicle accidents, which makes them more subject to diffuse axonal injury from shearing strain secondary to rotational forces. Younger children and infants are most likely to suffer head injury from falls and as a result of assault, which tend to be low-velocity events (Kraus et al., 1990).

The issue of whether or not younger children achieve better recovery from TBI than older children and adults has been debated for years. In reality, this question is phrased too broadly to ever achieve an answer beyond "it depends." Existing literature indicates that while age plays a role in predicting type and severity of cognitive morbidity, its influence is almost inextricably tied to other important variables, making isolation of the influence of age quite difficult. Specifically, one must parcel patients according to type of injury sustained (focal, lateralized, diffuse), age of injury, age of patient at time of assessment, and sensitivity of outcome measures used.

Brain plasticity refers to a hypothesized process in which brain injury is followed by reorganization in the unimpaired areas, allowing these to support cognitive functions. At times, recovery of functions may be due to this process. The concept of plasticity has been examined most commonly with regard to language processes. In support of greater brain plasticity in infants compared to older children and adults, Basser (1962) found that the children and adults in this sample, who all had onset of hemiplegia in infancy, did not show a significant relationship between side of hemispheric damage and language performance. Also, Gardner, Karnoch, McClure, and Gardner (1955), comparing the outcome of adults versus children undergoing hemispherectomies, found greater deficits in adults. These studies have been criticized, however, as not using sensitive measures of language functions (St. James-Roberts, 1979). Levin, Ewing-Cobbs, and Benton (1984) provide a critical review and reinterpretation of these previous studies and argue that these studies in fact do not show reliably different recovery rates in children versus adults.

Other studies have found that early brain damage to the left hemisphere does place the child at risk for language deficits more so than early damage to the right hemisphere. For example, Annett (1973) found that a larger proportion (41%) of hemiplegic children with early age of onset left hemisphere damage had language problems compared to those with early age right hemisphere damage (15%), indicating that even among young children damage to the left hemisphere is more likely to produce difficulties with later language development compared to when the early brain damage involved the right hemisphere. Dennis (1988) has pointed out that comparison of outcomes of brain damage in adults with outcomes in children in the hope of understanding something about plasticity has substantial weaknesses. She encourages a developmental context that emphasizes the interaction between developmental stage and injury. Dennis (1988) argues that, "the kind of brain damage that prevents the development of a skill appears to be different from the damage that disrupts the maintenance of that skill, once acquired" (p. 107). As a result, use of adults as a comparison group to children provides a weak model for understanding effects of brain damage.

TBI in children not only has the ability to disrupt previously acquired abilities, but also poses a threat to disruption of cognitive skills typically developed later in the maturational course. Longitudinal research has discovered that while a brain injury may not produce an observable deficit in cognitive performance in a child at one stage of development, testing at a later age may reveal deficits, suggesting that the early brain damage could only be appreciated at a time when later cognitive skills will normally develop (Fletcher, Miner, & Ewing-Cobbs, 1987). Also, to the extent that plasticity may occur, it is not equally likely throughout the brain. For example, damage to focal areas such as the visual tracts cannot be compensated for, while focal damage to cortical areas may have some hope of plasticity in the developing brain (Parker, 1990).

The type of brain lesion is of importance in predicting long-standing cognitive deficits. In the case of diffuse brain injury, Isaacson (1975) has argued that children show poorer recovery than do adults. Below, we briefly review neuropsychological outcome studies of traumatic brain injury in children across specific cognitive domains.

Intelligence

An association between intelligence, as measured by IQ tests, and severity of brain injury has been repeatedly demonstrated (Goldstein & Levin, 1985). For example, Levin, Huttenlocher, Banich, and Duda (1987) used CT scans to measure lesion size among a sample of children with either congenital or acquired hemiplegia, and found lesion size to be inversely correlated with VIQ, PIQ, and FSIQ from both populations. Levin and Eisenberg (1979a) found that the IQs of children who sustained TBI, when tested 6 months postinjury, were within the average range with the exception of those whose TBIs were rated as severe. These authors, however, go on to report that when comparisons were made between the children's performances on IQ tests and estimated premorbid ability, it appeared likely that even for many of the less than severe TBI children, there was likely some loss in abilities as measured on IQ tests.

Length of coma is also a predictor of IQ (Brink, Garrett, Hale, Woo-Sum, & Nickel, 1970). In the absence of a focal brain insult, the relationship between VIQ and PIQ following significant traumatic brain injury is that of relatively more impaired PIQ (Chadwick, Rutter, Shaffer, & Shrout, 1981; Rutter, 1982; Winogron, Knights, & Bawden, 1984). PIQ includes a substantial psychomotor speed component that is commonly diminished secondary to severe TBI (Spreen, Risser, & Edgell, 1995).

Language

While muteness and classical aphasia can occur during the acute stages of recovery from closed head injury, long-term sequelae of closed head injury more commonly involve subtle language deficits. Most common deficits are dysnomia, neologisms, paraphasias, and impaired auditory–verbal comprehension (Dennis, 1988). Verbal repetition is only rarely impaired (Levin & Eisenberg, 1979a).

For focal and lateralized brain injuries to the left hemisphere, there is evidence to indicate that very young children have less language impairment relative to older children (e.g., Annet, 1973; Woods & Carey, 1979). This is believed to be due to the young brain's ability to reorganize the anatomical underpinnings of language functions primarily by the right hemisphere taking over responsibility for language functions previously managed by the left hemisphere.

As already mentioned, for diffuse brain injuries, such as those typically sustained in TBI, the relationship between age and recovery of language function appears to point in the opposite direction. For example, Ewing-Cobbs, Fletcher, Landry, and Levin (1985) compared children and adolescents who had suffered TBI on language tests. As a group, age-related differences were found only on written language subtests, with the children showing more deficits than adolescents across the range of TBI severity.

Visual–Spatial

Impairment on visual–spatial tasks is a common finding across a variety of types of early brain injury (Witelson, 1987). The relationship between lesion site, age of onset, and consequent disruption in visual–spatial functions is not clear-cut (Dorman & Katzir, 1994). Among school-aged children, Meerwaldt and van Dongen (1988) found that the six children (age 8–15) in their sample with unilateral right hemisphere lesions showed impairments on tests of visual–spatial orientation and facial recognition, while the six children (7–15 years of age) in their sample with unilateral left hemisphere lesions did not show deficits on these tasks. The specialization of the right hemisphere for visual–spatial tasks at a very early age seems supported by a study by Stiles-Davis, Sugarman, and Nass (1985). They compared the performance of four children with right hemisphere lesions, ages 2 to 3 years, with four children with left hemisphere lesions in the same age range. All children obtained lesions prior to 3 months of age. They found that the right hemisphere lesion group had difficulties relative to the left hemisphere lesion patients and normal controls when performing a spatial grouping task (placing objects side by side).

Attention

Deficits on complex attentional tasks are common following TBI in children (Chadwick, Rutter, Brown, Shaffer, & Traub, 1981; Levin & Eisenberg, 1979b). Following the acute stage of recovery from TBI, simple attention and alertness are intact, while tests requiring selective attention, vigilance, psychomotor speed, and visuomotor speed are deficient. Continuous Performance Tests have been demonstrated to be sensitive to TBI (e.g., Timmermans & Christensen, 1991). Deficits in psychomotor–visuomotor speed are oftentimes displayed on tests such as the Trail Making Test, particularly part B, the Symbol Digit Modalities Test (Smith, 1982), and the coding subtest from the WISC-III.

Memory

Memory deficits may be the most commonly observed impairment following brain injury in children. For example, Levin and Eisenberg (1979a), using the Selective Reminding Test, found that almost one half of the 64 children in their sample had impaired verbal learning and memory, with increased impairment being related to severity of TBI. The children with left temporal lesions in the context of a TBI showed the most difficulty with storage and retrieval of verbal information.

Executive Functions

A recent study by Levin et al. (1994) found substantial relationships between severity of TBI among a sample of 6- to 16-year-old children and deficits on the Tower of London reasoning test. MRI-documented extent of damage to the frontal lobes was correlated with performance difficulties even after controlling for over-all severity of the head injury.

Sensorimotor

Even among children without gross motor deficits, finger tapping speed and manual dexterity are commonly slowed, with greater impairment occurring fol-lowing more severe injury (Bawden, 1985; Chadwick et al., 1981).

Academic Achievement Tests

Academic achievement testing usually involves at the minimum, evaluation of reading, spelling, and arithmetic (e.g., WRAT-3) abilities. Diminished perfor-mance on achievement tests can obviously occur secondary to TBI because of the multiple cognitive demands that these tests require. However, arithmetic is more sensitive to disruption than spelling and reading (Levin, Grafman, & Eisenberg, 1987). This is commonly believed to be due to the fact that arithmetic requires more fluid processing capacities than reading and spelling, and fluid processes are more easily disrupted by TBI than are retrieval abilities for previously acquired knowledge (spelling and reading).

Behavioral Changes

As with other functions, the extent of behavioral and emotional changes is correlated with extent of brain injury. The incidence of psychiatric disorders in children with known cerebral pathology is twice as high as that found among chil-dren with non-brain-based physical handicaps (Seidel, Chadwick, & Rutter, 1975). Multifocal bilateral lesions place children at most risk for development of significant behavioral difficulties (Eide & Tysnes, 1992). Mild closed head injury is not likely to produce drastic changes in personality or development of psychi-atric disturbance (Brown, Chadwick, Shaffer, Rutter, & Traub, 1981). In contrast, personality changes and development of psychiatric disturbance following a se-vere head injury are relatively common. Brown et al. (1981) reported that 50% of their sample of severe closed-head-injured children developed psychiatric dis-turbance at follow-up. The most prominent difficulty reported was that of disinhi-bition, leading to inappropriate comments and behavior, overtalkativeness, and decreased attention to personal hygiene.

Learning Disabilities

Difficulties in learning can be due to a host of problems, including sensory deficits (poor hearing or vision), poor academic learning opportunities, poor motivation, low intellectual level, or cognitive deficits secondary to a known brain injury. The term "learning disability," however, is used to define a circumscribed difficulty in learning that is not secondary to the above factors. The definition below has been put forth by the National Joint Committee for Learning Disabilities (1987):

> Learning disability is a generic term that refers to a heterogeneous group of disorders manifested by significant difficulties in the acquisition and use of listening, speaking, reading, writing, reasoning, or mathematical abilities. These disorders are intrinsic to the individual, and presumed to be due to central nervous system dysfunction. Even though an LD may occur concomitantly with other handicapping conditions (e.g., sensory impairment, mental retardation, social and emotional disturbance) or environmental influences (e.g., cultural differences, insufficient/inappropriate instruction, psychogenic factors) it is not the direct result of these conditions or influences (p. 107).

Learning disability is estimated to occur in 7 to 15% of the general population in the United States (Gaddes & Edgell, 1993), with the greatest magnitude of these LDs being a disruption in language-based learning (dyslexia) expressed mostly by reading and spelling difficulties. Other types of specific learning disabilities discussed in the literature include an arithmetic learning disorder (dyscalculia) and nonverbal learning disability (NLD). NLD includes dyscalculia as a prominent feature, but also proposes a syndrome consisting of additional neuropsychological deficits and maladaptive socioemotional adjustment. Some authors also discuss attention deficit hyperactivity disorder (ADHD) as being a type of learning disability, with the prominent cognitive deficits being that of impaired executive functions. For this chapter, we have chosen to discuss dyslexia in greater detail because of its high prevalence. We also will discuss the syndrome of NLD. Even though NLD is estimated to be relatively rare, it represents an area of relatively new and continuing growth in the field.

In simple terms, dyslexia is defined as unexpected reading and spelling difficulties that cannot be explained on the basis of deficient educational opportunities, sensory deficits, poor motivation, acquired brain damage, or generally low IQ (Pennington, 1991). The prevalence of dyslexia is estimated to be from 5 to 10% (Benton & Pearl, 1978). It is commonly believed that dyslexia is more prevalent among males than females (e.g., 4:1) (Pennington, 1991). This is certainly the case among clinical samples. However, recent family and epidemiological studies have suggested either an equal sex ratio or only a slightly increased prevalence for dyslexia among males (DeFries, 1989; Shaywitz, Shaywitz, Fletcher, & Escobar, 1990). There is a relatively small amount of longitudinal data on the long-term functioning of children with dyslexia. A broad range of outcomes is represented, but clearly dyslexia is associated with increased risk for poor adjustment in adulthood in many areas.

With regard to the neuropathology of dyslexia, there is evidence that the syndrome is frequently associated with a developmental anomaly of the left hemisphere. Several studies have pointed specifically to an unusual formation of the left planum temporale. Specifically, dyslexics are likely to have shorter left temporal planum length. Also, among nondyslexics, the left planum temporale is typically larger than the right. In contrast, dyslexics tend to show either no asymmetry in the size of the right–left temporal plana or they will show a right-sided superiority in size (Hynd, Semrud-Clikeman, Lorys, Novey, & Eliopulos, 1990).

A large amount of research has been conducted in an effort to understand the specific component of reading that is disrupted in dyslexia. The overwhelming conclusion is that dyslexia is a language-processing disorder, not a visual or spatial processing disorder (Pennington, 1991). Developmental dyslexia is characterized by difficulties in the phonological coding of written words. Reading tends to be slowed and labored due to difficulties in using phonological codes to recognize, pronounce, and spell words. The decreased automaticity of phonetic coding and phonetic decoding putatively requires more of the dyslexic's cognitive resources, leaving fewer resources that can be devoted to the comprehension process. As a result, dyslexics commonly show decreased comprehension as well as slow reading speed (Pennington, 1991).

Behavioral observations of dyslexic children's reading, spelling, and speech will typically reveal subtle language difficulties. Perhaps most common is slow and halting speech when reading out loud. Older children, however, may not display a significant dysfluency because of a larger, overlearned vocabulary. Dyslexics also commonly substitute function words such as "a" for "the." Visual errors involve substituting letters and words that are visibly similar (e.g., "car" for "cat"). Lexicalization errors occur on tests of nonwords. This occurs when a nonword is read as a real word (e.g., "boy" for "bym"). Reversal errors, in which letters are read or written in reverse (e.g., "bog" for "dog"), are actually relatively uncommon despite the notion in the lay population that these types of errors are almost pathognomonic for dyslexia (Pennington, 1991).

By most standards, the diagnosis of dyslexia requires formal testing with a standardized IQ test and a standardized achievement test that includes at least assessment of reading (word recognition), spelling, and computational math. In addition, it is useful to include further measures of reading, such as reading speed (e.g., word attack subtest from the Woodcock–Johnson) and reading comprehension (e.g., Peabody Individual Achievement Test Reading Comprehension subtest) (Markwardt, 1989). The typical dyslexic test pattern includes generally average FSIQ with a tendency toward VIQ being lower than PIQ. Reading and spelling performance is significantly below expectation relative to IQ, while computational arithmetic tends not to be impaired (Pennington, 1991). The diagnosis of dyslexia is most traditionally based on finding a substantial discrepancy between performance on the IQ test and on tests of reading abilities that is not believed to be due to limited educational opportunities, emotional disturbance, or acquired brain damage. There is substantial variation, however, in the specific standards employed with regard to how large the discrepancy should be before diagnosis of dyslexia is warranted. Reynolds (1990) provides a detailed review of these issues, including a discussion of the advantages and disadvantages of using different diagnostic criteria.

Nonverbal Learning Disability

NLD is a syndrome characterized primarily by specific deficits in math, poor visual–spatial–organizational abilities, and disturbed socioemotional development. This basic syndrome cluster has also been labeled as "right hemisphere" learning disability due to the presumed etiology of a developmentally based or early-age-acquired right hemisphere dysfunction (Pennington, 1991).

The research literature on NLD is much briefer than that found for dyslexia. The prevalence of NLD in the general population is not known but is estimated to be between 0.1 and 1.0% (cited in Pennington, 1991). Tentative estimates of sex ratio suggest a 1:1 ratio (Rourke, 1989), but again these are tentative estimates and epidemiological studies are needed.

NLD is a syndrome characterized by a specific pattern of strengths and weaknesses on neuropsychological tests and the presence of a specific difficulty in social and emotional functioning. The NLD syndrome has been associated with a number of medical syndromes, none of which are necessary or sufficient to produce NLD. For example, Turner's syndrome and fragile X syndrome are examples of genetic disorders that have been linked to NLD (e.g., Kemper, Hagerman, Ahmad, & Mariner, 1986; Pennington et al., 1985). Several other etiologies have been associated with NLD, including early closed head injury, poorly treated early hydrocephalus, childhood brain irradiation treatments, and agenesis of the corpus callosum (Rourke, 1989).

The neuropsychological test profile typically shows a significantly lower PIQ relative to VIQ (greater than 12 points). Computational arithmetic is substantially impaired relative to mostly intact reading and spelling. A tendency toward better verbal than nonverbal memory, better performance on auditory–verbal-based tasks than on visual constructive tasks, a mildly lateralized pattern on motor and tactile perceptual tests (right side better than left), and a tendency toward difficulties with conceptual reasoning.

In addition to cognitive deficits, the NLD syndrome is characterized by significant difficulties in socioemotional functioning. This is contrasted to dyslexics, who as a group are likely to experience more socioemotional difficulties than normal peers, but are quite heterogenous with regard to the nature of their socioemotional difficulties. Also, as many as half of dyslexics are likely to have no significant coexisting socioemotional difficulties. Socioemotional difficulties, particularly internalizing disorders, are so commonly associated with the neuropsychological and achievement test score pattern characteristic of NLD that

Rourke and colleagues have argued that the socioemotional difficulties result from the same underlying deficit in central processing that produce the cognitive deficits. Another difference noted between dyslexics and NLD children is that NLD children typically show worsening of psychopathology with increased age. This pattern of change is not characteristic of dyslexics as a group (Rourke, 1989).

Attention Deficit Hyperactivity Disorder

Historically, diagnosis of attention deficit hyperactivity disorder (ADHD) has been made by clinical assessment, relying heavily on descriptive information about the child's behavior obtained from interview of parents and teachers, as well as by having theses individuals complete behavioral checklists and rating scales. In more recent years, neuropsychological tests have been added to many clinician's ADHD assessment batteries in an attempt to quantify attentional disruption, impulsivity, and executive function deficits (Rapport, 1993).

ADHD is characterized by substantial levels of age-inappropriate inattentiveness, impulsivity, and hyperactivity. The specific criteria required for diagnosis by the DSM have changed over the years, primarily with regard to the emphasis placed on requiring hyperactivity as a core component of the disorder (Rapport, 1993). The DSM-IV, while citing data from field trials that "attention deficit" and "hyperactivity" are typically part of the same syndrome, has provided subtypes, allowing for more specific coding of each child's presentation: "combined, predominantly inattentive, predominantly hyperactive-impulsive."

ADHD rarely occurs in isolation. A variety of associated difficulties are commonly found that justify the use of broad-based clinical assessment when formally evaluating a child suspected of ADHD. Among young children, moodiness, temper tantrums, poor frustration tolerance, and social disinhibition are common (Rapport, 1993). Upon entering school, disturbed peer relationships, academic underachievement, learning disabilities, poor self-esteem, emotional disruption, and conduct problems are common (Barkley, 1981).

While the high comorbidity of ADHD with other difficulties makes clinical assessment by necessity complex and multifaceted, the picture is further complicated by the fact that children with ADHD have been found to be quite inconsistent in their test performance. This creates concern regarding the reliability of cognitive measures, and subsequently their diagnostic validity (Kinsbourne, 1984; Rapport, 1993).

The assessment of ADHD is best accomplished by employing a multimodal approach including information obtained from standardized interviews, behavioral checklists, intelligence testing, achievement testing, and neurocognitive assessment. Commonly use standardized interviews and broad-based behavioral rating scales were reviewed earlier in this chapter. There are numerous narrowband rating scales available that are designed to assess the specific features of ADHD. These have been reviewed by previous authors (e.g., Barkley, 1988).

Formal intellectual and achievement testing is vital to the evaluation of children suspected of ADHD, particularly when one considers that more than 50% of ADHD children will be found to have learning difficulties or underachievement (McGee & Share, 1988). While it is not clear that the overall IQs of ADHD children as a group differ significantly from normals, there is evidence to suggests that performance on certain neuropsychological tests may become increasingly deficient among ADHD children with increasing age (Massman, Nussbaum, & Bigler, 1988).

There are some misconceptions with regard to the relationship between ADHD and performance on IQ tests such as the WISC-R that should be mentioned. First, deficiency on the Freedom from Distractibility factor (arithmetic, coding, and digit span subscales) should not be considered as pathognomonic of ADHD. Difficulty on these subtests may be found among children with a variety of difficulties, and therefore is not specific to ADHD (Rapport, 1993). Second, findings of significant discrepancy between VIQ and PIQ as well as substantial intra- or intersubscale scatter have not been found to be specifically diagnostic of ADHD (Henry & Wittman, 1981; Kaufman, 1981).

Rapport (1993) and Barkley (1988) have reviewed commonly used neurocognitive instruments in the evaluation of children suspected of ADHD. These include the continuous performance test (CPT), the Matching Familiar Figures Test, the Underlining Test, and Mazes. These tests were briefly reviewed earlier in this chapter when we considered the assessment of attention. Below, we will focus primarily on CPTs because of their popularity.

There are various versions of CPTs available, differing the complexity of the task demands as well as specific stimulus presentation parameters, such as number of target stimuli presented, latency between stimulus presentation, and total test time. Klorman, Salzman, and Borgstedt (1988) note that there are three primary CPT models in use: The X version, the BX version, and the double-letter version. All three versions share in common the presentation of a single letter or number stimuli, lasting for a brief period of time (milliseconds to seconds), and presented in an unpredictable order.

The X version is the easiest type. These CPTs require the child to watch for a specific target letter (e.g., X) to be presented at which time the child is to immediately respond either by pressing a button or releasing a lever. The BX version requires the child to respond to the specified target letter (e.g., X) only when it is preceded by another designated letter, such as B. The child is instructed not to respond to presentation of letters not meeting these criteria. The double-letter version is the most difficult of the three models. This version requires the child to press the response key whenever any letter is presented twice in a row (Friedman, Vaughn, & Erlenmeyer-Kimling, 1978).

While the use of CPTs has become popular, the broad variety of specific CPTs available, with their various task demands and different stimulus and response parameters, makes it difficult to evaluate their usefulness as a group. In general, investigators have found that low-cognitive-demand CPTs such as the X version have not been sufficiently successful in discriminating among children with ADHD and normals (Schachar, Logan, Wachsmoth, & Chajczyk, 1988; Werry, Reeves, & Elkind, 1987). Even the more demanding CPTs tend to have poor discriminate validity for classifying ADHD children from normals when the total test duration is too short. Taken together, while CPTs show promise as a tool in the assessment process and perhaps for monitoring drug effects, they are not necessary nor sufficient for diagnosis of ADHD (Rapport, 1993).

The Matching Familiar Figures Task (MFFT) is described earlier in this chapter. This brief test considered to be a measure of impulsivity, although it is influenced by other variables such as attention, motivation, and intelligence (Douglas, 1988). Researchers have found that ADHD children usually make more errors and give their answers more quickly than normal controls (Rapport, Tucker, DuPaul, Merlo, & Stoner, 1986). Unfortunately, the MFFT has not been useful in differentiating ADHD children from children in other diagnostic groups (Werry, Reeves, & Elkind, 1987).

Maze performance has been used as a measure of impulsivity and sustained attention, with performance deficits being observed among ADHD children relative to normals (Milich & Kramer, 1984). Mazes have also been found to be sensitive to stimulant drug effects in ADHD children.

In recent yeas there has been increased interest in employing tests of executive functions in evaluation of children with suspected ADHD. Executive functions include one's planning abilities, ability to effectively choose desirable responses when given alternative choices, ability to effectively inhibit behavior, and overall complex behavioral regulation abilities. Inclusion of tests of executive functions is encouraged by a perspective that believes that many cases of ADHD are the result of dysfunction in the frontal lobes. The inference is made that because children with known frontal lobe damage tend to show deficits on executive function tests that children without brain damage but who show the same deficits on executive function tests may have frontal lobe dysfunction. This line of reasoning, by itself, is weak and requires empirical support to determine its meaningfulness. For example, the reasoning is analogous to stating, "All tires are round; some cheese is round; therefore, some tires are cheese." Empirical findings have emerged in recent years, however, to support the hypothesis that at least a subgroup of ADHD children may in fact have dysfunctional frontal systems. For example, Hynd et al. (1990, 1991) found that ADHD children tended to lack the typical asymmetry found between the size of the frontal lobes. Many of the ADHD children were also found to have smaller right frontal width and a smaller corpus callosum. In addition, Lou and colleagues (Lou, Henriksen, & Bruhn, 1984; Lou, Henriksen, Bruhn, Borner, & Nielsen, 1989) found that ADHD children showed hypoperfusion in part of the frontal lobes and caudate region. These findings were reversed by methylphenidate. Zametkin et al. (1990) used a positive emission tomography scan to study ADHD children and found reduced cerebral glucose utilization, especially in the frontal lobes.

Given these findings, it is reasonable to postulate that ADHD children should show deficits on cognitive tests putatively believed to be sensitive to frontal lobe dysfunction. To evaluate this question, Barkley and Grodzinsky (1994) examined the performance of 12 children with attention deficit disorder with hyperactivity (ADD + H), 12 children with attention deficit disorder without hyperactivity (ADD − H), 11 non-ADD LD children, and a normal community control group (*n* = 12), on the following tests of executive functions: CPT, F-A-S test, Hand Movements Scale, Porteus Mazes, Rey–Osterrieth Complex Figure, Stroop Color–Word Association Test, Trail Making Test, Wisconsin Card Sorting Test, and Grooved Pegboard Test. Results found that none of these tests resulted in adequate classification accuracy rates to distinguish between ADD + H and ADD − H. However, when the ADD groups were combined, acceptable levels of positive predictive power were found for the CPT and F-A-S (90% and above). Unfortunately, for these same tests, the negative predictive power was unacceptably low. As a result, while low scores on CPTs and F-A-S may be reasonably predictive of ADHD (relative to LD and normals), the presence of normal scores on these tests cannot be used to rule out ADHD. While these results argue against the use of these tests as screening measures (due to the high likelihood of false negatives), further research may find similar tests to be more useful. For example, in Barkley and Grodzinsky's study, a small sample was employed, which makes obtaining acceptable classifications rates more difficult. Second, in the clinical evaluation of children suspected of ADHD, many times the presence of LD can be ruled out. Therefore, if Barkley and Brodzinsky would have examined the classification rates comparing ADHD and normal controls, it is suspected that classification rates would have been better.

CURRENT ISSUES AND FUTURE DIRECTIONS

Child neuropsychological assessment may be performed in the service of several goals, including diagnosis of brain impairment, description of the type and severity of cognitive deficits, making predictions about functional capacities, and to inform treatment planning. Any combination of these goals may be emphasized in a given referral for neuropsychological assessment. Competence to practice child neuropsychology extends far beyond being familiar with the administration and scoring of a number of "neuropsychological tests." The child neuropsychologist must be well versed with regard to the reliability and validity of each of the tests used as they pertain to separate assessment goals (e.g., diagnosis, prediction of functional capacities, etc.). Grounding in clinical child psychology, developmental psychology, and the basics of pediatric neurology are required to select assessment tools, carry out, and complete a competent child neuropsychological examination. The International Neuropsychological Society has published general education and training guidelines for clinical neuropsychologists. However, specific training recommendations for child neuropsychologists have not been made. We suspect that child clinical neuropsychology will become a subspecialty just as child clinical psychology is generally considered to be a subspecialty within general clinical psychology.

Even for clinicians with a solid background in clinical child neuropsychology, the pace of changes in the knowledge base is rapid. Continued competency requires the clinician to keep current on the literature on brain–behavior relationships, changes in assessment tools, studies of test validity for the multiple goals of neuropsychological assessment, and advances in treatment. We suspect that the pace of new test development will continue to increase. We should caution, however, that marketing of new assessment tools commonly soars far in advance of the collection of needed empirical research examining their clinical utility. An open yet critical eye is most appropriate.

REFERENCES

Achenbach, T. M. (1986). *The direct observation form of the Child Behavior Checklist* (rev. ed). Burlington: University of Vermont, Department of Psychiatry.

Achenbach, T. M. (1991). *Manual for the youth self-report and 1991 profile.* Burlington: University of Vermont, Department of Psychiatry.

Achenbach, T. M., & Edelbrock, C. S. (1983). *Manual for the Child Behavior Checklist and revised Child Behavior Profile.* Burlington, VT: T. M. Achenbach.

Annett, M. (1973). Laterality of childhood hemiplegia and the growth of speech and intelligence. *Cortex, 9,* 4–33.

Barkley, R. A. (1981). *Hyperactive children: A handbook for diagnosis and treatment.* New York: Guilford Press.

Barkley, R. A. (1988). Attention. In M. G. Tramontana & S. R. Hooper (Eds.), *Assessment issues in child neuropsychology. Critical issues in neuropsychology* (pp. 145–176). New York: Plenum Press.

Barkley, R. A., & Grodzinsky, G. M. (1994). Are tests of frontal lobe functions useful in the diagnosis of attention deficit disorders? *The Clinical Neuropsychologist, 8,* 121–139.

Basser, L. S. (1962). Hemiplegia of early onset and the faculty of speech with special reference to the effects of hemispherectomy. *Brain, 85,* 427–460.

Bawden, H. N. (1985). Speeded performance following head injury in children. *Journal of Clinical & Experimental Neuropsychology, 7,* 39–54.

Beery, K. E., & Buktenica, N. A. (1989). *Developmental Test of Visual–Motor Integration.* Odessa, FL: Psychological Assessment Resources.

Beitchman, J. H., & Corradini, A. (1988). Self-report measures for use with children: A review and comment. *Journal of Clinical Psychology, 44,* 477–490.

Bender, L. (1938). *A visual motor gestalt test and its clinical use* (Research Monograph No. 3). New York: American Orthopsychiatric Association.

Benton, A. L., Hamsher, K. deS., Varney, N. R., & Spreen, O. (1993). *Contributions to neuropsychological assessment.* New York: Oxford University Press.

Benton, A. L., & Pearl, D. (1978). *Dyslexia.* New York: Oxford University Press.

Berg, R. A., Bolter, J. F., Ch'ien, L. T., Williams, S. J., Lancaster, W., & Cummins, J. (1984). Comparative diagnostic accuracy of the Halstead–Reitan and the Luria–Nebraska Neuropsychological Adults and Children's Batteries. *Clinical Neuropsychology, 6,* 200–204.

Bigler, E. D. (1988). The role of neuropsychological assessment in relation to other types of assessment with children. In M. G. Tramontana & S. R. Hooper (Eds.), *Assessment issues in child neuropsychology. Critical issues in neuropsychology* (pp. 67–91). New York: Plenum Press.

Boll, T. J. (1974). Behavioral correlates of cerebral damage in children aged 9–14. In R. M. Reitan & L. A. Davison (Eds.), *Clinical neuropsychology: Current status and applications* (pp. 91–120). Washington, DC: Winston.

Boll, T. J. (1981). The Halstead–Reitan Neuropsychology Battery. In S. B. Filskov & T. J. Boll (Eds), *Handbook of clinical neuropsychology* (pp. 577–607). New York: Wiley.

Boll, T. J. (1993). *Children's Category Test.* New York: The Psychological Corporation.

Boyd, T. A. (1988). Clinical assessment of memory in children: A developmental framework for practice. In M. G. Tramontana & S. R. Hooper (Eds.), *Assessment issues in child neuropsychology. Critical issues in neuropsychology* (pp. 177–204). New York: Plenum Press.

Brink, J., Garrett, A., Hale, W., Woo-Sum, J., & Nickel, V. (1970). Recovery of motor and intellectual function in children sustaining severe head injuries. *Developmental Medicine and Child Neurology, 12,* 565–571.

Brown, A. L. (1975). The development of memory, knowing, knowing about knowing, and knowing how to know. In H. W. Reese (Ed.), *Advances in child development and behavior* (Vol. 10, pp. 103–152). New York: Academic Press.

Brown, G., Chadwick, O., Shaffer, D., Rutter, M., & Traub, M. (1981). A prospective study of children with head injuries: Psychiatric sequelae. *Psychological Medicine, 11,* 63–78.

Brown, L., & Hammill, D. D. (1983). *Examiner's manual for the Behavior Rating Profile,* Austin, TX: PRO-ED.

Buschke, H. (1974). Components of verbal learning in children: Analysis by selective reminding. *Journal of Experimental Child Psychology, 18,* 488–496.

Butcher, J. N., Williams, C. L., Graham, J. R., Archer, R. P., Tellegen, A., Ben-Porath, Y. S., & Kaemmer, B. (1992). *MMPI-A: Manual for administration, scoring, and interpretation.* Minneapolis: University of Minnesota Press.

Bzoch, K. R., & League, R. (1971). *Receptive–Expressive Emergent Language Scale.* Gainesville, FL: Tree of Life Press.

Caplan, D. (1995). Language disorders. In R. L. Mapou & J. Spector (Eds.), *Clinical neuropsychological assessment: A cognitive approach* (pp. 83–113). New York: Plenum Press.

Carr, M. (1983). A test of clinical utility: The Luria–Nebraska Neuropsychological Battery, Children's Revision. (Doctoral dissertation, Boston University Graduate School, 1983). *Dissertation Abstracts International, 44,* 1586.

Carrow, E. (1985). *Test for Auditory Comprehension of Language—Revised.* Boston: Teaching Resources.

Chadwick, O., Rutter, M., Brown, G., Shaffer, D., & Traub, M. (1981). A prospective study of children with head injuries: II. Cognitive sequelae. *Psychological Medicine, 11,* 49–62.

Chadwick, O., Rutter, M., Shaffer, D., & Shrout, P. E. (1981). A prospective study of children with head injuries: IV. Specific cognitive deficits. *Journal of Clinical Neuropsychology, 3,* 101–120.

Chambers, W. J., Puig-Antich, J., Hirsch, M., Paez, P., Ambrosini, P. J., Tabrizi, A., & Davies, M. (1985). The assessment of affective disorders in children and adolescents by semistructured interview: Test–retest reliability of the Schedule for Affective Disorders and Schizophrenia for School-Age Children, Present Episode Version. *Archives of General Psychiatry, 42,* 696–702.

Chelune, G. J., & Thompson, L. L. (1987). Evaluation of the general sensitivity of the Wisconsin Card Sorting Test among younger and older children. *Developmental Neuropsychology, 3,* 81–89.

Clodfelter, C. J., Dickson, A. L., Newton-Wilkes, C., & Johnson, R. B. (1987). Alternate forms of selective reminding for children. *Clinical Neuropsychologist, 1,* 243–249.

Costello, A., Edelbrock, C., Kalas, R., Kessler, M., & Klaric, S. (1984). *NIMH Diagnostic Interview Schedule for Children (DISC).* Rockville, MD: National Institute of Mental Health.

Crary, M. A., Voeller, K. K. S., & Haak, N. J. (1988). Questions of developmental neurolinguistic assessment. In M. G. Tramontana & S. R. Hooper (Eds.), *Assessment issues in child neuropsychology. Critical issues in neuropsychology* (pp. 249–279). New York: Plenum Press.

Crawford, J. R., Stewart, L. E., & Moore, J. W. (1989). Demonstration of savings on the AVLT and development of a parallel form. *Journal of Clinical and Experimental Neuropsychology, 11,* 975–981.

Curry, J. F., Logue, P. E., & Butler, B. (1986). Child and adolescent norms for Russell's revision of the Wechsler Memory Scale. *Journal of Clinical Child Psychology, 15,* 214–220.

DeFries, J. C. (1989). Gender ratios in children with reading disability and their affected relatives: A commentary. *Journal of Learning Disabilities, 22,* 544–545.

Delis, D. C., Kramer, J., Kaplan, E., & Ober, B. A. (1994). *California Verbal Learning Test— Children's Version.* New York: The Psychological Corporation.

Dennis, M. (1988). Language and the young damaged brain. In T. Boll & B. K. Bryant (Eds.), *Clinical neuropsychology and brain function: Research, measurement, and practice. The master lecture series* (Vol. 7, pp. 89–123). Washington, DC: American Psychological Association.

Dennis, M. (1992). Word finding in children and adolescents with a history of brain injury. *Topics in Language Disorders, 13,* 66–82.

Denton, C. L., & McIntyre, C. W. (1978). Span of apprehension in hyperactive boys. *Journal of Abnormal Child Psychology, 6,* 19–24.

Dorman, C., & Katzir, B. (1994). *Cognitive effects of early brain injury.* Baltimore, MD: Johns Hopkins University Press.

Douglas, V. I. (1988). Cognitive deficits in children with attention deficit disorder with hyperactivity. In L. M. Bloomingdale & J. A. Sergeant (Eds.), *Attention deficit disorder: Criteria, cognition, intervention* (pp. 65–81). New York: Pergamon Press.

Duffy, J. B., Ritter, D. R., & Fedner, M. (1976). Developmental Test of Visual–Motor Integration and the Goodenough Draw-a-Man Test as predictors of academic success. *Perceptual and Motor Skills, 43,* 543–546.

Eide, P. K., & Tysnes, O. B. (1992). Early and late outcome in head injury patients with radiologic evidence of brain damage. *Acta Neurologica Scandinavica, 86,* 194–198.

Ernhart, C. B., Graham, F. K., Eichman, P. L., Marshall, J. M., & Thurston, D. (1963). Brain injury in the preschool child: Some developmental considerations. II. Comparison of brain injured and normal children. *Psychological Monographs, 77* (Whole No. 574), 17–33.

Ewing-Cobbs, L., Fletcher, J. M., Landry, S. H., & Levin, H. S. (1985). Language disorders after pediatric head injury. In J. K. Darby (Ed.), *Speech and language evaluation in neurology: Childhood disorders* (pp. 97–111). San Diego: Grune & Stratton.

Fenichel, G. M. (1988). *Clinical pediatric neurology.* Philadelphia: Saunders.

Fisk, J. L., & Rourke, B. P. (1979). Identification of subtypes of learning disabled children at three age levels: A neuropsychological, multivariate approach. *Journal of Clinical Neuropsychology, 1,* 29–31.

Fletcher, J. M. (1988). Brain-injured children. In E. J. Mash & L. G. Terdal (Eds.), *Behavioral assessment of childhood disorders* (Vol. 2, pp. 451–489). New York: Guilford Press.

Fletcher, J. M., Miner, M. E., & Ewing-Cobbs, L. (1987). Age and recovery from head injury in children: Developmental issues. In H. S. Levin, J. Grafman, & H. M. Eisenberg (Eds.), *Neurobehavioral recovery from head injury* (pp. 279–291). New York: Oxford University Press.

Fletcher, J. M., & Satz, P. (1980). Developmental changes in the neuropsychological correlates of reading achievement: A six-year longitudinal follow-up. *Journal of Clinical Neuropsychology, 2,* 23–37.

Fletcher, J. M., & Taylor, H. G. (1984). Neuropsychological approaches to children: Towards a developmental neuropsychology. *Journal of Clinical Neuropsychology, 6,* 24–37.

Fletcher, S. G. (1978). *The Fletcher Time-by-Count Test of Diadochokinetic Syllable Rate.* New York: Tigard, C. C. Publications.

Forehand, R. L., & Brody, G. (1985). The association between parental personal/marital adjustment and parent–child interactions in a clinic sample. *Behaviour Research & Therapy, 23,* 211–212.

Foster, S. L., & Cone, J. D. (1986). Design and use of direct observation procedures. In A. R. Ciminero, K. S. Calhoun, & H. E. Adams (Eds.), *Handbook of behavioral assessment* (2nd ed., pp. 253–324). New York: Wiley.

Frankenburg, W. K., Dodds, J. B., Fandel, A. W., Kazuk, E., & Cohrs, M. (1975). *Denver Developmental Screening Test.* Denver: LADOCA Project and Publishing Foundation.

Friedman, D., Vaughan, H., & Erlenmeyer-Kimling, L. (1978). Task related cortical potentials in children in two kinds of vigilance tasks. In D. A. Otto (Ed.), *Multidisciplinary perspectives in event-related brain potential research* (pp. 309–313). Washington, DC: US Government Printing Office.

Gaddes, W. H., & Edgell, D. (1993). *Learning disabilities and brain function* (3rd ed.). New York: Springer.

Gardner, W. J., Karnoch, I. J., McClure, C. C., & Gardner, A. K. (1955). Residual function following hemispherectomy for tumour and for infantile hemiplegia. *Brain, 78,* 487–502.

Gates, R. D. (1984). Florida Kindergarten Screening Battery. *Journal of Clinical Neuropsychology, 6,* 459–465.

Geary, D. C., & Gilger, J. W. (1984). The Luria–Nebraska Neuropsychological Battery—Children's Revision: Comparison of learning-disabled and normal children matched on full scale IQ. *Perceptual and Motor Skills, 58,* 115–118.

Glutting, J. J., & Kaplan, D. (1990). Stanford–Binet Intelligence Scale, fourth edition: Making the case for reasonable interpretations. In C. R. Reynolds & R. W. Kamphaus (Eds.), *Handbook of psychological and educational assessment of children* (pp. 277–295). New York: Guilford.

Golden, C. J. (1981). The Luria–Nebraska Children's Battery: Theory and formulation. In G. W. Hynd & J. E. Obrzut (Eds.), *Neuropsychological assessment and the school-age child: Issues and perspectives* (pp. 277–302). New York: Grune & Stratton.

Golden, C. J. (1988). The Nebraska Neuropsychological Children's Battery. In C. R. Reynolds & E. Fletcher-Janzen (Eds.), *Handbook of clinical child neuropsychology* (pp. 193–204). New York: Plenum Press.

Goldstein, F. C., & Levin, H. S. (1985). Intellectual and academic outcome following closed head injury in children and adolescents: Research strategies and empirical findings. *Developmental Neuropsychology, 1,* 195–214.

Goyette, C. H., Conners, C. K., & Ulrich, R. F. (1978). Normative data on revised Conners Parent and Teacher Rating Scales. *Journal of Abnormal Child Psychology, 6,* 221–236.

Gustavson, J. L., Golden, C. J., Wilkening, G. N., Hermann, B. P., Plaisted, J. R., MacInnes, W. D., & Leark, R. A. (1984). The Luria–Nebraska Neuropsychological Battery—Children's Revision: Validation with brain-damaged and normal children. *Journal of Psychoeducational Assessment, 2,* 199–208.

Halperin, J. M., Healey, J. M., Zeitchik, E., Ludman, W. L., & Weinstein, L. (1989). The development of linguistic and mnestic abilities in school-age children. *Journal of Clinical and Experimental Neuropsychology, 11,* 518–528.

Hammill, D. D., & Newcomer, P. L. (1982). *Test of language development.* Austin, TX: Pro-Ed.

Henry, S. A., & Wittman, R. D. (1981). Diagnostic implications of Bannatyne's recategorized WISC-R scores for identifying learning disabled children. *Journal of Learning Disabilities, 14,* 517–520.

Herjanic, B., & Campbell, W. (1977). Differentiating psychiatrically disturbed children on the basis of a structured interview. *Journal of Abnormal Psychology, 5,* 127–134.

Herjanic, B., & Reich, W. (1982). Development of a structured psychiatric interview for children: Agreement between child and parent on individual symptoms. *Journal of Abnormal Child Psychology, 10,* 307–324.

Hetherington, E. M., & Martin, B. (1979). Family interaction. In H. C. Quay & J. S. Werry (Eds.), *Psychopathological disorders of childhood* (2nd ed., pp. 247–302). New York: Wiley.

Hodges, K., McKnew, D., Cytryn, L., Stern., L., & Kline, J. (1982). The Child Assessment Schedule (CAS) diagnostic interview: A report of reliability and validity. *Journal of the American Academy of Child Psychiatry, 21,* 468–473.

Hynd, G. W. (1988). *Neuropsychological assessment in clinical child psychology.* Newbury Park, CA: Sage.

Hynd, G. W., Semrud-Clikeman, M., Lorys, A. R., Novey, E. S., & Eliopulos, D. (1990). Brain morphology in developmental dyslexia and attention deficit disorder/hyperactivity. *Archives of Neurology, 47,* 919–926.

Hynd, G. W., Semrud-Clikeman, M., Lorys, A. R., Novey, E. S., Eliopulos, D., & Lyytinen, H. (1991). Corpus callosum morphology in attention deficit-hyperactivity disorder (ADHD): Morphometric analysis of MRI. *Journal of Learning Disabilities, 3,* 141–146.

Isaacson, R. L. (1975). The myth of recovery from early brain damage. In N. Ellis (Ed.), *Aberrant development in infancy* (pp. 1–26). London: Wiley.

Kagan, J., Rosman, B., Day, D., Albert, J., & Phillips, W. (1964). Information processing in the child: Significance of analytic and reflective attitudes. *Psychological Monographs, 78* (1, Whole No. 578).

Kail, R. (1975). *Interrelations in children's use of mnemonic strategies.* Unpublished doctoral dissertation, University of Michigan.

Kail, R., & Hagen, J. W. (1982). Memory in childhood. In B. Wolman, G. Stricker, S. Ellman, P. Keith-Spiegel, & D. Palermo (Eds.), *Handbook of developmental psychology* (pp. 350–366). Englewood Cliffs, NJ: Prentice-Hall.

Kaufman, A. S. (1981). The WISC-R and learning disabilities assessment: State of the art. *Journal of Learning Disabilities, 14,* 520–526.

Kemper, M. B., Hagerman, R. J., Ahmad, R. S., & Mariner, R. (1986). Cognitive profiles and the spectrum of clinical manifestations in heterozygous fragile X females. *American Journal of Medical Genetics, 23,* 139–156.

Kinsbourne, M. (1984). Beyond attention deficit: Search for the disorder in ADD. In L. Bloomingdale (Ed.), *Attention deficit disorder; Diagnostic, cognitive, and therapeutic understanding* (pp. 133–162). New York: Spectrum Publications.

Kistner, J. A., & Torgesen, J. K. (1987). Motivational and cognitive aspects of learning disabilities. In B. B. Lahey & A. E. Kazdin (Eds.), *Advances in clinical child psychology* (Vol. 10, pp. 289–333). New York: Plenum Press.

Klee, S. H., & Garfinkel, B. D. (1983). The Computerized Continuous Performance Task: A new measure of inattention. *Journal of Abnormal Child Psychology, 11,* 487–496.

Klorman, R., Salzman, L. F., & Borgstedt, A. D. (1988). Brain event-related potentials in evaluation of cognitive deficits in attention deficit disorder and outcome of stimulant therapy. In L. M. Bloomingdale (Ed.), *Attention deficit disorder: Vol. 3. New research in attention, treatment, and psychopharmacology* (pp. 49–80). Oxford: Pergamon Press.

Kolb, B., & Whishaw, I. (1985). *Fundamentals in human neuropsychology* (2nd ed.). New York: Freeman.

Kovacs, M. (1982). *The longitudinal study of child and adolescent psychopathology: I. The Semi-Structured Psychiatric Interview Schedule for Children (ISC).* Unpublished manuscript, Western Psychiatric Institute.

Kovacs, M. (1985). The Children's Depression Inventory (CDI), *Psychopharmacology Bulletin, 21,* 995–998.

Kraus, J. F., Rock, A., & Hemyari, P. (1990). Brain injuries among infants, children, adolescents, and young adults. *American Journal of Disabilities in Children, 144,* 684–691.

Kreutzer, M., Leonard, C., & Flavell, J. (1975). An interview study of children's knowledge about memory. *Monographs of the Society for Research in Child Development, 40,* (1, Whole No. 159).

Lachar, D. (1982). *Personality Inventory for Children (PIC).* Los Angeles: Western Psychological Services.

Lachar, D. (1990). Objective assessment of child and adolescent personality: The Personality Inventory for Children (PIC). In C. R. Reynolds & R. W. Kamphaus (Eds.), *Handbook of psychological and educational assessment of children* (pp. 298–323). New York: Guilford Press.

Lachar, D., & Gruber, C. P. (1994). *A manual for the Personality Inventory for Youth (PIY): A self-report comparison to the Personality Inventory for Children (PIC)*. Los Angeles: Western Psychological Services.

Lee, L. L. (1971). *Northwestern Syntax Screening Test*. Evanston, IL: Northwestern University Press.

Levin, H. S., Aldrich, E. F., & Saydjari, C. (1992). Severe head injury in children: Experience of the traumatic coma data bank. *Neurosurgery, 32,* 435–443.

Levin, H. S., & Eisenberg, H. M (1979a). Neuropsychological impairment after closed head injury in children and adolescents. *Journal of Pediatric Psychology, 4,* 389–402.

Levin, H. S., & Eisenberg, H. M. (1979b). Neuropsychological outcome of closed head injury in children and adolescents. *Child's Brain, 5,* 281–292.

Levin, H. S., Ewing-Cobbs, L., & Benton, A. L. (1984). Age and recovery from brain damage: A review of clinical studies. In S. W. Scheff (Ed.), *Aging and recovery of function in the central nervous system* (pp. 169–205). New York: Plenum Press.

Levin, H. S., Grafman, J. & Eisenberg, H. M. (1987). *Neurobehavioral recovery from brain injury*. New York: Oxford University Press.

Levin, H. S., Mendelsohn, D., Lilly, M. A., Fletcher, J. A., Culhane, K. A., Chapman, S. B., Harward, H., Kusnerik, C., Bruce, D., & Eisenberg, H. M. (1994). Tower of London performance in relation to magnetic resonance imaging following closed head injury in children. *Neuropsychology, 8,* 171–179.

Levine, S. C., Huttenlocher, P., Banich, M. T., & Duda, E. (1987). Factors affecting cognitive functioning of hemiplegic children. *Developmental Medicine and Child Neurology, 29,* 27–35.

Lindgren, S. D., & Benton, A. L. (1980). Developmental patterns of visuospatial judgment. *Journal of Pediatric Psychology, 5,* 217–225.

Lou, H. C., Henriksen, L., & Bruhn, P. (1984). Focal cerebral hypoperfusion in children with dysphasia and/or attention deficit disorder. *Archives of Neurology, 41,* 825–829.

Lou, H. C., Henriksen, L., Bruhn, P., Borner, H., & Nielsen, J. B. (1989). Striatal dysfunction in attention deficit and hyperkinetic disorder. *Archives of Neurology, 46,* 48–52.

Markwardt, F. C. (1989). *Peabody Individual Achievement Test—Revised*. Circle Pines, MN: American Guidance Service.

Massman, P. J., Nussbaum, N. L., & Bigler, E. D. (1988). The mediating effect of age on the relationship between Child Behavior Checklist hyperactivity scores and neuropsychological test performance. *Journal of Abnormal Child Psychology, 16,* 89–95.

McConaughy, S. H., & Achenbach, T. M. (1988). *Practical guide for the Child Behavior Checklist and related materials*. Burlington: University of Vermont, Department of Psychiatry.

McConaughy, S. H., & Achenbach, T. M. (1990). *Guide for the Semistructured Clinical Interview for children aged 6–11*. Burlington: University of Vermont, Department of Psychiatry.

McGee, R., & Share, D. L. (1988). Attention deficit disorder-hyperactivity and academic failure: Which comes first and what should be treated? *Journal of the American Academy of Child & Adolescent Psychiatry, 27,* 318–325.

Meerwaldt, J. D., & van Dongen, H. R. (1988). Disturbances of spatial perception in children. *Behavioral Brain Research, 31,* 131–134.

Menyuk, P., & Bernholts, N. (1969). Prosodic features and children's language. *Quarterly Progress Report of Research Laboratory of Electronics, 93,* 216–219.

Milich, R., & Kramer, J. (1984). Reflections on impulsivity: An empirical investigation of impulsivity as a construct. *Advances in Learning and Behavioral Disabilities, 3,* 57–94.

Morgan, S. F. (1982). Measuring long-term memory, storage, and retrieval in children. *Journal of Clinical Neuropsychology, 4,* 77–85.

National Joint Committee for Learning Disabilities. (1987). Perspectives in dyslexia. *Journal of Learning Disabilities, 20,* 107–108.

Nolan, D. R., Hammeke, T. A., & Barkley, R. A. (1983). A comparison of the patterns of the neuropsychological performance in two groups of learning-disabled children. *Journal of Clinical Child Psychology, 12,* 13–21.

Parker, R. S. (1990). *Traumatic brain injury and neuropsychological impairment.* New York: Springer-Verlag.

Pennington, B. F. (1991). *Diagnosing learning disorders: A neuropsychological framework.* New York: Guilford Press.

Pennington, B. F., Heaton, R. K., Karzmark, P., Pendleton, M. G., Lehman, R., & Shucard, D. W. (1985). The neuropsychological phenotype in Turner syndrome. *Cortex, 21,* 391–404.

Puig-Antich, J., & Chambers, W. (1978). *The Schedule for Affective Disorders and Schizophrenia for School-Aged Children.* New York: New York State Psychiatric Institute.

Quay, H. C., & Peterson, D. R. (1983). *Interim manual for the Revised Behavior Problem Checklist.* Unpublished manuscript, University of Miami.

Rapport, M. D. (1993). Attention deficit hyperactivity disorder. In T. H. Ollendick & M. Hersen (Eds.), *Handbook of child and adolescent assessment. General psychology series* (Vol. 167, pp. 269–291). Boston: Allyn & Bacon.

Rapport, M. D., Tucker, S. B., DuPaul, G. J., Merlo, M., & Stoner, G. (1986). Hyperactivity and frustration: The influence of control over and size of rewards in delaying gratification. *Journal of Abnormal Child Psychology, 14,* 191–204.

Reed, H. B. C., Reitan, R. M., & Klove, H. (1965). Influence of cerebral lesions on psychological test performance of older children. *Journal of Consulting Psychology, 29,* 247–251.

Reitan, R. M. (1969). *Manual for administration of neuropsychological test batteries for adults and children.* Indianapolis, IN: Author.

Reitan, R. M. (1974). Psychological effects of cerebral lesions in children of early school age. In R. M. Reitan & L. A. Davison (Eds.), *Clinical neuropsychology: Current status and applications* (pp. 53–90). Washington, DC: Winston.

Reitan, R. M., & Boll, T. J. (1973). Neuropsychological correlates of minimal brain dysfunction. *Annals of the New York Academy of Sciences, 205,* 65–88.

Reynolds, C. R. (1990). Conceptual and technical problems in learning disability diagnosis. In C. R. Reynolds & R. W. Kamphaus (Eds.), *Handbook of psychological and educational assessment of children* (pp. 571–592). New York: Guilford Press.

Reynolds, C. R., & Bigler, E. (1994). Tests of memory and learning. Los Angeles: Western Psychological Services.

Reynolds, C. R., & Richmond, B. O. (1985). *Revised Children's Manifest Anxiety Scale (RCMAS).* Los Angeles: Western Psychological Services.

Reynolds, W. M. (1986). *Reynolds Adolescent Depression Inventory.* Odessa, FL: Psychological Assessment Resources.

Richman, L. C., & Lindgren, S. D. (1981). Verbal mediation deficits: Relation to behavior and achievement in children. *Journal of Abnormal Psychology, 90,* 99–104.

Riley, G., & Riley, J. (1985). *Oral motor assessment and treatment: Improving syllable production.* New York: Tigard, C. C. Publications.

Rourke, B. P. (1982). Central processing deficiencies in children: Toward a developmental neuropsychological model. *Journal of Clinical Neuropsychology, 4,* 1–18.

Rourke, B. P. (1989). *Nonverbal learning disabilities: The syndrome and the model.* New York: Guilford Press.

Rourke, B. P., & Finlayson, M. A. J. (1978). Neuropsychological significance of variations in patterns of academic performance: Verbal and visual–spatial abilities. *Journal of Abnormal Child Psychology, 6,* 121–133.

Rourke, B. P., & Gates, R. D. (1980). *Underlining Test: Preliminary norms.* Windsor, Ontario: Author.

Rourke, B. P., & Gates, R. D. (1981). Neuropsychological research and school psychology. In G. W. Hynd & J. E. Obrzut (Eds.), *Neuropsychological assessment of the school-age child: Issues and procedures* (pp. 3–25). New York: Grune & Stratton.

Rourke, B. P., & Orr, R. (1977). Prediction of the reading and spelling performances of normal and retarded readers: A four-year follow-up. *Journal of Abnormal Child Psychology, 5,* 9–20.

Rudel, R. G. (1978). Neuroplasticity: Implications for development and education. In J. S. Chall & A. F. Mirsky (Eds.), *Education and the brain (Part II).* Chicago: University of Chicago Press.

Rutter, M. (1982). Developmental neuropsychiatry: Concepts, issues, and prospects. *Journal of Clinical Neuropsychology, 4,* 91–115.

Ryckman, D. B., & Rentfrow, R. K. (1971). The Beery Developmental Test of Visual–Motor Integration: An investigation of reliability. *Journal of Learning Disabilities, 4,* 333–334.

Schachar, R., Logan, G., Wachsmoth, R., & Chajczyk, D. (1988). Attaining and maintaining preparation: A comparison of attention in hyperactive, normal, and disturbed control children. *Journal of Abnormal Child Psychology, 16,* 361–378.

Seidel, U. P., Chadwick, O., & Rutter, M. (1975). Psychological disorders in crippled children: A comparative study of children with and without brain damage. *Developmental Medicine and Child Neurology, 17,* 563–573.

Shallice, T. (1982). Specific impairments of planning. In D. E. Broadbent & L. Weiskrautz (Eds.), *The neuropsychology of cognitive function* (pp. 199–209). London: The Royal Society.

Shallice, T. (1988). *From neuropsychology to mental structure.* Cambridge, England: Cambridge University Press.

Shapiro, K., & Smith, L. P. (1993). Special considerations for the pediatric age group. In P. R. Cooper (Ed.), *Head Injury* (3rd ed., pp. 427–458). Baltimore: Williams & Wilkins.

Shaywitz, S. E., Schnell, C., Shaywitz, B. A., & Towle, V. R. (1986). Yale Children's Inventory (YCI): An instrument to assess children with attentional deficits and learning disabilities: I. Scale development and psychometric properties. *Journal of Abnormal Child Psychology, 14,* 347–364.

Shaywitz, S. E., Shaywitz, B. A., Fletcher, J. M., & Escobar, M. D. (1990). Prevalence of reading disabilities in boys and girls: Results of the Connecticut Longitudinal Study. *Journal of American Medical Association, 264,* 998–1002.

Sheslow, D., & Adams, W. (1990). *Wide Range Assessment of Memory and Learning.* Wilmington, DE: Jastak Associates.

Slomka, G. T., & Tarter, R. E. (1993). Neuropsychological assessment. In T. H. Ollendick & M. Hersen (Eds.), *Handbook of child and adolescent assessment. General psychology series* (Vol. 167, pp. 208–223). Boston: Allyn & Bacon.

Smith, A. (1982). *Symbol Digit Modalities Test.* Los Angeles: Western Psychological Services.

Snow, J. H., & Hynd, G. W. (1985a). A multivariate investigation of the Luria–Nebraska Neuropsychological Battery—Children's Revision with learning-disabled children. *Journal of Psychoeducational Assessment, 3,* 101–109.

Snow, J. H., & Hynd, G. W. (1985b). Factor structure of the Luria–Nebraska Neuropsychological Battery—Children's Revision. *Journal of School Psychology, 23,* 271–276.

Snow, J. H., Hynd, G. W., & Hartlage, L. C. (1984). Difference between mildly and more severely learning-disabled children on the Luria–Nebraska Neuropsychological Battery—Children's Revision. *Journal of Psychoeducational Assessment, 2,* 23–28.

Spreen, O., Risser, A. H., & Edgell, D. (1995). *Developmental neuropsychology.* New York: Oxford University Press.

St. James-Roberts, I. (1979). Neurological plasticity, recovery from brain insult, and child development. In H. W. Reese & L. P. Lipsitt (Eds.), *Advances in child development and behavior* (pp. 253–319). New York: Academic Press.

Stevenson, H., Parker, T., & Wilkinson, A. (1975). *Ratings and measures of memory processes in young children.* Unpublished manuscript, University of Michigan.

Stiles-Davis, J., Sugarman, S., & Nass, R. (1985). The development of spatial and class relations in four young children with right-cerebral-hemisphere damage: Evidence for an early spatial constructive deficit. *Brain & Cognition, 4,* 388–412.

Stone, W. L., & LeManek, K. L. (1990). Developmental issues in children's self-reports. In A. M. La Greca (Ed.), *Through the eyes of the child: Obtaining self-reports from children and adolescents* (pp. 18–56). Boston: Allyn & Bacon.

Tarter, R. E., Van Theil, D. H., & Edwards, K. L. (Eds.). (1988). *Medical neuropsychology: The impact of disease on behavior. Critical issues in neuropsychology* (pp. 75–97). New York: Plenum Press.

Taylor, H. G., & Fletcher, J. M. (1990). Neuropsychological assessment of children. In G. Goldstein, & M. Hersen (Eds.), *Handbook of psychological assessment* (pp. 228–255). New York: Pergamon Press.

Teasdale, G., & Jennett, B. (1974). Assessment of coma and injured consciousness: A practical scale. *Lancet, 2,* 81–83.

Templin, M., & Darley, F. (1969). *Templin–Darley Tests of Articulation* (2nd ed.). Iowa City: Burea of Educational Research and Services, University of Iowa.

Thompson, L. L., Heaton, R. K., Mathews, C. G., & Grant, J. (1987). Comparison of preferred and nonpreferred hand performance on four neuropsychological motor tasks. *Clinical Neuropsychology, 1,* 324–334.

Thorndike, R. L., Hagen, E. P., & Sattler, J. M (1986). *Stanford–Binet Intelligence Scale: Fourth Edition.* Chicago: Riverside.

Timmermans, S. R., & Christensen, B. (1991). The measurement of attention deficits in TBI children and adolescents. *Cognitive Rehabilitation, 9,* 26–31.

Tramontana, M. G., & Hooper, S. R. (1988). Child neuropsychological assessment: Overview of current status. In M. G. Tramontana & S. R. Hooper (Eds.), *Assessment issues in child neuropsychology. Critical issues in neuropsychology* (pp. 3–38). New York: Plenum Press.

Tramontana, M. G., Sherrets, S. D., & Wolf, B. A. (1983). Comparability of the Luria–Nebraska and Halstead–Reitan neuropsychological batteries for older children. *The International Journal of Clinical Neuropsychology, 5,* 186–190.

van Zomeren, A. H., & Brouwer, W. H. (1994). *Clinical neuropsychology of attention.* New York: Oxford Press.

Wechsler, D. (1991). *Wechsler Intelligence Scale for Children—Third Edition.* New York: The Psychological Corporation.

Wechsler, D. (1992). *Wechsler Individual Achievement Test.* New York: The Psychological Corporation.

Wechsler, D. (1995). *Children's Memory Scale.* San Antonio, TX: The Psychological Corporation.

Werry, J. S., Reeves, J. C., & Elkind, G. S. (1987). Attention deficit, conduct, oppositional, and anxiety disorders in children: III. Laboratory differences. *Journal of Abnormal Child Psychology, 15,* 409–428.

Wiig, E. H. (1982a). *Let's talk: Developing prosocial communication skills.* Columbus, OH: Charles E. Merrill.

Wiig, E. H. (1982b). *Let's talk inventory for adolescents.* Columbus, OH: Charles E. Merrill.

Wiig, E. H., & Bray, C. M. (1983). *Let's talk for children.* Columbus, OH: Charles E. Merrill.

Wilkening, G. N., Golden, C. J., MacInnes, W. D., Plaisted, J. R., & Hermann, B. P. (1981, August). *The Luria–Nebraska Neuropsychological Battery—Children's Revision: A preliminary report.* Paper presented at the meeting of the American Psychological Association, Los Angeles, CA.

Wilkinson, G. S. (1993). *The Wide Range Achievement Test* (3rd ed.). Wilmington DE: Jastak. D. C., Zorn, G. L., & Kirklin, J. K. (1995). *Neurocognitive and emotional deficits in lung transplant candidates.* Unpublished manuscript.

Winogron, H. W., Knights, R. M., & Bawden, H. N. (1984). Neuropsychological deficits following head injury in children. *Journal of Clinical Neuropsychology, 6,* 269–286.

Witelson, S. F. (1987). Neurobiological aspects of language in children. *Child Development, 58,* 653–688.

Witken, H. A., Oltman, P., Raskin, E., & Karp, S. (1971). *Manual for the Children's Embedded Figures Test.* Palo Alto, CA: Consulting Psychologists Press.

Woodcock, R. W., & Johnson, M. B. (1989). *Woodcock–Johnson Psycho-Educational Battery—Revised.* Allen, TX: DLM Teaching Resources.

Woods, B. T., & Carey, S. (1979). Language deficits after apparent clinical recovery from childhood aphasia. *Annals of Neurology, 6,* 405–409.

Zametkin, A. J., Nordahl, T. E., Gross, M., King, A. C., Semple, W. E., Rumsey, J., Hamburger, S., & Cohen, R. (1990). Cerebral glucose metabolism in adults with hyperactivity of childhood onset. *New England Journal of Medicine, 323,* 1361–1366.

9

Recent Developments in Neuropsychological Assessment of the Elderly and Individuals with Severe Dementia

PAUL D. NUSSBAUM AND DANIEL ALLEN

INTRODUCTION

The United States is experiencing a demographic revolution in which individuals 65 years of age and older are comprising a larger percentage of the general population. Indeed, although 12% of the population is now considered elderly (defined as 65 and older), this number will increase to approximately 20% by the year 2030 (La Rue, 1992). The "baby boom generation," which represents 76 million individuals, will begin to turn 65 years of age in the year 2010. The demographic revolution will place tremendous pressure on the health care system, something we are not prepared to address at the current time.

Clinical neuropsychology must begin to prepare for the increased needs of the older adult population (Nussbaum, in press). Defining geriatrics as a specialization within neuropsychology might represent a logical approach to training clinicians to care for older adults. Additionally, clinical research is needed to better define normal aging, develop normative data, and assist in increasing the knowledge base in multiple areas of aging. The field of geriatric neuropsychology is relatively new. As a result, our understanding of basic aspects of the aging process is only beginning to be appreciated. Indeed, health care has generally not

PAUL D. NUSSBAUM • Aging Research and Education Center, Lutheran Affiliated Services, Mars, Pennsylvania 15044; and University of Pittsburgh, School of Medicine, Pittsburgh, Pennsylvania 15260   DANIEL ALLEN • Department of Veterans Affairs Medical Center, Pittsburgh, Pennsylvania 15206 defined normal aging, particularly for those individuals older than age 85. There is little doubt that age correlates with dementia and that neuropsychologists play an important role in the assessment and care of older adults with damage to the central nervous system. Unfortunately, the field has not produced enough information pertaining to assessment of elderly individuals with moderate to severe dementia. This chapter provides an overview of assessment of persons with mild, moderate, and severe dementia, with the goal of creating widespread interest in this important but heretofore neglected area of neuropsychology.

CONSIDERATIONS WHEN ASSESSING ELDERLY INDIVIDUALS WITH DEMENTIA

When evaluating individuals with dementia, clinicians need to consider several factors unique to the patient group in order to provide valid and accurate assessments. These derive from two sources including: (1) those that are the result of the normal aging process, and (2) those that are the result of significant brain damage. Some of these considerations are listed in Table 1. As the majority of the items in Table 1 are self-explanatory, we will not provide in-depth explanations of all of them. We will mention a few of the factors that we feel are of particular relevance when assessing individuals who are older and have concomitant cognitive impairment. Storandt (1994), Zarit, Eiler, and Hassinger (1985), and Crook (1979) provide excellent summaries of the special considerations necessary when assessing older individuals. Readers are encouraged to consult these sources for an in-depth review.

In regard to subject variables, one important factor to consider is individual variability when comparing the young-old to the old-old. Storandt (1994) points out that individuals typically considered "old" can be separated by one or even two generations. Because of this age span, elders in our society have broad and varied life, educational, vocational, and sociopolitical experiences. Based on these varied experiences, elders may bring vastly different perspectives to evaluation sessions. As with all individuals, examiners must consider the unique perspectives brought to evaluation sessions by elders, how these perspectives influence test performance, and how their unique views should be integrated into the conclusions derived from test performance.

Similarly, individuals working with elders need to consider the impact that physical illness has on test performance. Storandt (1994) points out that chronic illness is quite prevalent among individuals over the age of 65, with some studies indicating that 80% of these individuals have at least one chronic medical condition. Moreover, the number of chronic medical conditions increases with age as does the level of disability caused by these conditions, so that by age 85, 29% of the elderly are severely disabled (Kunkel & Applebaum, 1992). Adams and Benson (1992) report that the 10 most common health problems of adults over the age of 65 are arthritis (48%), hypertension (37%), hearing impairments (32%), heart

TABLE 1. Variables to Consider when Assessing
Elderly Individuals

Client characteristics
    Variability between young-old and old-old
    Chronic illness
    Medication effects
    Sensory impairment (visual, auditory, tactile)
    Physical disability
    Increased response time
    Decreased information processing speed
    Circumstantial and verbose responses
    Personality variables
    Fatigue
    Psychiatric disorders (depression, anxiety, dementia)
Instrument and test environment characteristics
    Face validity
    Criterion-related validity (concurrent, predictive)
    Contextual validity
    Construct validity
Examiner characteristics
    Experience evaluating elders
    Stereotypes
    Transference and countertransference

---

conditions (30%), orthopedic impairments (18%), cataracts (17%), sinusitis (14%), diabetes (10%), tinnitus (8%), and varicose veins (8%). Of these conditions, probably the most important to consider when assessing elderly individuals with severe dementia are: (1) those that can cause damage to the cerebrum (e.g., cerebrovascular accident caused by hypertension), and/or (2) those that can cause impairment in sensory and motor processes, which in turn can negatively influence test performance (e.g., peripheral neuropathy caused by diabetes, visual and hearing impairments, or arthritic pain). Finally, the effects of medications on cognitive performances should always be considered when assessing elderly individuals because of the prevalence of medication usage in this group. As would be expected, medication use increases with age. Therefore, the type and combinations of medications and how these change from one assessment session to the next should always be considered when assessing elderly individuals.

Probably one of the most significant factors regarding test development that can influence neuropsychological evaluations centers on the validity of the assessment instruments. Most neuropsychological tests were developed for use with middle-aged, Caucasian individuals. It has been relatively recently that cognitive tests and test batteries designed specifically for the elderly (e.g., Golding, 1989; Smith et al., 1994) or elderly norms for existing neuropsychological tests (e.g., Heaton, Grant, & Matthews, 1991; Ivnik et al., 1992a–c) have become available. Still, in many cases, adequate reliability and validity data are not available, particularly for the old-old. Because of this, it is often not possible to account for the impact that, for example, decreased information processing speed and increased response time have on the assessment of specific cognitive abilities, such as visuospatial and memory abilities.

Along these same lines, Crook (1979) suggests that, just as specialized tests have been developed to assess the intellectual functioning of children because of the realization that intelligence in children is qualitatively different than in adults, tests should also be developed for elderly individuals, whose life tasks are often significantly different than those of middle-aged individuals. Tests developed specifically for the elderly could measure abilities relevant to everyday tasks required to live successfully after the age of 60 or 65. This suggestion is in concert with the more general movement toward ecological validity in the field of neuropsychological assessment. Crook also points out that the issue of face validity may be even more relevant for elderly individuals than it is for younger individuals, because lack of face validity appears to have a greater negative impact on level of motivation in the elderly than it does in younger people.

Examiner characteristics can also influence evaluation outcome. Probably the most important examiner variable is experience working with and evaluating elderly individuals. Also, experience with employing specific measures is necessary for accurate and valid assessments to occur. Experience is of even greater necessity when evaluating elders who have significant cognitive impairment, because they are often less able to cooperate and will have decreased tolerance for slow or clumsy administrations of tests. Other issues such as stereotypical views of elders and transference–countertransference issues can impinge on the evaluation process. However, it is our experience that many of the stereotypes that limit or skew psychologists' views of elders, as well as possible transference and countertransference issues, can be addressed within the context of gaining experience under appropriate supervision.

If not adequately accounted for during evaluation of elders, the aforementioned variables may interact to cause significant differences in test results from one examination to the next. With patients who are severely cognitively impaired, greater onus lies with the examiner to ensure that patients are able to provide optimal levels of performance. We emphasize this point, because the client variables listed in Table 1 are often more difficult to assess in patients with severe dementia than in other neurologically impaired individuals. This is because issues that may be readily apparent in individuals without cognitive impairment may not be readily apparent in individuals with severe cognitive impairment. For example, sensory impairments may not be readily apparent in individuals with significant cognitive impairment because they may not spontaneously report decreased visual acuity or hearing deficits to the examiner. Similarly, it may be difficult to determine if severely impaired individuals are paying attention or are able to understand what examiners are asking. If attention and comprehension are not adequate, patients will provide answers that are irrelevant and inappropriate, because the responses result from hearing only portions of test questions or misunderstanding directions. Also, patients with severe dementia will not be able to inform examiners of changes in medications and will often have little awareness of how these changes affect their cognitive processing. Therefore, examiners must take extra care to ensure that decrements in test performance are the result of actual declines in cognitive functioning that result from progression of the underlying neuropathology, rather than the result of one or more of these factors.

During clinical evaluations, examiners can help ensure optimal levels of test performance by making allowances for at least two problems inherent in testing individuals with severe dementia. First, these individuals often have limited attention spans and exhibit decreased task persistence. It generally has been our experience that these patients must be redirected frequently during the course of assessment. Also, they cannot be expected to continue with a task for more than 15–20 minutes (Albert & Cohen, 1992; Saxton, McGonigle-Gibson, Swihart, & Boller, 1993). As such, examiners should be attentive to lapses in attention and should structure examination sessions so that they can be conducted in no more than 15–20 minutes. Second, rapport is often difficult to establish with these patients because of their diminished cognitive and perceptual capacities. However, rapport is often more important with these patients than with patients who are less impaired, because severely impaired patients often have lower frustration tolerances and higher levels of impulsivity. We suggest that if an examiner feels that adequate rapport has not been established prior to testing, the evaluation should not be conducted, regardless of the properties of the assessment instrument or the skill of the examiner. It is highly unlikely that proceeding under these circumstances will yield valid test results. On the other hand, it is quite probable that proceeding will serve to irritate the patient.

SCREENING FOR COGNITIVE IMPAIRMENT IN INDIVIDUALS WITH DEMENTIA

Because the primary purpose of this chapter is to discuss the instruments developed to assess severely demented patients, the majority of the ensuing discussion has been dedicated to that topic. However, we will also review the instruments currently available that are used to assess patients who are mildly to moderately impaired. These instruments generally have a longer history of use, because instruments for assessing the cognitive function of patients in the end stages of dementia have only recently been developed.

Screening for Impairment in Mild and Moderate Dementia

In discussing these instruments, we have divided them into two categories, including: (1) brief cognitive screening instruments, and (2) intermediate cognitive screening instruments. Brief cognitive screening instruments typically take 10 minutes or less to administer, while intermediate-length screening procedures may take as long as 45 minutes. Also, brief screens usually provide an overall score that classifies patients as cognitively impaired or unimpaired. Intermediate-length tests generally provide a more specific assessment of a broader range of cognitive abilities and may also provide information pertinent to differential diagnosis. Brief and intermediate-length screening procedures for early detection of dementia and mild–moderate cognitive impairment in dementia have received the most attention in the literature. This review is not intended to be exhaustive; rather, it focuses on those instruments that tend to be the most widely used.

Brief Cognitive Screening Instruments

Table 2 contains reliability and validity data on some of the most popular brief cognitive screening measures including the Mini-Mental State Examination (Folstein, Folstein, & McHugh, 1975), the Short Portable Mental Status Questionnaire (Pfeiffer, 1975), the Blessed Information–Memory–Concentration test (Blessed, Tomlinson, & Roth, 1968), and an abbreviated version of the Blessed Information–Memory–Concentration test, the Short Orientation–Memory–Concentration test (Katzman et al., 1983). Sensitivity and specificity estimates are provided in Table 2. Sensitivity reflects the proportion of cognitively impaired individuals who are identified by the instrument as cognitively impaired, while specificity is the percentage of individuals without cognitive impairment who are identified as such by the instrument.

By far, the most widely studied and widely used brief cognitive screening instrument is the Mini-Mental State Examination (MMSE) (Folstein et al., 1975). Since its publication, it has been used in well over 600 published studies. It consists of 19 questions that yield a score between 0 and 30. The MMSE items assess orientation, registration, attention, calculation, verbal memory, language, and visual construction. The standard cutoff for impairment is 23 or below (Folstein et al., 1975). Some authors use the following cutoff scores to provide a more precise classification of cognitive functioning: 24–30 = no cognitive impairment; 18–23 = mild cognitive impairment; 11–17 = moderate cognitive impairment; and 0–10 = severe cognitive impairment (Albert & Cohen, 1992; Tombaugh & McIntyre, 1992). The majority of the studies addressing the reliability and validity of the MMSE focus on distinguishing elderly individuals with dementia or delirium from elderly individuals who are not cognitively impaired. Most of these studies suggest that the MMSE has adequate reliability. Reliability studies based on patients with cognitive impairment or combinations of cognitively and noncognitively impaired individuals generally tend to produce higher reliability coefficients than studies examining only cognitively intact individuals, probably because there is greater variability in the range of MMSE scores when the test is used with cognitively impaired individuals or combined samples of cognitively

TABLE 2. Brief Cognitive Screening Instruments for Mild to Moderate Dementia

Test	References	Sample	n	Age	Reliability	Sensitivity	Specificity	Validity
Mini-Mental State Examination (MMSE)	Holzer et al (1984)	Community	4917	18–85+	.77[a]			
	Morris et al. (1989)	1. Community	278	M = 68	.38[b]			
		2. Mild DAT*	200	M = 72	.74[b]			
		3. Moderate DAT*	132	M = 72	.79[b]			
		4. Community & DAT*	632	M = 70>	>.92[a]			.85;.80;.74–.89[c]
	O'Connor et al (1989)	1. Cognitively Intact	285	75+	.63[b]			
		2. Demented or delirious	196	75+	.83[b]			
		3. Unspecified	10	75+	.97[d]			
		4. Samples 1 & 2	481	75+	.84[b]	.86	.92	
	Baker et al. (1993)	Community	55	M = 78		.70	.93	
	Weiler et al. (1994)	Mild-Very Severe DAT*	201	M = 77	.90[a]			
Short Portable Mental Status Questionnaire	Pfeiffer (1975)	1. Unspecified	30	65+	.82[b]			
		2. Unspecified	29	65+	.83[b]			
		3. Psychiatric referrals	133	65+		.68	.96	
	Erkinjuntti et al. (1987)	1. Community	119	M = 73		.68;.68;1.0[e]	1.0;1.0;1.0[e]	
		2. Medical inpatients	282	M = 76		.76;.86;1.0[e]	1.0;.99;.89[e]	
	Albert et al. (1991)	Normal & DAT*	467	65+		.34	.94	
	Roccaforte et al. (1994)	Nondemented & demented	100	M = 79	.83[b]	.74;.74[f]	.79;.91[f]	.73;.81[g]
Information	Thal et al. (1986)	DAT*	40	50–90	.82–.90[h]		−.73–−.83[i]	
Memory	Salmon et al. (1990)	DAT*	92	M = 72			−.88;−.79[j]	
Concentration test (IMC)	Weiler et al. (1994)	Mild-very severe DAT*	201	M = 77	.94[a]			

(continued)

TABLE 2. (*Continued*)

Test	References	Sample	n	Age	Reliability	Sensitivity	Specificity	Validity
Short Orientation Memory Concentration Test (SOMC)	Davous et al. (1987)	1. Demented	18	†	.83[b]		−.93[k]	
		2. Nondemented & demented	133	37–94			−.33−−.84;.09[m]	
	Fillenbaum et al. (1987)	DAT*	36	M = 65		.87	.94	
		DAT*	24	M = 64	.77[b]		−.83[n]	
	Morris et al. (1989)	Community & DAT*	632	M = 70	>.92[a]			−.84;−.84; −.77;−.89[o]

*DAT = Dementia of the Alzheimer type. Includes diagnoses of probable and possible DAT (McKhann et al., 1984).
†This information was not reported by the authors.
[a]Internal consistency.
[b]Test-retest reliability.
[c]The four correlations represent MMSE's correlations with the Consortium to Establish a Registry for Alzheimer's disease (CERAD; Morris et al., 1989) Word List Memory, CERAD Word List Recall, CERAD Word List Recognition, and the Short Orientation-Memory-Concentration Test (Katzman et al., 1983), respectively.
[d]Kappa coefficient based on ratings of 10 interviews made by 5 to 9 raters (n = 54 ratings for 10 interviews).
[e]The three percentages reported represent sensitivities and specificities when cutoff scores of four, three, or two errors are used, respectively.
[f]Sensitivities and specificities were calculated using the criteria of seven or greater errors. The authors administered the SPMSQ initially on the phone and then face to face. The two estimates of sensitivity and specificity reflect phone and face-to-face interviews, respectively.
[g]Correlation with MMSE for phone and face-to-face interviews, respectively (see "f" for more information).
[h]Range of test-retest reliability coefficients for four test administrations conducted at 0, 1, 3, and 6 weeks.
[i]Range of correlations between the MMSE and the IMC across four separate evaluations.
[j]The two correlations represent IMC total score correlations with the MMSE and Mattis Dementia Rating Scale (Mattis, 1976, 1988), respectively.
[k]Correlation with MMSE scores for all groups.
[l]Range of correlations with the Wechsler Memory Scale.
[m]Correlation with the Ravens Progressive Matrices.
[n]Correlation with MMSE total score.
[o]The four correlations represent SOMC's correlations with the Consortium to Establish a Registry for Alzheimer's Disease (CERAD; Morris et al., 1989) Word List Memory, CERAD Word List Recall, CERAD Word List Recognition, and the MMSE (Folstein et al., 1975), respectively.

impaired and cognitively unimpaired individuals. As can be seen from Table 2, the MMSE has good interrater and test–retest reliabilities.

The studies presented in Table 2 that examine the validity of the MMSE support its concurrent and construct validity. As would be expected, scores on the MMSE decline significantly over a 1-year interval in patients with dementia of the Alzheimer's type (DAT) (Becker, Huff, Nebes, Holland, & Boller, 1989). Also, MMSE scores are significantly correlated ($r = .93, p < .001$) with physicians' ratings of Alzheimer's patients' competency to make decisions regarding their medical treatments (Marson, Herfkens, Brooks, Ingram, & Harrell, 1995). The studies in Table 2 suggest that the MMSE has adequate specificity when classifying individuals as impaired. However, clinicians should be aware that a normal score on the MMSE does not indicate normal cognitive functioning. In fact, at least two reports suggest that individuals can have significant cognitive impairment and still obtain perfect or near-perfect scores on the MMSE (Benedict & Brandt, 1992; Yue, Fainsinger, & Bruera, 1994). This appears particularly true for patients with dense amnesia who are often able to perform perfectly on the MMSE memory items (Benedict & Brandt, 1992). In cases of less severe impairment, authors have also criticized the MMSE for being unable to distinguish between patients without cognitive impairment and those with mild dementia (Albert, Smith, Scherr, Taylor, & Funkenstein, 1991; see also Tombaugh & McIntyre, 1992). Some authors have attempted to modify the MMSE in order to increase its sensitivity and specificity. While some of the modifications have increased reliability and validity of the MMSE (Teng, Chiu, Schneider, & Erickson-Metzger, 1987), they have either significantly altered the content and format of the original test or added additional tests that require substantially longer administration (Pfeffer et al., 1981).

Some authors suggest that the MMSE should be adjusted based on education so that a cutoff score of 20 and below is used for individuals with 8 or fewer years of education. This is because individuals with 8 or fewer years of education typically perform more poorly than individuals with more than 8 years of education (Anthony, LeResche, Niaz, VonKorff, & Folstein, 1982). One recent study examined the effects of multiple conditions, including age, education, socioeconomic status, sensory impairment, medical conditions, and psychiatric conditions in a large sample ($N = 3974$) of community-dwelling elderly (Launer, Dinkgreve, Jonker, Hooijer, & Lindeboom, 1993). Factors that were found to negatively influence MMSE performance included decreased visual acuity, Parkinson's disease, stroke, depression, diabetes, increased age, and less education. Moreover, the influence of age and education on MMSE performance was generally independent of other conditions (such as medical conditions) that negatively influenced MMSE performance (Launer et al., 1993). Out of concern over the impact of age and education on MMSE performance, Marshall and Mungas (1995) developed a statistical technique for adjusting MMSE scores based on education and age. Marshall and Mungas report that this adjustment increased the overall sensitivity of the MMSE without affecting its specificity. If replicated, this statistical adjustment technique may prove to be the most efficient method for controlling for the effects of age and education on MMSE performance.

The Short Portable Mental Status Questionnaire (SPMSQ) (Pfeiffer, 1975) consists of 10 items that assess orientation, remote memory, and concentration. It has been used with community, medical, and psychiatric samples. Based on the studies presented in Table 2, the SPMSQ appears to have adequate test–retest reliability and internal consistency. However, when the standard cutoff of four or more errors is used, the sensitivity of the SPMSQ to cognitive impairment is limited. Some authors suggest lowering the cutoff score to three for dementia and two for delirium in order to increase sensitivity (Erkinjuntti, Sulkava, Wikström, & Autio, 1987). These same authors report that the SPMSQ appears to be better in screening for dementia than for delirium. Of the studies presented in Table 2, Albert et al. (1991) report the lowest sensitivity. This is probably because they attempted to detect cases of probable DAT in a group of individuals who were unimpaired, impaired for reasons other than DAT, or impaired as a result of DAT. Based on Albert and co-workers (1991) report, it is not expected that the SPMSQ will distinguish between different types of dementia. Another criticism of the SPMSQ is that it does not contain any items that assess learning, which is particularly important when assessing patients with dementia. Also, at least one investigation examining the SPMSQ's relation to clinical diagnosis and neuropsychological test performance in a sample of psychiatric and neurological patients indicated that the SPMSQ was not significantly related to either clinical or neuropsychological diagnosis (Dalton, Pederson, Blom, & Holmes, 1987). Because of this, some authors suggest that a normal score on the SPMSQ should not be taken to mean that there is an absence of cognitive impairment. Finally, the original report by Pfeiffer (1975) indicated that cutoff scores should be adjusted based on education and race, although this assertion has not been consistently supported (Erkinjuntti et al., 1987).

The Blessed Information–Memory–Concentration test (IMC) (Blessed et al., 1968) is composed of three of the four subscales that make up the Blessed Dementia Scale (Blessed et al., 1968). These three subscales are Information, Memory, and Concentration. The remaining Blessed subscale is a behavioral rating scale rather than a direct measure of cognitive functioning. It assesses changes in day-to-day activities, habits, and personality variables. The three cognitive scales originally consisted of 30 items that assessed knowledge of basic personal information, orientation, memory (remote and delayed recall), attention, and concentration. However, the test has been modified for use in the United States (Fuld, 1978; Katzman et al., 1983). the US version contains 26 items that assess similar abilities as the original version. Items that were revised or replaced were not relevant to individuals living in the United States, e.g., "What is the name of the Prime Minister?" For the US version, scores range from 1 to 33. Higher scores indicate greater impairment. Investigators report excellent test–retest reliabilities (Thal, Grundman, & Golden, 1986) and internal consistencies (Weiler, Chiriboga, &

Black, 1994) for the IMC. Salmon, Thal, Butters, and Heindel (1990) report significant correlations between the IMC total score and scores on the MMSE and Mattis Dementia Rating Scale (Mattis, 1976, 1988), which provide support for the validity of the IMC. Also, several authors report significant increases in the IMC scores of patients who have DAT and who are followed longitudinally (Salmon et al., 1990; Stern et al., 1992). However, it also appears that the IMC loses its sensitivity to change in cognitive deterioration when used with patients who initially have severe dementia (Katzman et al., 1988; Salmon et al., 1990).

The Short Orientation–Memory–Concentration test (SOMC) was originally developed by Katzman and colleagues (1983). It is a six-item version of the IMC test (Blessed et al., 1968). In developing the SOMC, Katzman and co-workers analyzed data collected on four samples composed of individuals in a skilled nursing facility ($n = 321$; mean age $= 87.0$), an additional 170 individuals in a skilled nursing facility, 52 members of a senior citizen center, and 42 patients from an inpatient unit specializing in the treatment of dementia. Although reliability and validity coefficients were not calculated in the original report, the six SOMC items accounted for 88.6–92.6% of the variance in the Blessed IMC, and correlated significantly ($r = .54$, $p < .001$) with temporal, parietal, and frontal cortex plaque counts of 38 autopsied patients. As with the IMC, a higher score on the SOMC indicates more severe impairment. At least one large-scale study indicated that the SOMC correlates comparably to the MMSE with tests of memory and is highly correlated with the MMSE (Morris et al., 1989). Also, Davous, Lamour, Debrand, and Rondot (1987) suggest that he SOMC is as effective as the MMSE when used to screen for dementia.

Brief cognitive screening instruments have several advantages:

1. They are particularly valuable when only gross screening is possible.
2. They can be administered by technicians or other staff with minimal training, are easy to score, and require little interpretation.
3. At least one report indicates that performance on brief mental status examinations, such as the MMSE (Folstein et al., 1975) and the IMC (Blessed et al., 1968), significantly predicts activities of daily living (ADL) capacity and rated level of care by caregivers for patients with Alzheimer's disease (Weiler et al., 1994). It also appears that items representing specific ability domains differentially predict specific aspects of ADL functioning. For example, Weiler and colleagues used factor analysis to determine the factor structure of the combined IMC and MMSE items. They extracted five underlying factors. Two of these factors (General Cognitive Functioning and Orientation) were significant predictors of ADL dependency in patients with DAT. This type of study has yet to be conducted with most neuropsychological tests designed to assess severe impairment.
4. It appears that the MMSE and IMC are impervious to significant practice when repeatedly administered to patients who have DAT (Thal et al.,

1986). Thal and co-workers reported that there were no significant practice effects when the IMC and MMSE were administered to patients with DAT four times over the course of 6 weeks.

5. Based on the specificity and sensitivity estimates for these instruments, clinicians and researchers can be assured that individuals scoring in the "impaired range" are probably cognitively impaired. (We make this statement keeping in mind that the scores in the impaired range are obtained in the absence of other conditions that could adversely influence test performance, such as decreased visual acuity or bilateral hearing impairment).

However, one limitation of these instruments is that they have lower sensitivity than specificity. As a result, performance in the "normal range" does not indicate the absence of significant cognitive deficits. This point was highlighted in a recent study by Albert and co-workers (1991), who were investigating the prevalence of DAT in a sample of community-dwelling elderly individuals. They found that between 3 and 3.7% of individuals who performed in the unimpaired range on the SPMSQ (Pfeiffer, 1975) and on a brief verbal memory test were found to have probable DAT on more thorough evaluation. A second limitation is that it is not possible to draw conclusions regarding the etiology of the underlying neuropathology and/or medical conditions based solely on the results on one of these measures. Third, it appears that for brief cognitive screening instruments, age and education can significantly affect test performance, so that individuals who are younger and have more education preform better than older, less educated individuals. This issue has been the most thoroughly examined in the MMSE, and techniques have been suggested to deal with the effects of age and education on MMSE test performance. While studies exist that support the reliability and validity of all of the tests presented in Table 2, the MMSE obviously has the most support and validation data of all the brief cognitive screening instruments. Based on this observation, we suggest that the MMSE be used for screening purposes unless there is a specific reason why it would be inappropriate (e.g., in cases of suspected amnestic disorder or when time constraints require a briefer technique).

Intermediate-Length Cognitive Screening Instruments

Table 3 summarizes reliability and validity data for two intermediate-length cognitive screening instruments: the Mattis Dementia Rating Scale (DRS) (Mattis, 1976, 1988) and the Middlesex Elderly Assessment of Mental State (Golding, 1989). The DRS has the longest history of use and is one of the most popular intermediate-length screening batteries. It was designed specifically to assess patients with neurological conditions and, more specifically, patients with degenerative dementias. The DRS contains 36 different tasks that contribute to five subscales. These five subscales are Attention, Initiation/Perseveration, Construction,

TABLE 3. Intermediate-Length Cognitive Screening Instruments for Mild to Moderate Dementia

Test	References	Sample	n	Age	Reliability	Sensitivity	Specificity	Validity
Mattis Dementia Rating Scale (DRS)	Coblentz et al. (1973)	1. DAT*	30	†	.97a			
		2. OMS**	20	58–71				.75b
	Gardner et al. (1981)	CI***	25	M = 82	.90c			
	Salmon et al. (1990)	DAT	92	M = 73				.82d; −.79e
Middlesex Elderly Assessment of Mental State	Golding (1989)	1. MDD****	22	†	.98f			
		2. MDD	28	†	.91g			
		3. MDD	120	M = 80		.91	.95	
	Powell et al. (1993)	1. Dementia	12	M = 78	.82g			
		2. Normal controls	12	†	.95g			

*DAT = Dementia of the Alzheimer type. Included diagnoses of probable and possible DAT (McKhann et al., 1984).
**OMS = Organic mental syndrome.
***CI = Cognitively impaired.
****MDD = Mixed sample of patients with depression or dementia.
†This information was not specified.
aTest–retest reliability coefficient.
bCorrelation between DRS total scores and Wechsler Adult Intelligence Scale (Wechsler, 1955) Full Scale IQ scores.
cSplit-half reliability coefficient.
dCorrelation with MMSE.
eCorrelation with IMC.
fInterrater reliability.
gAlternate form reliability.

Conceptualization, and Memory. Scores range from 0 to 144. Scores of 122 and below (2 SD below the mean) are considered indicative of impairment. However, most individuals who are not cognitively impaired obtain scores between 140 and 144 (Granholm, Wolfe, & Butters, 1985; Moss, Albert, Butters, & Payne, 1986). In addition to the split-half and test–retest reliabilities reported in Table 3, Vitaliano, Breen, Albert, Russo, and Prinz (1984a) reported that the DRS subscales have alpha coefficients ranging between .75 and .95 when they are used with patients who have DAT.

In regard to validity, the DRS is much more sensitive to changes in cognitive deterioration in patients with DAT than brief measures, such as the IMC and MMSE (Salmon et al., 1990). This is because the DRS contains many items with low levels of difficulty, which decreases the floor effects that often limit the utility of other instruments. Also, investigators report that the DRS total score is significantly correlated ($r = .79$, $p < .05$) with physicians' rating of DAT patients' competency to make decisions regarding their medical treatment (Marson et al., 1995). Marson and colleagues reported that of the five DRS subscales, the Perseveration/Initiation and Memory subscales were significantly correlated with patient competency ($r = .90$, $p < .002$; and $r = .80$, $p < .05$, respectively). This finding is similar to previous research indicating that the Initiation/Perseveration subtest distinguishes individuals with mild dementia from those with no cognitive impairment, while all of the DRS subscales distinguish between individuals with mild and moderate dementia (Mattis, 1988; see also Vitaliano et al., 1984b).

Further evidence for the validity of the Initiation/Perseveration subtest was provided by the finding that it was directly related to frontal release signs in patients with dementia (Vieweg, Brashear, Sautter, & Tabscott, 1993). In addition, two studies suggest that the Attention subtest differentiates patients who exhibit mild impairment of functional abilities from those with more severe functional impairment (Shay et al., 1991); Vitaliano et al., 1984a). The sensitivity of the Initiation/Perseveration, Memory, and Attention subscales of the DRS to cognitive and functional impairment reflect the importance of these cognitive domains for determining independent, day-to-day functioning, as well as their central roles in detecting cognitive deterioration resulting from progressive dementia. Based on recent factor analytic work, it appears that when used with patients who have DAT, the DRS is composed of three underlying factors that assess: (1) conceptualization/organization abilities; (2) visual–spatial abilities; and (3) memory and orientation (Colantonio, Becker, & Huff, 1993). The test manual (Mattis, 1988) provides more information on the reliability and validity of the DRS.

The Middlesex Elderly Assessment of Mental State (MEAMS) (Golding, 1989) was devised to detect significant cognitive deficits in elderly individuals. It is composed of 54 items that contribute to 12 different subtest scores. These subtests are entitled Orientation, Name Learning, Naming, Comprehension, Remembering Pictures, Arithmetic, Spatial Construction, Fragmented Letter Perception, Unusual Views, Usual Views, Verbal Fluency, and Motor Perseveration. The Unusual Views and Usual Views subtests assess individuals' abilities to perceive and identify photographs of objects taken from unusual angles and usual angles. These two subtests are purported to distinguish between sensory deficits and perceptual deficits. Also, there are two equivalent forms of the MEAMS to control for practice effects if the test is administered more than once to the same individuals. Total scores range from 0 to 12 with scores of 10, 11, and 12 considered normal. Scores of 8 and 9 are considered borderline, while scores of 7 and below are considered impaired. Because the original version of the MEAMS contained 10 subtests that did not assess memory functioning, it was supplemented with two subtests (Name Learning and Remembering Pictures) adapted from the Rivermead Behavioral Memory Test (Wilson, Cockburn, & Baddeley, 1991).

Initial validity data on the MEAMS suggest that it is able to distinguish between depression and dementia [both DAT and multi-infarct dementia (MID)]. Also, individuals with DAT performed significantly worse on 6 of the 10 subtests relative to patients with MID. However, the authors suggest that subscale differences noted between DAT and MID groups may have been due to extraneous factors, such as disease severity, rather than the MEAMS ability to distinguish between these groups. Since the time of the original report, there have been three other investigations utilizing the MEAMS (McKenna et al., 1990; Powell, Brooker, & Papadopolous, 1993; Shiel & Wilson, 1992). One of these studies used the MEAMS to investigate cognitive impairment in patients with schizophrenia (McKenna et al., 1990). The authors did not report reliability or validity data supporting the psychometric characteristics of the MEAMS. On the other hand, Powell and colleagues reported that when the MEAMS was used with a sample of 12 dementia patients and 12 normal controls, there was a version effect for the dementia patients but not for the controls (i.e., differences in levels of performance were present due to the test form administered; this suggests that the alternate forms have differing levels of difficulty). Subtests that appeared to contribute to this difference included Fragmented Letters, Unusual Views, and Verbal Fluency. Patients appeared to score higher on alternate version B on these three subtests. Given the limited sample sizes, these results should be considered tentative at best. Shiel and Wilson (1992) reported additional data based on the MEAMS performance of 38 patients who had either right or left hemisphere strokes. Expected patterns of performance based on lateralization of strokes were noted (i.e., patients who had left hemisphere strokes failed more tests requiring language abilities, while patients with right hemisphere strokes failed more tests requiring visuospatial abilities). Patients with right hemisphere lesions had significantly higher total scores than patients with left hemisphere lesions. The authors suggest that left and right hemisphere patients in their study tended to perform better than the patients with MID on the MEAMS, although this may be been the result of an age effect.

Reliability and validity data reported by Golding (1989) and Powell and co-workers (1993) suggest that the MEAMS has adequate reliability and validity. However, the data presented in the manual are limited primarily because all of the

MEAMS subtests were not administered to the same groups of patients. Because the original version of the MEAMS was supplemented with two memory tests, validity and reliability information for the memory subtests were collected on different samples than the original validation sample reported in the manual. Also, more studies are required to clarify normal performance on the MEAMS. We calculated the sensitivity and specificity estimates for the MEAMS that are reported in Table 3. These estimates are based on information from the MEAMS test administration manual (Golding, 1989). The sensitivity and specificity estimates reflect the MEAMS ability to differentiate patients with depression from patients with dementia. One would expect that when the MEAMS is used to distinguish between cognitively impaired and normal controls, estimates of sensitivity and specificity would increase.

In addition to intermediate-length cognitive screening instruments that assess only cognitive abilities, there are instruments that combine behavioral ratings of psychiatric status and functional abilities, self-report depression items, and tests of cognitive abilities. One such instrument is the Canberra Interview for the Elderly (CIE) (Social Psychiatry Research Unit, 1992). The CIE has recently been developed to differentially diagnose cases of dementia, amnestic syndrome, dysthymia, delirium, and depression according to World Health Organization ICD-10 Diagnostic Criteria for Research (as cited in Social Psychiatry Research Unit, 1992) and the *Diagnostic and Statistical Manual of Mental Disorders,* 3rd edition, revised (DSM-III-R) (American Psychiatric Association, 1987). It consists of two sections: the first is administered to patients, and the second to informants who have adequate knowledge of patients' behaviors. This test assesses a broad range of abilities, but does so by incorporating items and subtests from currently existing tests, such as the Symbol Digit Modalities Test (Smith, 1982), Wechsler Memory Scale (Wechsler, 1945), Wechsler Adult Intelligence Scale—Revised (Wechsler, 1981), and the MMSE (Folstein et al., 1975). Initial data on the CIE suggest that its diagnoses are as accurate as diagnoses derived by clinical interviews and by other psychiatric interview methods. However, the patient portion takes on the average 69 minutes to administer (range = 18–130) and the informant section takes an average of 37 minutes (range = 16–220) to administer. Its length makes it prohibitive for use with the severely impaired.

Of the two intermediate-length cognitive screening instruments reviewed in this section, the DRS is the most well established and should continue to prove useful in clinical and research endeavors focusing on assessing elderly patients with cognitive impairment. On the other hand, the MEAMS appears to be a promising instrument in that initial validity and reliability studies support its psychometric properties. Further research is needed to determine if the MEAMS is a sensitive as the DRS to cognitive impairment, particularly at the more severe levels. In contrast to brief screening instruments, future research may show that the DRS and MEAMS are sensitive to differences in cognitive performance resulting from dementias with differing etiologies, and thus assist in differential diagnosis.

However, both brief and intermediate-length instruments are limited by the fact that they are unsuitable for assessing individuals with severe dementia. The ensuing discussion focuses on elucidating the reasons why many existing instruments are of limited utility. We also present information on scales that are useful in assessing individuals with severe impairment.

Assessment of Severe Dementia

Before discussing specific measures of severe cognitive impairment, some clarification of what is meant by severe dementia is needed. Also, discussion of those factors contributing to the recent interest in evaluating patients with severe dementia is in order.

Clinicians and researchers use several approaches to determine whether or not individuals have "severe dementia." One of the most popular approaches is to diagnose dementia and its severity according to medical categorical classification systems, such as the DSM-IV (American Psychiatric Association, 1994). In this approach, mental disorders such as dementia are distinguished and diagnosed through the application of specific sets of criteria. Typically, each disorder is characterized by several cardinal features or defining symptoms. These defining symptoms help to differentiate between disorders. However, because some heterogeneity of symptomatology always exists within any type of mental disorder, categorical systems often provide lists of additional symptoms. Individuals are diagnosed as having a mental disorder when they exhibit a predetermined number and pattern of symptoms. The diagnosis of severity is then based on the number of symptoms exhibited by the individual in excess of the minimum number required to meet diagnostic criteria and/or the extent to which these symptoms impair occupational and social functioning. Also in the DSM-IV system, emphasis is placed on specifying the etiology of the dementia. For example, according to the DSM-IV, dementia is primarily characterized by the onset of multiple cognitive deficits (one of which is memory impairment) that significantly interfere with occupational and/or social functioning. Individuals who are diagnosed with mild dementia exhibit few symptoms and experience only minor impairment in functioning, while those who are diagnosed with severe dementia exhibit many symptoms that significantly interfere with occupation and/or social functioning.

Other authors have relied on ratings provided by standardized methods developed to stage severity levels of dementia. We will discuss these global staging methods later in this chapter. Briefly, these methods assess the deterioration of cognitive abilities and functional behaviors through ratings provided by interviews with patients or caregivers. A specific number is then assigned that corresponds to a level of severity (e.g., 1 = no impairment, 7 = severe impairment). Severity of dementia and cognitive impairment have also been established through the application of neuropsychological tests. When specific patterns of cognitive loss are of interest, clinicians and researchers will often administer extensive neuropsychological test batteries. Deviation from expected levels of performance, as determined by normative information, is then used to classify the severity of cognitive impairment. However (as will be discussed later), several factors limit the use of these batteries with severely impaired individuals. As an alternative to the use of extended neuropsychological batteries, some authors report using MMSE scores within a specific range to classify individuals as severely demented. Most authors have typically focused on assessing individuals with MMSE scores below 10 or 12. These scores are considered to reflect severe cognitive impairment. Using the MMSE in this fashion certainly does not address the issues of etiology, pattern of cognitive deficits, or level of functional impairment. However, it does provide an estimate of the severity of cognitive impairment, which is of central importance when developing tests designed to assess severity of dementia.

Each of these methods to classify individuals as severely demented has distinct advantages and disadvantages. All have been used by authors of cognitive tests for the severely impaired. However, most authors of tests designed to assess severe cognitive impairment report patients' scores according to an MMSE classification.

While many of the tests in Tables 2 and 3 have been widely used to detect and monitor the progress of dementia varying in severity from mild to moderate, most tests are significantly limited because they cannot be used to assess patients with severe dementia. At least two general factors limit their usage with patients who have severe dementia: (1) instructions are worded in such a way as to make them incomprehensible to individuals with severe cognitive impairment due to impaired language abilities, and (2) the items are often too difficult or inappropriate for individuals with severe impairment. Because of these factors, several authors note significant floor effects when using standard cognitive screening procedures with severely impaired patients (Mohs, Kim, Johns, Dunn, & Davis, 1986; Reisberg et al., 1989; Wilson, & Kaszniak, 1986). Other authors suggest that currently available dementia screening tests are insensitive to cognitive changes that occur in patients with severe dementia (Katzman et al., 1988; Salmon et al., 1990). As a result, many patients with severe dementia until recently have been considered untestable (Lopez, Boller, Becker, Miller, & Reynolds, 1990). Limitations of the currently available neuropyschological assessment techniques have contributed to the increased interest in developing new measures appropriate for individuals who are severely impaired. In addition to these general factors, more specific empirical and clinical considerations have fueled the current movement toward developing instruments to assess individuals with severe cognitive impairment.

From the empirical side, these factors include: (1) the need to increase the emphasis on clarifying the relation between changes in the cerebrum noted at autopsy and cognitive functioning prior to death (Fairburn & Hope, 1988; Proctor, Francis, Strattman, & Bowen, 1992); (2) the need for appropriate outcome measures when conducting trials of new medications designed to treat severely demented individuals (Davidson & Stern, 1991; Kanowski, Fischhof, Hiersemenzel, Röhmel, & Kern, 1989); (3) the need to clarify the rate and pattern of cognitive deterioration in severe dementia (Panisset, Roudier, Saxton, & Boller, 1994; Saxton, McGonigle-Gibson, Swihart, Miller, & Boller, 1990) and to assist in the longitudinal study of progressive dementias, such as DAT (Panisset et al., 1994); and (4) the need to assess patients who are otherwise untestable using more complex neuropsychological instruments because of floor effects (Lopez et al., 1990). As Ward, Dawe, Proctor, Murphy, and Weinman (1993) suggest, research in these areas would be assisted if standardized methods of assessing patients with severe dementia were available.

In addition to furthering empirical investigations into the natural history of dementia, some authors have suggested clinical utility in assessing patients who are severely impaired:

1. Several investigators (Anthony, Proctor, Silverman, & Murphy, 1987; Ward et al., 1993) suggest that assessments conducted before and after patients are moved to new environments may indicate how much the change in environment impacts patients' levels of confusion, mood, and general well-being. This type of assessment may, in turn, lead to environmental manipulations that could increase adjustment and decrease problematic behaviors that often accompany increased confusion and dysphoria in elderly individuals with severe dementia.

2. Others suggest that the level of cognitive function in severely demented patients may have implications for treatment planning, e.g., type of cognitive stimulation, environmental complexity, and so forth (Panisset et al., 1994; Sclan, Foster, Reisberg, Franssen, & Welkowitz, 1990). Along these same lines, J. Saxton (personal communication, January 18, 1995) suggests that information gained from tests of severe impairment can be used by treatment staff (e.g., activities directors, occupational therapists) in devising individualized programming based on patients' preserved abilities. As a caveat, Beatty and colleagues (1988) reported one case that highlights the possible preservation of abilities in patients with severe dementia. They reported the case of an 81-year-old pianist who was able to continue to play difficult piano pieces despite marked impairment in most ability areas including the ability to identify well-known songs. While this case is an exception to the rule, uneven deterioration of cognitive abilities is quite common during the courses of progressive dementias.

3. Results from tests of severe impairment may have implications for placement decisions (Saxton et al., 1990) (i.e., determining the level of care individuals will require).

4. Results of these tests can be used to provide feedback to staff and family members about patients' levels of awareness and recognition. When this type of information is provided to caregivers, it may influence patients' well-being by increasing the amount of attention given to patients by their caregivers (Sclan et al., 1990). This is because the quantity and quality of

attention given to patients by caregivers may be a direct result of care-givers' perceptions of patients' awareness of their environments as well as their awareness of the attention being given by the caregivers (Sclan et al., 1990).

Because of the lack of available instruments to quantify cognitive impairment in patients with severe dementia, some authors have attempted to use behavioral rating scales to assess the progression of dementias in their severe stages. There is even one report of the use of a coma scale to quantify the cognitive functioning of severely demented patients (Benesch, McDaniel, Cox, & Hamill, 1993). Over the past 5 years, several new behavioral rating scales have emerged. Other exist-ing rating scales have been applied to patients with severe dementia. Finally, five neuropsychological tests have been developed that directly assesses the cog-nitive functioning of patients who are severely impaired. In the following sections, we will discuss the strengths and weaknesses of several of the behavioral rating scales and all of the neuropsychological tests of severe impairment. The majority if the discussion focuses on neuropsychological measures of severe impairment. However, we will also mention several behavioral rating scales because of their widespread use and the contributions these scales have made to understanding be-havior and cognition in individuals with severe impairment.

Behavior Rating Scales

Although behavior rating scales are quite popular and have been developed for use with many different populations, it has been only recently that investiga-tors have made a concerted effort to develop scales specifically for patients with dementia and/or to examine the properties of existing scales when used with pa-tients who have dementia (Drachman, Swearer, O'Donnell, Mitchell, & Maloon, 1992: Ritchie & Ledesert, 1991). Behavioral rating scales used to assess individ-uals with dementia sample several classes of symptoms, including functional sta-tus, behavioral excesses or deficiencies, cognition, and psychiatric conditions. Some scales focus on one specific class of symptoms (such as psychiatric), while other scales are multidimensional. Behavioral rating scales are valuable because they allow the quantification of symptoms associated with severe dementia. Many of these symptoms reflect underlying neuropathology in the cerebrum, and can therefore be viewed as correlates of cerebral pathology. When conceived of in this manner, one envisions many clinical and empirical applications for behavioral rat-ing scales. Possible clinical applications include quantification of behavioral and psychiatric disturbances in order to facilitate and expedite communication be-tween professionals. Monitoring of these quantified symptoms can help clinicians and researchers evaluate the efficacy of treatments. Also, these scales may allow for examination of specific cerebral pathology as it relates to prevalent sympto-matology. This may be useful in differentiating specific types of dementia or subtypes within a specific type of dementia. These scales may be useful in studying brain–behavior relationships at autopsy, since many of the scales can be administered close to the time of death.

However, behavioral rating scales are also significantly limited. While they may provide a range of scores reflecting behavioral changes in severely demented patients, behavioral rating scales and coma scales do not directly assess cognitive functioning as would a mental status examination. Rather, clinicians rate patients' abilities (e.g., memory abilities) based on their knowledge of patients' behaviors and/or based on interviews with caregivers who are familiar with patients' levels of functioning. Our emphasis in reviewing these scales is to provide the reader with a general overview of some of the recent scales that have been used to assess patients with dementia. As such, we do not attempt to summarize all of the existing scales. Rather, we have selected scales that have been developed recently, have recent reliability and validity data, and/or have recently been applied to patients with dementia. We should also point out that there is great variation between the behavioral and psychiatric domains that these scales are designed to assess. In Table 4, we provide examples of several scales, cite major references that contain information on their development and validation, and describe the specific domains they assess. The text that follows describes the development and psychometric characteristics of the scales.

The London Psychogeriatric Rating Scale (LPRS) (Hersch, Kral, & Palmer, 1978) is a 36-item, factor analytically derived behavioral rating scale designed to assess behavioral functioning of elderly patients as an alternative to standard mental status evaluations. It is completed by a caregiver who rates the frequency of various behaviors on a scale of 1 to 3 (never, occasionally, frequently). A total score and a score for each of the four subscales can be calculated. These subscales include Mental Disorganization/Confusion, Physical Disability, Socially Irritating Behavior, and Disengagement. Several studies report information on the validity and reliability of the LPRS (Hersch, Csapo, & Palmer, 1978; Hersch, Kral, & Palmer, 1978; Hersch, Mersky, & Palmer, 1980; Reid, Tierney, Zorzitto, Snow, & Fisher, 1991; Rozenbilds, Goldney, Gilchrist, Martin, & Connelly, 1986). To summarize, these studies indicate that the LPRS is able to distinguish: (1) patients with dementia from patients with schizophrenia and bipolar disorder, (2) inpatients with dementia and outpatients with dementia, (3) patients with DAT and patients with other dementing disorders, and (4) patients with dementia and normal controls (Reid et al., 1991). As would be expected, LPRS scores of patients with dementia indicate more severe impairment when compared to normal control groups. Inpatients with dementia exhibit more severe impairment than outpatients with dementia. Patients with DAT exhibited higher scores on the LPRS scales assessing Mental Disorganization/Confusion compared to other patients with dementia. When used to classify individuals as demented or nondemented, the LPRS provided significantly more incremental predictive validity ($p < .001$) than a brief mental status examination (Reid et al., 1991). In addition, the LPRS total score

TABLE 4. Behavior Rating Scales Used to Access Patients with Dementia

Rating scales	Reference	Subjects	Test characteristics	Domains assessed
Neurobehavioral Rating Scale (NRS)	Sultzer et al., (1992)	61 DAT* and 22 MID**; M Age = 73 ± 7.5; M education = 13 ± 3.4; M MMSE = 12 ± 9.0	28 Items[a]; administration time = 30–40 minutes; structured interview with patient	Cognition/Insight, Agitation/Disinhibition, Behavioral Retardation, Anxiety/Depression, Verbal Output Disturbance, Psychosis
Echelle Comportement et Adaptation	Ritchie & Ledesert (1991)	246 mixed dementias; M age = 83.9 ± 7.2; M education 8.9 ± 3.2	32 items; administration time not specified; patient observation and interview.	Social Integration, Occupation and Orientation, Language, Physical Independence, Mobility
Nurses' Observation Scale for Geriatric Patients	Spiegel et al. (1991)	485 normal and demented[b,c]	30 items; time to complete <10 minutes; patient observation	Memory, IADL, Self-care (ADL), Mood, Social Behavior, Disturbing Behavior
London Psychogeriatric Rating Scale	Reid et al. (1991)	274 normal and demented[c]	36 items; time to complete <10 minutes; informant rating scale	Mental Disorganization/Confusion, Physical Disability, Socially Irritating Behaviors, Disengagement

*DAT = Dementia of the Alzheimer type.
**MID = Multi-infarct dementia.
[a]Sultzer et al. (1992) added an additional item to the original 27 NRS items to assess fluent aphasia.
[b]The N = 485 includes subjects from three separate studies conducted at different sites. Results of these three studies were reported by Spiegel et al. (1991).
[c]Aged and education were not specified although it is assumed that all patients are elderly.

correlated significantly ($r = -.79, p < .0001$) with performance on a mental status examination (Reid et al., 1991). Reliability studies indicate high internal consistency (alpha $= .96$) (Reid et al., 1991). Also, certain items on LPRS are highly predictive of whether or not psychogeriatric patients will be discharged from the hospital (Hersch et al., 1980).

However, it does appear than even though the LPRS was derived using factor analysis, the four LPRS subscales are not independent. A factor analysis conducted by Reid and co-workers (1991) produced a three-factor solution in which Disengagement, Socially Irritating Behaviors, and Physical Disability factors were extracted. Items from the Mental Disorganization/Confusion factor were scattered across the three extracted factors. Overall, these studies suggest that the LPRS is a reliable and valid measure of behavioral symptomatology associated with dementia, particularly when the total score is used. Factor analysis indicates that some caution is required when interpreting individual subscale scores, particularly the Disorientation/Confusion subscale. Finally, although the LPRS was reported to differentiate between patients with DAT and patients with other types of dementia, the differences between the two patient groups were relatively small, which significantly limits the usefulness of the LPRS to make differential diagnoses (Reid et al., 1991).

The original version of the Neurobehavioral Rating Scale (NRS) (Levin et al., 1987) contained 27 items and was used to assess behavioral sequelae arising from head injury. Items were scored on a seven-point scale according to level of severity (Not Present to Extremely Severe), with a higher score indicating greater severity. While the NRS has most often been used with individuals who exhibit cognitive dysfunction resulting from head injuries (Corrigan, Dickerson, Fisher, & Meyer, 1990; Levin et al., 1987; Levin, Van Horn, & Curtis, 1993; Vilkki et al., 1994), at least two studies report the use of the NRS with patients who have dementia (Sultzer, Levin, Mahler, High, & Cumings, 1992, 1993). Of these two studies, one examined the psychometric properties of the NRS (Sultzer et al., 1992). In this study, principal components analysis was used to generate six factors (see Table 4) from the original 27 NRS items. The authors also examined the relationship between NRS factors and measures of cognitive function, functional abilities, and depression. Significant correlations were present between the NRS Cognition/Insight Factor and the MMSE ($r = -.95, p < .0001$). Similarly, the Cognition/Insight factor was significantly related to a functional ability scale ($r = .85, p < .004$). The Hamilton Rating Scale for Depression (Hamilton, 1967) correlated significantly with NRS factors Anxiety/Depression ($r = .54, p < .0001$), Psychosis ($r = .40, p < .0002$). Agitation/Disinhibition ($r = .35, p < .0012$), and Cognition/Insight ($r = .34, p < .008$). Three of the NRS factors (Cognition/Insight, Agitation/Disinhibition, and Verbal Output Disturbance) differentiated patients with severe dementia (MMSE < 10; $n = 35$) from those with mild to moderate dementia (MMSE ≥ 10; $n = 26$). Although the authors did not report information on the reliability of the NRS when used with patients who have dementia, other studies examining patients with cognition impairment resulting from head injuries indicate that the NRS has good test–retest and interrater reliabilities (Corrigan et al., 1990; Levin et al., 1987). Because patients representing all levels of dementia severity were evaluated by Sultzer and colleagues (1992), the NRS appears to be appropriate for use with patients who have severe dementia. Also, because NRS scores are only minimally based on information gained from the patient (Sultzer et al., 1992), one would not expect patient fatigue to interfere with the evaluation process. However, in some cases, depending on how much information is derived from the patient, the length of the structured interview process used to derive ratings for each of the NRS items may be prohibitive. Also, fluctuations in behavioral disturbances may not be reflected in the NRS score (Sultzer et al., 1992). Obtaining information from caregivers may help increase the sensitivity of the NRS to behavioral fluctuations and increase the accuracy of estimating typical levels of functioning.

The Echelle Comportement et Adaptation (ECA) is a behavioral rating scale that primarily assesses the capacity or ability to perform certain adaptive behaviors (as opposed to the opportunity to perform or actual performance of the behaviors). It was developed for French-speaking patients, but has been translated into English (Ritchie & Ledesert, 1991). We report on the ECA because of its careful construction, extensive normative group, and emphasis on assessment of severe dementia. The ECA assesses behaviors classified by the World Health Organization as "principal survival roles" (World Health Organization, 1980), which include physical independence, mobility, social integration, occupation, and orientation. The test authors also included an assessment of language abilities. In the original experimental version of the ECA, nursing home staff members rated 21 patients on two occasions using 52 items. The authors reported high interrater reliabilities for this experimental version. Items that did not have significant ($p < .05$) test–retest reliabilities were excluded, leaving 32 items in the final version of the scale. Scoring of items is variable, with some items being dichotomous and others ranging from 0 to 8. Total scores range from 0 to 163.

The 32-item version of the ECA was then administered to 322 individuals diagnosed with dementia. Of the original 322 patients, 42.7% were classified as severely demented according to the Clinical Dementia Rating Scale (Hughes, Berg, Danziger, Coben, & Martin, 1982) and 72% carried diagnoses of DAT. Those patients with questionable dementia were excluded. An additional 32 patients (mean age = 82.3, mean education = 8.6) without dementia but with other physical disabilities were included as a comparison group. Ritchie and Ledesert (1991) present reliability and validity data for the remaining 246 patients who were unquestionably demented. Alpha coefficients for each of the five ECA subscales ranged between .40 and .70. The authors also provide cutoffs for differentiating between severity levels of dementia as follows: severe dementia ≤ 55, moderate dementia ≤ 80, and mild dementia ≤ 95. In contrast to these scores, individuals in the comparison group obtained scores between 110 and 150. The ECA total score and the MMSE total score were significantly correlated ($r = .40$,

$p < .0009$). Individuals who scored zero on the MMSE (20% of the patients with dementia) exhibited a wide range of scores on all of the ECA subscales with the exception of the Occupation and Orientation subscale. This suggests that the ECA is not subject to floor effects reported for instruments such as the MMSE. No significant effects for age, education, or dementia type were present among the group with dementia. It is also important to note that the ECA differentiated between cognitively intact patients with disabilities and patients with dementia. Based on this finding, it appears that the ECA is not primarily assessing the physical disability of patients with severe dementia, but is evaluating behavioral symptomatology associated with the dementing process. When subjected to factor analysis, the ECA subscales fared relatively well in that most of the factors extracted emulated those originally proposed by the authors. The validation study of the ECA provides information, suggesting that the scale is both reliable and valid. Alpha coefficients for some of the ECA subscales are moderately low, possibly reflecting heterogeneity of subscale content. This shortcoming may be resolved if the ECA items are reorganized according to the results of the factor analysis. This scale awaits further validation with an English-speaking population.

The Nurses' Observation Scale for Geriatric Patients (NOSGER) (Spiegel et al., 1991) is also a European measure. It was devised as a brief behavioral rating scale that could be completed by untrained caregivers. To form the initial version of the test, the authors selected items from two behavioral rating scales. Items selected assessed six categories of behaviors that were originally specified as domains of interest for the NOSGER. There are five items in each subscale and each item is rated on a scale of 1 to 5. Ratings reflect the frequency of specific behaviors during the past 2 weeks. The NOSGER yields separate subscale scores. The test authors present reliability and validity information that was gathered across three separate studies. Information regarding the reliability and validity of the NOSGER suggest that it is psychometrically sound. For example, across the three samples, interrater reliabilities ranged from .53 to .89 for the Disturbing Behavior subscale, to .74 to .91 for the Memory subscale. The low reliability for the Disturbing Behavior subscale appears to be due to a restriction of range in one of the study sample; in that sample, behaviors classified as disturbing were rare. Test–retest reliabilities were also high, generally falling between .80 and .90 for the six subscales across three different samples. These reliability coefficients are quite impressive when one considers that many of the raters were untrained.

Validity estimates are also impressive. Spiegel and colleagues (1991) performed multiple correlations between the NOSGER subscales and measures thought to assess similar domains of functioning. Measures included neuropsychological tests of memory functioning (e.g., the Rey Auditory Verbal Learning Test, Rey, 1964), self-report measures of affective state (e.g., the Geriatric Depression Scale, Yesavage et al., 1983), and behavioral rating scales (e.g., Geriatric Rating Scale, Plutchik et al., 1970). Correlations typically ranged between .50 and .80, supporting the construct validity of the NOSGER. Also, the

NOSGER subscales assessing memory, instrumental ADL (IADLs), and disturbing behaviors proved to be the most sensitive to changes in patients with mild to moderate dementia (Tremmel & Spiegel, 1993). A factor analysis of the NOSGER conducted by Brunner and Spiegel (as cited in Spiegel et al., 1991) indicated that one factor accounted for most of the total variance. The authors suggest that this factor is a general index of cognitive deterioration. This factor solution may argue for the use of an overall score, in addition to the subscales scores, as an estimate of severity. Spiegel and co-workers provide a copy of the revised NOSGER (NOSGER II), which clarifies several ambiguously worded questions while retaining the content of the original version. The authors report that studies are being conducted in European and North American centers to determine if the NOSGER is sensitive to change in behavior based on treatment or dementia progression. The NOSGER is available in German, French, and English. While the fact that the NOSGER can be administered by untrained caregivers may be viewed as a strength, it may also be that individuals who are trained in the administration of the test may produce higher reliability scores.

In addition to those instruments listed in Table 4, there are also global staging methods used to specify severity and progression of dementia. Rather than providing estimates of functioning across several areas (e.g., social interaction, language, dress, and grooming), global staging methods assign a particular number based on the extent of overall impairment. Because staging methods are often used in research, we briefly mention them here. Two scales used as global measures of impairment to stage levels of impairment in patients with dementia are the Clinical Dementia Rating Scale (CDR) (Heyman et al., 1987; Hughes et al., 1982) and the Global Deterioration Scale (GDS) (Reisberg, Ferris, de Leon, & Crook, 1982, 1988).

The GDS provides a classification of dementia severity based on the following seven point rating system: $1 =$ no cognitive decline, $2 =$ very mild cognitive decline, $3 =$ mild cognitive decline, $4 =$ moderate cognitive decline, $5 =$ moderately severe cognitive decline, $6 =$ severe cognitive decline, and $7 =$ very severe cognitive decline (Reisberg et al., 1982, 1988). Information used to assign global ratings of impairment is derived through interviews with patients and caregivers. GDS scores correlate significantly with psychometric measures, clinical ratings of cognitive status, computed tomography scans assessing ventricular dilation and sulcal enlargement, and decreased glucose metabolism in specific brain regions as evinced by positron emission tomography (Reisberg et al., 1982). Test–retest and interrater reliabilities of the GDS have generally been greater than .90, suggesting good reliability (see Reisberg et al., 1988; Kluger & Ferris, 1991). An additional test, the Functional Assessment Staging Test (FAST), has been developed to be used in conjunction with the GDS (Reisberg, 1988). The FAST is composed of 16 items designed to stage the typical pattern of functional loss in patients with DAT. Items are arranged in order of increasing severity so that they coincide with stages of the GDS. Reisberg (1988) reported that the FAST score significantly correlates with psychometric tests and with clinical assessments. The FAST has also been used successfully to describe deterioration of functioning in patients with advanced Alzheimer's disease (Franssen, Kluger, Torossian, & Reisberg, 1993).

The second global staging method, the CDR assigns severity ratings based on information from six areas of functioning including memory, orientation, judgment and problem solving, community affairs, home and hobbies, and personal care (Hughes et al., 1982). A semistructured interview conducted with the patient and an appropriate caregiver is used to derive information needed to establish impairment ratings for each category. In the original version, impairment was rated in each area of functioning according to the following system: 0 = none, 0.5 = questionable, 1 = mild, 2 = moderate, and 3 = severe. Scores from the six categories are then used to establish a global rating of impairment as follows: CDR 0 = none, CDR 0.5 = questionable, CDR 1 = mild, CDR 2 = moderate, and CDR 3 = severe. Heyman and colleagues (1987) have suggested that the CDR be expanded to include ratings of profound impairment (advanced; CDR 4) and terminal stages (vegetative; CDR 5) to help the scale distinguish between levels of severe impairment. The CDR has undergone modifications since its initial publication in an effort to decrease ambiguities that were present between levels of severity within specific categories. Morris (1993) provides a summary of these modifications and a copy of the new version of the CDR. Several studies have provided information supporting the reliability and validity of the CDR (Burke et al., 1988; Davis, Morris, & Grant, 1990; Forsell, Fratiglioni, Grut, Viitanen, & Winbald, 1992; Morris, McKeel, Fulling, Torach, & Berg, 1988).

The GDS and CDR were designed to assess degenerative dementias and primarily DAT. Special care was taken to assure that the GDS and CDR stages coincided with the progression of symptoms in patients with progressive dementia. Detailed descriptions of the behaviors noted at each stage have been provided for both the GDS (Reisberg et al., 1988) and the CDR (Morris, 1993). Some authors suggest that the GDS differentiates the earlier stages of dementia better than the CDR (Kluger & Ferris, 1991). The addition of the FAST to the GDS also gives it some advantages over the CDR, particularly for investigators interested in staging dementia severity and impairment of functional ability simultaneously. While sensitive to all levels of dementia severity, these instruments provide gross estimates of functional and overall levels of impairment. Fine-grained analyses of behavioral and psychiatric symptoms require more extensive behavior rating scales such as the NRS, ECA, NOSGER, and LPRS.

It is also important to emphasize that behavioral rating scales and global staging scales are not designed to provide differential diagnoses, although some behavioral rating scales do appear to distinguish between patients with dementia of varied etiology (Sultzer et al., 1993). Further research and refinement is needed in order to establish the utility of these scales (if any) in differentially diagnosing dementias. Parenthetically, some scales do assist in differential diagnosis. Cummings and Benson (1986) developed the DAT Inventory to differentiate between DAT and other forms of dementia. The results of retrospective and prospective studies of the DAT Inventory indicate that it has excellent specificity (.94–.95) and sensitivity (.98–1.00) when used with patients in the moderate to severe stages of the disorder (Coen et al., 1994; Cummings & Benson, 1986). However, inclusion of patients with mild DAT significantly decreases the inventories sensitivity. Some authors also suggest that behavioral rating scales may be of limited usefulness in assessing severely demented patients because of the physical disability (and resulting in decreased behavioral repertoires) often noted inpatients with severe dementia (Ward et al., 1993; Ward, Murphy, & Proctor, 1991). Comparisons between patients with disabilities who are not demented and patients with severe dementia (e.g., Ritchie & Ledesert, 1991) may help elucidate possible differences in the presentation of physical disabilities in these two groups. Finally, it is important to recognize that multidimensional scales do not evaluate all behaviors commonly seen in patients with dementia. As a result, information produced by these scales may need to be supplemented based on the specific reason for their use.

Tests of Cognitive Abilities

In contrast to assessment batteries focusing on early detection of dementia and quantification of cognitive functioning in patients with mild to moderate levels of cognitive impairment, researchers have only recently reported the development of instruments designed to assess cognitive functioning in individuals with severe dementia. These instruments have been designed to fill an obvious gap in the assessment literature. The importance of these new tests is not fully realized clinically or empirically. However, the obvious contribution of cognitive measures of severe impairment to current assessment approaches is based on the fact that, prior to their development, researchers and clinicians were often unable to directly investigate (in a standardized manner) the level of cognitive impairment and the progression of cognitive deficits in patients during the latter stages of dementia.

After an extensive review of the literature, we located five neuropsychological tests for severe impairment that have some initial reliability and validity data. These include the Severe Impairment Battery (SIB) (Saxton et al., 1990, 1993), Test of Severe Impairment (TSI) (Albert & Cohen, 1992), Guy's Advanced Dementia Schedule (GADS) (Ward et al., 1993), Severe Cognitive Impairment Profile (SCIP) (Peavy, Salmon, Rice, & Butters, 1995), and Rush Advanced Dementia Scale (RADS) (Gilley, Wilson, Bernard, Stebbins, & Fox, 1990). Of these tests, the SIB has received the most attention in the literature. Because there is more information available on the validity and reliability of the SIB, we will devote the majority of the current discussion to the SIB. However, we will also review the published articles on the TSI, GADS, SCIP, and RADS. In addition to tests specifically designed to assess individuals with severe cognitive impairment, we will review one report of the use of a pediatric test (the Ordinal Scales of Psychological Development) (Uzgiris & Hunt, 1975) with patients who exhibit severe cognitive impairment (Sclan et al., 1990).

The Severe Impairment Battery (SIB) (Saxton et al., 1990, 1993) was specifically developed to assess cognitive functioning of individuals with severe dementia. It has undergone two revisions since the initial report of its reliability and validity. The original experimental version of the SIB yielded a score of 0–152 (Saxton et al., 1990). However, after initial results were obtained, the test authors removed those items that could not be performed by any of the patients or changed items so they were easier to answer. For example, in the original version, examiners asked patients to tell them the current date. No patients with MMSE scores of less than 10 could answer this question, so the question was dropped. Other orientation questions (e.g., current month) were changed so that patients could receive partial credit if they were able to identify the correct answer from three alternatives (J. Saxton, personal communication, January 18, 1995). Following the first revision, the total number of points decreased from 152 to 133. In the second revision of the SIB (Saxton et al., 1993), changes focused on modifying scoring criteria so that some items were not weighted too heavily in the total score. For example, instead of assigning one point to each correct response during the verbal fluency portion of the SIB, patients receive two points for four or more correct responses and one point for one to three correct responses.

The final version of the SIB (Saxton et al., 1993) contains 40 questions and takes approximately 20 minutes to administer. Scores range from 1 to 100. The SIB yields six major subscale scores that reflect the six cognitive domains often assessed in individuals with mild to moderate levels of dementia. As such, the test extends standard neuropsychological assessment techniques to the severely impaired. The abilities assessed by these six subscales include attention, orientation, language, memory, visuospatial perception, and construction. Less extensive assessments of praxis, patient's ability to orient to his or her name when spoken, and social interactions are also included. There is no cutoff for "normal" because of the nature of the scale. Individuals scoring less than 63 on the SIB are classified as very severely impaired. Subjects without dementia or other forms of cognitive impairment almost always receive perfect scores on the SIB (Panisset, Roudier, Saxton, & Boller, 1992). In order to facilitate administration with severely impaired subjects, SIB items are one-step commands that can be repeated as needed to ensure comprehension. These commands are accompanied by gestures that are intended to help patients understand what they are to do. Also, the SIB authors designed the test so that it is presented in a smooth, flowing style, similar in some ways to a structured clinical interview.

To date, at least seven articles describe the psychometric characteristics of the SIB (Panisset et al., 1992, 1994; Parlato, et al., 1992; Reglà et al., in press; Saxton et al., 1990; Wild & Kaye, in press; Wild, Lear, & Kaye, 1995) in addition to the reliability and validity information reported in the SIB test administration manual (Saxton et al., 1993). Four of these studies report the use of the SIB with non-English-speaking populations; two of the studies reported the use of the SIB with French-speaking populations (Panisset et al., 1992, 1994), one reported the use of an Italian version of the SIB (Parlato et al., 1992), and another reported the use of the SIB with Spanish-speaking individuals (Reglà et al., in press). The results of all of the studies providing reliability and validity data for the SIB are presented in Table 5.

In the initial report, Saxton and colleagues (1990) administered the experimental version of the SIB to 41 patients with dementia. They calculated interrater reliability and test–retest reliabilities using subsets of this group of patients. Interrater reliability correlations ranging between .87 and 1.00 were obtained for the various subtests. The Praxis subtest received interrater correlation of .87, while the remaining subtests ranged between .97 and 1.00. A test–retest correlation of .85 was obtained for the total SIB score. For the various SIB subscales, test–retest correlations ranged between .22 (Construction) and .86 (Praxis). Initial information on the construct validity of the SIB was also derived by comparing patients' performances on the SIB Total Score to their MMSE performances. A correlation of .74 was obtained when all of the subjects' SIB and MMSE scores were compared (SIB range, 15–136; MMSE range, 0–13). For the 31 patients scoring 9 or below on the MMSE, the correlation between SIB and MMSE scores was .71. These results provided initial evidence supporting the reliability and validity of the SIB.

Panisset and colleagues (1994) provided further support for the validity and reliability of the SIB, using the first revision. They assessed 69 French patients who had diagnoses of probable DAT. Diagnoses of DAT were made according to National Institute of Neurologic and Communicative Diseases and Stroke/ Alzheimer's Disease and Related Disorders Association criteria (McKhann et al., 1984). An additional 22 patients with orthopedic problems who were similar in age and educational level to the DAT group were included as controls. As in their previous study, the SIB was compared to the MMSE. Also, patients with DAT were divided into four groups based on severity of impairment. Severity of impairment was determined by their MMSE scores. The groups were formed as follows: group 1, MMSE from 0 to 5; group 2, MMSE from 6 to 11; group 3, MMSE from 12 to 17; group 4, MMSE > 17. The results confirmed the SIB sensitivity to severe impairment. Those patients in the group who scored 0–5 on the MMSE obtained scores ranging between 7 and 81. Furthermore, patients receiving MMSE scores of 0 ($n = 8$) obtained SIB total scores ranging between 7 and 65. Similarly, the primary author of the SIB reported that individuals who have progressive dementia and MMSE scores of 8 or 9 can be followed for at least 2 years using the SIB. During this time, declines in SIB scores will be noted (J. Saxton, personal communication, January 18, 1995). The sensitivity of the SIB to severe impairment is also supported by the finding that significant differences were present between the SIB total scores of group 1 and group 2, although no significant differences were present between groups 2, 3, and 4 (Panisset et al., 1994). Panisset and co-workers were also able to reassess 26 of the original 69 dementia patients 10–52 weeks after the initial assessment (mean = 34.58 ± 12.88 weeks). As would be expected in patients with progressive dementia, SIB follow-up scores were significantly lower than initial scores (mean = 81.23 ± 38.30 and 91.19 ± 33.80, respectively). However, while

TABLE 5. Severe Impairment Battery (SIB) Reliability and Validity Data

Study	Sample	n	Age	Validity	Test–retest interval	Test–retest reliability	Interrater reliability
Saxton et al. (1990)	Severe dementia; M education = 11.6 ± 3.0; M MMSE = 6.6 ± 4.0	41	M = 72.2 ± 7.8	.74 (n = 41)c; .16–.77b	6–30 days; M = 14.3 days	.85 (n = 14)c; .22–.86d	1.00 (n = 11)c; .87–1.00d
Panisset et al. (1992)	DAT*; M MMSE = 10.11 ± 6.38	54	M = 83.2 ± 6.4	Not specified	Not specified	.87c (n = 17)	.996c (n = 36)
Parlato et al. (1992)	DAT*; M MMSE = 5.89 ± 4.86	55	M = 68.5 ± 8.7	Not specified	Not specified	†	††
Saxton et al. (1993)	69 DAT*; 1 MID**; M education = 11.5; M MMSE = 6.0 ± 3.8	70	M = 72.7 ± 7.8	.77 (n = 70)c; .88 (n = 55)e	Not specified	.90 (n = 22)c; .06–.87d	.99 (n = 24)c; .89–1.00d
Panisset et al. (1994)	69 DAT* (M MMSE = 10.7 ± 6.1; Primary education); 22 nondemented controls (M MMSE = 28.4 ± 0.8; primary education)	91	DAT M = 83.0 ± 5.7; control M = 81.5 ± 6.5	.82 (n = 69 DAT)a	7 days	.87 (n = 17 DAT)c	.996c (n = 36 DAT)

*DAT = Dementia of the Alzheimer type. Includes patients with diagnoses of probable and possible DAT (McKhann et al., 1984).
**MID = Multi-infarct dementia.
†Authors reported significant (p < .001) test–retest reliabilities for SIB total score (n = 15), although the exact coefficient was not reported.
††Authors reported significant interrater reliabilities for SIB total score. Sample size and exact correlation coefficient were not reported.
aCorrelation between MMSE total scores and SIB total scores.
bRange of correlations between MMSE total scores and SIB subtest scores.
cCorrelation for SIB total score.

(continued)

TABLE 5. (*Continued*)

Study	Sample	n	Age	Validity	Test–retest interval	Test–retest reliability	Interrater reliability
Wild & Kaye (in press)	43 DAT*; 3 MID**; 4 other dementias; *M* education = 13.0 ± 2.9; *M* MMSE = 9.0 ± 4.9	50	*M* = 71.1 ± 10.0				.79[a]; −.55[f]; −.40[g]; −.76[h]
Reglà et al. (in press)	46 DAT*; 12 MID**; *M* MEC[i] = 10.76 ± 6.41	58	*M* = 74.5 ± 7.8	.83 (n = 41)[j]; .29–.80[k]	7–14 days	.98 (n = 17)[c]; .76–.97[d]	.999 (n = 12)[c]; .995–1.00[d]

[a]Range of correlations for SIB subtest scores.
[c]Correlation between DRS total score and SIB total score.
[d]Correlation between SIB total score and ADL score.
[f]Correlation between SIB total score and IADL score.
[g]Correlation between SIB total score and Clinical Dementia Rating Scale score (CDR; Hughes et al., 1982).
[h]Correlation between SIB total score and MMSE.
[i]The MEC (Mini-Examen Cognoscitivo) is the Spanish adaptation of the MMSE.
[j]Correlation between the SIB total score and the MEC.
[k]Range of correlations between the SIB subscale scores and the MEC.

the majority of these patients exhibited significantly decreased scores over the time lapse ($n = 17$), one patient's score remained the same and four patients exhibited significant improvement. These differences in performance across time probably reflect the natural variability in cognitive status during the course of DAT.

Studies examining SIB performances in non-English- and English-speaking populations report very similar results. Interrater reliabilities appear consistently lower for the Praxis subtest (reliabilities of .87, .89, and .95, reported by Saxton et al., 1990, Saxton et al., 1993, and Reglà et al., in press, respectively) than for other subtests. However, these interrater reliabilities are quite high. It may be that due to increased subjectivity, particular emphasis should be placed on standard administration and scoring of the Praxis subtest. In regard to test–retest reliabilities, some consistencies are also noted across studies. The higher test–retest correlations have been reported for the Language subtest (reliabilities of .79, and .87, and .97, reported by Saxton et al., 1990, Saxton et al., 1993, and Reglà, in press, respectively), while the lowest were generally reported for the Orientation subtest (reliabilities of .06, .36, and .78, reported by Saxton et al., 1990, Saxton et al., 1993, and Reglà et al., in press, respectively) and the Construction subtest (reliabilities of .22 and .76, reported by Saxton et al., 1990, and Reglà et al., in press, respectively). It is also worth noting that the interrater and test–retest reliabilities for the SIB subtests appear to have improved as the test was revised. The language subtest also appears to consistently correlate strongly with MMSE scores across studies.

Other reports of the SIB's validity have been equally consistent. Wild and co-workers (1995) reported significant decline in the SIB scores of 20 patients with dementia who were assessed twice (mean assessment interval = 12 months; range = 4–26 months). Additionally, Wild and Kaye (in press) reported that when an SIB cutoff score of 50 was used to classify their most severely impaired patients (i.e., those patients with CDR ratings of 3), the sensitivity and specificity of the SIB were .89 and .97, respectively. Wild and Kaye also confirmed the original reports of the sensitivity of the SIB to severe cognitive impairment. They suggest that the sensitivity of the SIB relative to other cognitive screening instruments is seen when noting the range of scores obtained on the SIB as compared to, for example, the MMSE. In this regard, Wild and Kaye (in press) reported that patients who receive scores ranging between 0 and 16 on the MMSE score between 4 and 95 on the SIB. Sensitivity of the SIB to cognitive impairment is further supported by the fact that the scores of those individuals classified as the most severely cognitively impaired (as determined by MMSE scores) were significantly different than scores of the less impaired patients (Wild & Kaye, in press).

In the only study examining the relationship of the SIB to measures of ADLs and IADLs as well as the Clinical Dementia Rating Scale (CDR) (Hughes et al., 1982), Wild and Kaye (in press) reported significant correlations between the SIB and all of these measures (see Table 5). Analyses of the relationships between SIB subscales and a measure of ADLs indicated that the Construction, Attention, Visuospatial Skills, and Memory subscales were significantly correlated with scores of the ADL measure. All of the SIB subtests correlated significantly with CDRs, with the exception of Orientation to Name. The weakest correlation was noted between the SIB and the IADL measure. This may have been the results of the restricted range of IADL scores (range = 0–14; mean = 11.4; *SD*; = 2.8). This restricted range is consistent with the fact that most patients with severe dementia need full assistance with activities that IADL scales assess (e.g., managing money). Finally, Wild and Kaye reported that the SIB is not significantly correlated with age or education.

These initial studies suggest that patients who are severely impaired and have traditionally been considered untestable do exhibit a wide range of performances on the SIB. In fact, the SIB has the most sensitivity in subjects with the most significant cognitive impairment. This suggests that there is not a floor effect when the SIB is used with severely impaired patients. Wild and Kaye (in press) also point out that the relationships noted between the SIB test scores and measures of functional ability provide initial support for the idea that cognitive functioning is a predictor of functional abilities, a relationship that has not always been supported in previous studies of patients with dementia. Relationships between specific cognitive abilities and specific functional abilities may also be present, and the SIB may allow for an exploration of these relationships in patients with severe dementia. Another strength of the SIB it that versions are available in English, Spanish, French, and Italian. The strong reliability and validity coefficients reported for the initial experimental version have been replicated across these ethnolinguistic groups, adding further support for the tests excellent psychometric properties.

The SIB does, however, have several limitations:

1. The instrument was developed primarily with research applications in mind, and as a result, the clinical applications of the test have not been investigated.
2. While the population on which the initial reliability and validity data were gathered generally had MMSE scores of less than 10, it was made up of outpatients who were maintained in the community with help from significant others. As a result, the original group appears to be significantly different than institutionalized patients who are considered severely impaired (J. Saxton, personal communication, January 18, 1995). This may be true even when MMSE scores of the two groups are equal. The primary author of the SIB reported that data have been gathered on more severely impaired nursing home populations, although it has not been published as of this writing (J. Saxton, personal communication, January 18, 1995). At this juncture, the impact of institutionalization and the limitations it may cause for tests such as the SIB are not fully understood.
3. The SIB is appropriate for patients who could be described as moderately severely impaired, rather than those who are severely severely impaired. The primary test author validly points out that the cognitive abilities of se-

verely severely impaired individuals (i.e., those who are vegetative, non-verbal, and/or respond only to pain stimuli) are not testable regardless of the test employed because they are unable to respond in a meaningful way (J. Saxton, personal communication, January 18, 1995). These individuals are most appropriately assessed with behavioral rating scales.

4. While there does not appear to be a floor effect for the SIB, there is a ceiling effect. In this regard, J. Saxton suggests that the SIB should be used with care when assessing individuals who score 11–13 or greater on the MMSE, because individuals functioning at or above these levels may become irritated with the ease of the test.

5. The high interrater reliabilities obtained by investigators will not be achieved unless examiners have adequate training. While this is obviously true with all neuropsychological instruments, we make special mention of it here because the SIB may be more difficult to master than other tests. This is because it is meant to be administered in a flowing manner accompanied by appropriate gestures. Also, individuals with severe dementia are often unable to tolerate clumsy or slow administrations.

There is very little published information currently available on the four remaining scales for assessing severe dementia. In fact, for the Test of Severe Impairment (Albert & Cohen, 1992) and the Guy's Advanced Dementia Scale (Ward et al., 1993), the only published information consists of the initial articles reporting scale development, reliability data, and validity data. For the Severe Cognitive Impairment Profile (Peavy et al., 1995) and the Rush Advanced Dementia Scale (Gilley et al., 1990), only published abstracts of papers presented at conventions are available. The results of these studies are presented in Table 6.

The Test of Severe Impairment (TSI) (Albert & Cohen, 1992) was designed as both a clinical and research tool. It consists of 24 items and takes approximately 10 minutes to administer. Albert and Cohen (1992) report that the 24 TSI items contribute to six subscales that assess the following abilities: " . . . well learned motor performance, language comprehension, language production, immediate and delayed memory, general knowledge, and conceptualization" (p. 450). The TSI requires minimal verbal responding; only 3 of 24 items require a verbal response. Principal components analysis revealed that three factors accounted for approximately 40% of the total variance. These factors appeared to assess: (1) memory, (2) verbal production of well-learned information, and (3) identification and manipulation of body parts (Albert & Cohen, 1992). Initial data on the TSI suggest that it has good test–retest reliability, internal consistency, and high correlation with the MMSE when it is used with individuals who have severe dementia. Also, TSI scores were not significantly correlated with the level of education or the age of their subjects. Albert and Cohen suggest that the TSI has several advantages over the SIB, including that it takes less time to administer and that its subscales have higher test–retest reliability coefficients.

TABLE 6. Tests for Severely Impaired Patients

Test	Study	Sample	n	Age	Validity	Test–retest reliability	Interrater reliability	Internal consistency
Rush Advanced Dementia Scale	Gilley et al. (1990)	Outpatients with DAT*	135	†	.81[a]			
Test for Severe Impairment (TSI)	Albert & Cohen (1992)	Institutionalized patients with severe dementias; M MMSE = 6.4 ± 3.2	40	72–98	.83[b]	.96[c] .74–.97[d]; (n = 19)		.91[e]
Guy's Advanced Dementia Schedule (GADS)	Ward et al. (1993)	Institutionalized patients with moderate–severe dementias; M MMSE = 2.63 ± 4.76	41	M = 78 ± 6	††	>.6[f]	>.7[g]	
Severe Cognitive Impairment Profile (SCIP)	Peavy et al. (1995)	Patients with severe dementia	33	†	.95[h]	.97[i]	.99	

*DAT = Dementia of the Alzheimer type.
†This information was not reported.
††Ward et al. (1993) report significant correlations between GADS scores and scores on the MMSE and teh Clifton Assessment Procedures for Elderly behavior rating scale (Pattie & Gilleard, 1979), although exact correlations are not specified.
[a]Correlation between the RADS total score and patients' MMSE scores ≦ 10.
[b]Correlation between MMSE total scores and TSI total scores.
[c]Test-retest reliability for TSI total score. Test–retest interval of 1 week.
[d]Range of test–retest reliabilities for TSI subtests. Test–retest interval of 1 week.
[e]Coefficient alpha.
[f]Exact reliability coefficient was not specified. Test–retest interval of 1 week.
[g]Exact reliability coefficient was not specified.
[h]Correlation between SCIP and DRS.
[i]Test–retest was not specified.

The Guy's Advanced Dementia Scale (GADS) (Ward et al., 1993) was primarily designed for research applications in patients with severe dementia, although the authors do suggest that it may have clinical applications. It consists of several objects (e.g., harmonica, baby rattle, comb) and two words (*table* and *stand*). As with other tests of confrontational naming, such as the Boston Naming Test, the GADS includes objects and words whose usage varies in frequency of occurrence. Those objects that have lower frequency of usage are thought to be more difficult, while words that are used more often are thought to be easier. Objects are presented to patients, and their responses, either verbal or nonverbal, are recorded. Also, patients are presented with candy as an incentive to maintain or increase motivation periodically throughout the test. Responses to the candy presentation are record. After subjects have had a chance to identify objects, they are prompted to name the objects and show how they are used. When patients are not able to show how objects are used, the examiner demonstrates their use and requests the patients to then show how the objects are used. Scores range from 1 to 40 and are derived based on five categories of responding including reading, naming, using, taking, and eating candy. Also, a score ranging from 0 to 48 is derived based on the number of prompts, although it is not clear from the article how this score is calculated. The GADS was able to differentiate between a severely impaired patient group and a less severely impaired group as determined by MMSE scores (Folstein et al., 1975). In the same groups, the Glasgow Coma Scale (Teasdale, Knill-Jones, & Van der Sande, 1978) was unable to distinguish between the severely and less severely impaired patients. The GADS also distinguished between patients scoring 0 on the MMSE. Finally, when 31 of the original 41 subjects were tested with the GADS 6 months after the initial testing, significant decreases in performance were noted, which is consistent with the course of progressive dementias. However, the authors did not specify the diagnoses of the 31 patients who completed the evaluations at 6 months, which obscures the interpretation of their results.

The Severe Cognitive Impairment Profile (SCIP) (Peavy et al., 1995) was developed for both clinical and experimental applications. The number of items and administration time of the SCIP were not specified in the only existing report. The SCIP items contribute the eight subscales that assess Comportment, Attention, Language, Memory, Motor Function, Conceptualization, Arithmetic, and Visuospatial Abilities. As can be seen from Table 6, test–retest and interrater reliability estimates are quite good for the initial sample. The significant correlation reported between the Dementia Rating Scale and the SCIP provides initial support for the validity of the SCIP. Also, when patients with the greatest level of cognitive impairment were examined (DRS score < 50), approximately 66% had meaningful SCIP scores. Floor effects were noted when standard neuropsychological measures were used with this same group.

The Rush Advanced Dementia Scale (RADS) was initially reported by Gilley and colleagues (1990). It is composed of 33 items that are primarily linguistic. Administration time was not specified in the published presentation abstract. Published information is not currently available on the reliability of the RADS. However, the strong correlation reported between RADS scores and MMSE scores provides initial evidence supporting the validity of the RADS. Also, some variability in RADS scores was present in patients scoring 0 on the MMSE, suggesting that it is less subject to the floor effects often noted when typical neuropsychological evaluation techniques are used to assess patients who have severe dementia.

Finally, Sclan and colleagues (1990) used a scale originally designed to assess mental functions (as proposed by Piaget). The authors hypothesized that tests designed to evaluate children in the sensoimotor stage of cognitive development would be useful with individuals who have severe dementia, because these tasks do not require higher symbolic functions such as those used in language or abstract reasoning. Subtests selected from the Ordinal Scale of Psychological Development (OSPD) (Sclan et al., 1990) assessed visual pursuit, object permanence, means–ends reasoning, operational causality, construction, and the ability to develop schemes for relating to objects. Some modification of the standard administration and scoring procedure for the OSPD subtests was necessary to make the subtests appropriate for individuals with severe dementia. Twenty-six patients who completed the assessment were divided into two groups (severely impaired and very severely impaired) based on Global Deterioration Scale scores (Reisberg et al., 1982, 1988). All of these patients obtained scores of zero or close to zero on typical brief screening measures of cognitive functioning, including the MMSE and the Blessed Information–Memory–Concentration test. However, the OSPD subtests were sensitive to differences ($p < .05$) in cognitive functioning between the severely impaired and very severely impaired groups (mean scores of 28.87 ± 19.54 and 9.67 ± 11.83, respectively). Split-half reliability coefficients for the individual OSPD subscales ranged between .94 and .99. The authors also reported correlations coefficients ranging between $-.53$ and $-.57$ ($p < .01$) when the OSPD subtests were correlated with a behavioral rating scale that assessed ADLs. Based on these results, the authors suggest that the OSPD subscales, as well as other tests designed to assess infant and neonate cognition, may be useful in assessing patients with severe dementia.

Of the available neuropsychological assessment procedures for severe dementia, the SIB appears superior for several reasons. First, it has been the most widely used, and as a result, has the most extensive reliability and validity data. Second, when compared to the TSI, RADS, and GADS, the SIB assesses a broader range of cognitive abilities. In addition to those cognitive abilities assessed by the TSI, the SIB assesses attention, praxis, visuospatial perception, and construction. Language is also assessed more thoroughly by the SIB than the other tests. The GADS is limited because it primarily assesses language abilities and praxis. Similarly, the RADS is described as primarily assessing linguistic abilities. It does appear that the SCIP assesses four cognitive domains (arithmetic, motor function, conceptualization, and comportment) that are not assessed by the SIB. On the other hand, the SIB assesses orientation, praxis, construction, social skills, and specific language abilities that the SCIP does not assess. It is not possible to ascertain the overlap between these SCIP and SIB subscales based on the information provided in the SCIP abstract. The very limited information available on the construction, validity, and reliability of the SCIP significantly limits its usefulness. Second, the SIB is more appropriate for assessing individuals with severe dementia than tests initially developed for assessing infants or neonates because these tests lack construct, concurrent, and content validity when applied to the elderly. Theoretically, it is not clear whether or not the cognitive deterioration noted in progressive dementias represents a reversal of cognitive developmental stages that Piaget and others noted in infants. Also, it is difficult to interpret the meanings of test scores developed for infants (such as the OSPD) and to determine the relationships between infant tests and standard neuropsychological test scores.

We suggest that clinicians and researchers use the SIB until more information is available for the other measures, unless there is a compelling reason not to use the SIB. In this regard, the TSI may be particularly useful in patients who have limited verbal production abilities because it requires so few verbal responses. Also, because the TSI takes less time to administer than the SIB, it may be more useful for patients with decreased frustration tolerance and attentional abilities. The initial report on the GADS suggests that the sample it was used with was more severely impaired that those studied with the SIB. However, before firm conclusions can be drawn about the relative merits of these neuropsychological measures of severe impairment, research must be conducted comparing them in the same populations. This type of research would help determine if there is an overlap in the abilities assessed by these tests. However, a more interesting finding might be that these scales assess unique cognitive domains. This type of research would also help clarify the relative difficulty level of each of the tests.

CONCLUSION

Tests for severe cognitive impairment have had limited use. Some validity data exist for all of the tests, but this typically involves correlating the tests with a cognitive screening measure such as the MMSE. More extension validity data are required. This information could be obtained in several ways including: (1) making comparisons between each of the currently available tests of severe impairment in the same populations; (2) calculating sensitivity and specificity estimates based on categorization of patients according to levels of severe impairment; and (3) estimating strength of relationships between tests of severe impairment and measures of functional ability (ADL and IADL scales), dementia staging scales and more extensive tests of neuropsychological function. Also, there is a need to determine the relationships, if any, between performance on tests of severe impairment and the severity of neuropathology at autopsy. One would expect that because significant relationships have been reported for quite some time between estimates of neuropathology derived by autopsy and screening measures of cognitive function (Blessed et al., 1968; Katzman et al., 1983), these relationships would also exist with more specific and extensive measures of cognitive functioning. Along these same lines, tests such as the SIB and SCIP that assess multiple cognitive domains may help clarify previous findings by allowing for more precise examination of brain–behavior relationships. Scores on these measures may be related to volume loss or number of plaques and tangles in specific regions of the cerebrum. While tests initially developed for infants exhibit some utility in assessing individuals with severe impairment, these tests do not appear to have any advantages over tests designed specifically for assessing patients with severe dementia.

Available data on the validity of the neuropsychological measures of severe impairment reviewed in the chapter suggest that they are sensitive to changes in cognitive impairment in cases of severe dementia. The sensitivity of these tests to severe cognitive impairment may help resolve some controversies regarding the progression of dementias from mild through severe stages. For example, some authors suggest that floor effects are responsible for the differential rates of decline in cognitive abilities over the course of DAT, while others suggest that differential rates of cognitive decline reflect an interaction between neuronal degeneration and cognitive status (Wild et al., 1995). Neuropsychological tests designed for patients with severe dementia may help resolve this controversy by allowing for assessment of cognitive abilities at severe levels of dementia without floor effects.

The relationship between behavioral rating scales and neuropsychological measures of severe impairment are not clearly defined. It has yet to be determined if there is a strong relationship between behavioral rating scales (including dementia staging techniques) and mental status examinations for severely impaired patients with the exception of the SIB. Depending on the strength of this relationship, it may be that behavioral rating scales are appropriate for most instances that require an individual with severe dementia to be assessed. One would expect that as the sophistication and psychometric properties of behavioral rating scales continue to improve, instruments that assess multiple domains of functioning (e.g., cognition, behavioral excesses and deficiencies, psychiatric status, etc.) may begin to allow for clear distinctions between dementias of varying etiology and course. Additionally, localization of neuropathology may be accomplished. Some steps have already been made in this direction. For example, investigators report significant differences between the patterns of psychiatric, behavioral, and cognitive disturbances in patients with multi-infarct dementia compared to patients with dementia of the Alzheimer's type (Cummings, Miller, Hill, & Neshkes, 1987; Sultzer et al., 1993). Similarly, some authors report variation in behavioral and cognitive disturbances based on severity of dementia (Cooper, Mungas, & Weiler, 1990; Teri, Larson, & Reifler, 1988). However, these distinctions have not been consistently supported.

Neuropsychological scales may prove to provide better discrimination of dementias with differing etiologies than behavioral rating scales, as well as to enable the investigators to follow more closely different presentations within specific types of dementias. Further research is necessary to determine if these measures of severe cognitive impairment are sensitive enough to reflect the expected differences in patterns of cognitive performance based on the type of dementia. Investigations could begin by attempting to distinguish between prototypic dementia syndromes such as cortical dementias (e.g., Alzheimer's disease) and subcortical dementias (e.g., Huntington's disease), using measures of severe impairment. At this time, it is not clear whether any of the available instruments are sensitive enough or assess a broad enough range of abilities to make these distinctions. Clinicians and researchers may want to use neuropsychological tests for severe impairment in conjunction with behavioral rating scales, particularly when there is a question regarding how cognitive impairment impacts functional abilities.

Availability of standardized tests, such as the SIB and NOSGER, that can be administered to multiple ethnolinguistic groups may assist in developing a standard international test battery that could then expedite comparisons between internationally conducted pharamcotherapy trials, studies examining the prevalence of dementia, autopsy investigations of brain–behavior relationships in individuals with severe dementia, and studies describing the cognitive and behavioral deficits that occur during the course of dementias. The need for this type of battery has been pointed out (Schmage, Boehme, Dycka, & Schmitz, 1989).

From our review, it is clear that there are very few instruments to assess the cognition of individuals with severe dementia. As would be expected, there is also a dearth of information to support the clinical utility of instruments assessing severe impairment, such as the SIB. The implications of applying these tests in a clinical setting need to be examined. For instance, it does appear that performance on the SIB is significantly correlated with ratings of functional abilities. As such, SIB scores may be helpful in determining level of disability and care. There is a need to address important questions regarding these implications: For example, is it true, as some investigators suggest, that knowledge of cognitive functioning influences the attention caregivers provide to severely impaired patients? If the education of caregivers regarding cognitive functioning of severely impaired patients does significantly impact the attention given to the patients, tests of severe impairment would make direct and indirect contributions to the patients' qualities of life. Also, is there any basis to the assertion that assessment of severe dementia can assist in treatment planning by providing information about preserved cognitive abilities? There is currently no published information available to support this claim. However, if neuropsychological assessment of the severely cognitively impaired did contribute to treatment planning, it would again have the potential to significantly influence patients' qualities of life.

For patients with severe-severe impairment, evaluation options are limited. Although CDR criteria have been expanded to encompass end-stage Alzheimer's disease by adding advanced (CDR-4) and vegetative (CDR-5) categories, global staging methods (including the CDR and GDS) provide only gross estimations of dementia severity and provide little information about cognitive functioning. Those scales reviewed that are designed to assess severe dementia are not appropriate for the assessment of individuals in the vegetative stage of the disorder, and they may not be appropriate for individuals in the advanced stage of dementia as defined by CDR criteria. For these patients, there currently exists little information that characterizes their cognitive functioning. It may be that only gross distinctions are possible between these groups, such as those reported by Benesch and co-workers (1993), who used the Glasgow Coma Scale and rudimentary neurological functions (e.g., primitive reflexes, myoclonus, extensor plantar responses) to distinguish between CDR-4 and CDR-5 patients. Distinctions at these levels of severity would primarily be made for research purposes.

REFERENCES

Adams, P. F., & Benson, V. (1992). *Current estimates from the national health interview survey, 1991* (Vital and Health Statistics, Series 10 No. 184). Hyattsville, MD: National Center for Health Statistics.

Albert, M., & Cohen, C. (1992). The Test for Severe Impairment: An instrument for the assessment of patients with severe cognitive dysfunction. *Journal of the American Geriatrics Society, 40,* 449–453.

Albert, M., Smith, L. A., Scherr, P. A., Taylor, J. O., & Funkenstein, H. H. (1991). Use of brief cognitive tests to identify individuals in the community with clinically diagnosed Alzheimer's disease. *International Journal of Neurosciences, 57,* 167–178.

American Psychiatric Association. (1987). *Diagnostic and statistical manual of mental disorders* (3rd ed., rev.). Washington, DC: Author.

American Psychiatric Association. (1994). *Diagnostic and statistical manual of mental disorders* (4th ed.). Washington, DC: Author.

Anthony, J. C., LeResche, L., Niaz, U., VonKorff, M. R., & Folstein, M. F. (1982). Limits of the "Mini-Mental State" as a screening test for dementia and delirium among hospital patients. *Psychological Medicine, 12,* 397–408.

Anthony, K., Proctor, A. W., Silverman, A. M., & Murphy, E. (1987). Mood and behavior problems following the relocation of elderly patients with mental illness. *Age and Ageing, 16,* 355–365.

Baker, F. M., Robinson, B. H., & Stewart, B. (1993). Use of the Mini-Mental State Examination in African American elders. *Clinical Gerontologist, 14,* 5–13.

Beatty, W. W., Zavadil, K. D., Bailly, R. C., Rixen, G. J., Zavadil, L. E., Farnham, N., & Fisher, L. (1988). Preserved musical ability in a severely demented patient. *International Journal of Clinical Neuropsychology, 4,* 158–164.

Becker, J. T., Huff, F. J., Nebes, R. D., Holland, A., & Boller, F. (1989). Neuropsychological function in Alzheimer's disease: Pattern of impairment and rates of progression. *Archives of Neurology, 45,* 263–268.

Benedict, R. H., & Brandt, J. (1992). Limitations of the Mini-Mental State Examination for the detection of amnesia. *Journal of Geriatric Psychiatry and Neurology, 5,* 233–237.

Benesch, C., McDaniel, K. D., Cox, C., & Hamill, R. W. (1993). Endstage Alzheimer's disease: Glasgow Coma Scale and the neurologic examination. *Archives of Neurology, 50,* 1309–1315.

Blessed, G., Tomlinson, E., & Roth, M. (1968). The association between quantitative measures of dementia and senile change in the cerebral grey matter of elderly subjects. *British Journal of Psychiatric Medicine, 114,* 797–811.

Burke, W., Miller, J. P., Rubin, E., Morris, J. C., Coben, L. A., Ducheck, J., Wittels, I. G., & Berg, L. (1988). Reliability of the Washington University Clinical Dementia Rating (CDR). *Archives of Neurology, 45,* 31–32.

Coblentz, J. M., Mattis, S., Zingesser, L., Kasoff, S. S., Wisniewski, H. M., & Katzman, R. (1973). Presenile dementia: Clinical aspects and evaluation of cerebral spinal fluid dynamics. *Archives of Neurology, 29,* 299–308.

Coen, R. F., O'Mahoney, D., Bruce, I., Lawlor, B. A., Walsh, J. B., & Coakley, D. (1994). Differential diagnosis of dementia: A prospective evaluation of the DAT Inventory. *Journal of the American Geriatrics Society, 42,* 16–20.

Colantonio, A., Becker, J., & Huff, F. J. (1993). Factor structure of the Mattis Dementia Rating Scale among patients with probable Alzheimer's disease. *The Clinical Neuropsychologist, 7,* 313–318.

Cooper, J. K., Mungas, D., & Weiler, P. G. (1990). Relation of cognitive status and abnormal behaviors in Alzheimer's disease. *Journal of the American Geriatrics Society, 38,* 867–870.

Corrigan, J. D., Dickerson, J., Fisher, E., & Meyer, P. (1990). The Neurobehavioral Rating Scale: Replication in an acute inpatient rehabilitation setting. *Brain Injury, 4,* 215–222.

Crook, F. H. (1979). Psychometric assessment in the elderly. In A. Raskin & L. F. Jarvik (Eds.), *Psychiatric symptoms and cognitive loss in the elderly: Evaluation and assessment techniques* (pp. 207–220). Washington, DC: Hemisphere.

Cummings, J. L., & Benson, D. F. (1986). Dementia of the Alzheimer type. An inventory of diagnostic clinical features. *Journal of the American Geriatrics Society, 34,* 12–19.

Cummings, J. L., Miller, B., Hill, M. A., & Neshkes, R. (1987). Neuropsychiatric aspects of multi-infarct dementia and dementia of the Alzheimer type. *Archives of Neurology, 44,* 389–393.

Dalton, J. E., Pederson, S. L., Blom, B. E., & Holmes, N. R. (1987). Diagnostic errors using the Short Portable Mental Status Questionnaire with a mixed clinical population. *Journal of Gerontology, 42,* 512–514.

Davidson, M., & Stern, R. G. (1991). The treatment of cognitive impairment in Alzheimer's disease: Beyond the cholinergic approach. *Psychiatric Clinics of North America, 14,* 461–481.

Davis, P. B., Morris, J. C., & Grant, E. (1990). Brief screening tests versus clinical staging in senile dementia of the Alzheimer type. *Journal of the American Geriatrics Society, 38,* 129–135.

Davous, P. L. Y., Lamour, Y., Debrand, E., & Rondot, P. (1987). A comparative evaluation of the Short Orientation Memory Concentration Test of cognitive impairment. *Journal of Neurology, Neurosurgery, and Psychiatry, 50,* 1312–1317.

Drachman, D. A., Swearer, J. M., O'Donnell, B. F., Mitchell, A. L., & Maloon, A. (1992). The Caretaker Obstreperous-Behavior Rating Assessment (COBRA) scale. *Journal of the American Geriatrics Society, 40,* 463–470.

Erkinjuntti, T., Sulkava, R., Wikström, J., & Autio, L. (1987). Short Portable Mental Status Questionnaire as a screening test for dementia and delirium among the elderly. *Journal of the American Geriatrics Society, 35,* 412–416.

Fairburn, C. G., & Hope, R. A. (1988). Changes in behaviour in dementia: A neglected research area. *British Journal of Psychiatry, 152,* 406–407.

Fillenbaum, G. G., Heyman, A., Wilkinson, W. E., & Haynes, C. S. (1987). Comparison of two screening tests in Alzheimer's disease: The correlation and reliability of the Mini-Mental State Examination and the Modified Blessed Test. *Archives of Neurology, 44,* 924–927.

Folstein, M. F., Folstein, S. E., & McHugh, P. R. (1975). Mini-Mental State. A practical method for grading the cognitive state of patients for the clinician. *Journal of Psychiatric Research, 12,* 189–198.

Forsell, Y., Fratiglioni, L., Grut, M., Viitanen, M., & Winbald B. (1992). Clinical staging of dementia in a population survey: Comparison of DSM-III-R and the Washington University Clinical Dementia Rating Scale. *Acta Psychiatrica Scandinavica, 86,* 49–54.

Franssen, E. H., Kluger, A., Torossian, C. L., & Reisberg, B. (1993). The neurologic syndrome of severe Alzheimer's disease: Relationship to functional decline. *Archives of Neurology, 50,* 1029–1039.

Fuld, P. A. (1978). Psychological testing in the differential diagnosis of dementias. In R. Katzman, R. D. Terry, & K. L. Bick (Eds.), *Alzheimer's disease: Senile dementia and related disorders* (pp. 185–193). New York: Raven Press.

Gardner, R., Oliver-Muñoz, S., Fisher, L., & Empting, L. (1981). Mattis Dementia Rating Scale: Internal reliability study using a diffusely impaired population. *Journal of Clinical Neuropsychology, 3,* 271–275.

Gilley, D. W., Wilson, R. S., Bernard, B. A. Stebbins, G. T., & Fox, J. H. (1990). Scaling of severe dementia. *Journal of Clinical and Experimental Neuropsychology, 12,* 19.

Golding, E. (1989). *The Middlesex Elderly Assessment of Mental State: Description and validation.* Fareham, England: Thames Valley Test Company.

Granholm, E., Wolfe, J., & Butters, N. (1985). Affective arousal factors in the recall of thematic stories by amnesic and demented patients. *Developmental Neuropsychology, 1,* 317–333.

Hamilton, M. (1967). Development of a rating scale for primary depressive illness. *British Journal of Social and Clinical Psychiatry, 6,* 278–296.

Heaton, R. K., Grant, I., & Matthews, C. G. (1991). *Comprehensive norms for an expanded Halstead–Reitan Battery: Demographic corrections, research findings, and clinical applications.* Odessa, Florida: Psychological Assessment Resources.

Hersch, E. L., Csapo, K. G., & Palmer, R. B. (1978). Guidebook to the London Psychogeriatric Rating Scale. *London Psychiatric Hospital Research Bulletin, 1,* 3.

Hersch, E. L., Kral, V. A., & Palmer, R. B. (1978). Clinical value of the London Psychogeriatric Rating Scale. *Journal of the American Geriatrics Society, 26,* 348–354.

Hersch, E. L., Mersky, H., & Palmer, R. B. (1980). Prediction of discharge from a psychogeriatric unit: Development and evaluation of the LPRS Prognosis Index. *Canadian Journal of Psychiatry, 25,* 234–241.

Heyman, A., Wilkinson, W. E., Hurwitz, B. J., Helms, M. J., Haynes, B. A., Utley, C. M., & Gwyther, L. P. (1987). Early onset Alzheimer's disease: Clinical predictors of institutionalization and death. *Neurology, 37,* 980–984.

Holzer, C. E., III, Tischler, G. L., Leaf, P. J., & Myers, J. K. (1984). An epidemiologic assessment of cognitive impairment in a community population. In J. R. Greenley (Ed.), *Research in community mental health* (vol. 4, pp. 3–32). London, England: JAI Press.

Hughes, C. P., Berg, L., Danziger, W., Coben, L., & Martin, R. (1982). A new clinical scale for the staging of dementia. *British Journal of Psychiatry, 140,* 566–572.

Ivnik, R. J., Malec, J. F., Smith, G. E., Tangalos, E. G., Petersen, R. C., Kokmen, E., & Kurland, L. T. (1992a). Mayo's older Americans normative studies: WAIS-R norms for ages 56–97. *The Clinical Neuropsychologist, 6, (Suppl),* 1–30.

Ivnik, R. J., Malec, J. F., Smith, G. E., Tangalos, E. G., Petersen, R. C., Kokmen, E., & Kurland, L. T. (1992b). Mayo's older Americans normative studies: WMS-R norms for ages 56–97. *The Clinical Neuropsychologist, 6 (Suppl),* 49–82.

Ivnik, R. J., Malec, J. F., Smith, G. E., Tangalos, E. G., Petersen, R. C., Kokmen, E., & Kurland, L. T. (1992c). Mayo's older American normative studies: Updated AVLT norms for ages 56–97. *The Clinical Neuropsychologist, 6 (Suppl),* 83–104.

Kanowski, S., Fischhof, P., Hiersemenzel, R., Röhmel, J., & Kern, U. (1989). Therapeutic efficacy of Nootropic drugs—A discussion of clinical phase III studies with nimodipine as a model. In M. Bergener & B. Reisberg (Eds.), *Diagnosis and treatment of senile dementia* (pp. 339–349). Berlin: Springer-Verlag.

Katzman, R., Brown, T., Fuld, P., Peck, A., Schechter, R., & Schimmel, H. (1983). Validation of a Short Orientation Memory Concentration Test of cognitive impairment. *American Journal of Psychiatry, 140,* 734–739.

Katzman, R., Brown, T., Thal, L. J., Fuld, P. A., Aronson, M., Butters, N. Klauber, M. R., Wiederholt, W., Pay, M., Renbing, X., Ooi, W. L., Hofstetter, R., & Terry, R. D. (1988). Comparison of rate of annual change of mental status score in four independent studies of patients with Alzheimer's disease. *Annals of Neurology, 24,* 384–389.

Kluger, A., & Ferris, S. H. (1991). Scales for the assessment of Alzheimer's disease. *Psychiatric Clinics of North America, 14,* 309–326.

Kunkel, S. R., & Applebaum, R. A. (1992). Estimating the prevalence of long-term disability for an aging society. *Journal of Gerontology, 47,* S253–S260.

La Rue, A. (1992). *Aging and neuropsychological assessment.* New York: Plenum Press.

Launer, L. J., Dinkgreve, M. A. H. M., Jonker, C., Hooijer, C., & Lindeboom, J. (1993). Are age and education independent correlates of the Mini-Mental State Exam performance of community-dwelling elderly? *Journal of Gerontology, 48,* P271–P277.

Levin, H. S., High, W. M., Goethe, K. E., Sisson, R. A., Overall, J. E., Rhoades, H. M., Eisenberg, H. M., Kalisky, Z., & Gary, H. E. (1987). The Neurobehavioral Rating Scale: Assessment of the behavioral sequelae of head injury by the clinician. *Journal of Neurology, Neurosurgery, and Psychiatry, 50,* 183–193.

Levine, M. J., Van Horn, K. R., & Curtis, A. B. (1993). Developmental models of social cognition in assessing psychosocial adjustments in head injury. *Brain Injury, 7,* 153–167.

Lopez, O., Boller, F., Becker, J. T., Miller, M., & Reynolds, C. F. (1990). Alzheimer's disease and depression: Neuropsychological impairment and progression of the illness. *American Journal of Psychiatry, 147,* 855–860.

Marshall, S. C., & Mungas, D. (1995). Age and education correction for the Mini-Mental State Exam. *Journal of the International Neuropsychological Society, 1,* 166.

Marson, D., Herfkens, K., Brooks, A., Ingram, K., & Harrell, L. (1995). Relevance of dementia screening instruments to physicians competency judgments in Alzheimer's disease. *Journal of the International Neuropsychological Society, 1,* 143.

Mattis, S. (1976). Mental status examination for organic mental syndrome in the elderly patient. In R. Bellak & B. Karasa (Eds.), *Geriatric psychiatry* (pp. 77–121). New York: Grune & Stratton.

Mattis, S. (1988). *DRS: Dementia Rating Scale Professional manual.* New York: Psychological Assessment.

McKenna, P. J., Tamlyn, D., Lund, C. E., Mortimer, A. M., Hammond, S., & Baddeley, A. D. (1990). Amnesic syndrome in schizophrenia. *Psychological Medicine, 20,* 967–972.

McKhann, G., Drachman, D., Folstein, M., Katzman, R., Price, D., & Stadlan, E. M. (1984). Clinical diagnosis of Alzheimer's disease: Report of the NINCDS-ADRDA Work Group under the auspices of the Department of Health and Human Services Task Force on Alzheimer's disease. *Neurology, 34,* 939–944.

Mohs, R., Kim, G., Johns, C., Dunn, D., & Davis, K. (1986). Assessing changes in Alzheimer's disease: Memory and language. In L. Poon (Ed.), *Handbook for clinical memory assessment* (pp. 149–155). Washington, DC: American Psychological Association.

Morris, J. C. (1993). The Clinical Dementia Rating (CDR): Current version and scoring rules. *Neurology, 43,* 2412–2414.

Morris, J. C., Heyman, A., Mohs, R. C., Hughes, J. P., van Belle, G., Fillenbaum, G., Mellits, E. D., Clark, S., & the CERAD Investigators. (1989). The consortium to establish a registry for Alzheimer's disease (CERAD). Part I. Clinical and neuropsychological assessment of Alzheimer's disease. *Neurology, 39,* 1159–1164.

Morris, J. C., McKeel, D. W., Fulling, K., Torack, R. M., & Berg, L. (1988). Validation of clinical diagnostic criteria for Alzheimer's disease. *Annals of Neurology, 24,* 17–22.

Moss, M. B., Albert, M. S., Butters, N., & Payne, M. (1986). Differential patterns of memory loss among patients with Alzheimer's disease, Huntington's disease, and alcoholic Korsakoff syndrome. *Archives of Neurology, 43,* 239–246.

Nussbaum, P. D. (in press). Neuropsychological assessment of the elderly. In A. E. Puente, E. Bigler, & G. Goldstein (Eds.), *Handbook of human brain function: Assessment and rehabilitation.* New York: Plenum Press.

O'Connor, D. W.,Pollitt, P. A., Hyde, J. B., Fellows, J. L., Miller, N. D., Brook C. P. B., & Reiss, B. B. (1989). The reliability and validity of the Mini-Mental State in a British community survey. *Journal of Psychiatric Research, 23,* 87–96.

Panisset, M., Roudier, M., Saxton, J., & Boller, F. (1992). Validation d'une batterie d'évaluation neuropsychologique pour des patients avec démence sévère [Validation of a neuropsychological evaluation battery for patients with severe dementia]. *La Presse Mèdicale, 21,* 1271–1274.

Panisset, M., Roudier, M., Saxton, J., & Boller, F. (1994). Severe Impairment Battery: A neuropsychological test for severely demented patients. *Archives of Neurology, 51,* 41–45.

Parlato, V., Iavaronnem, A., Galeone, F., Boller, F., Saxton, J., Carlomagno, S., & Bonavita, V. (1992). La Severe Impairment Battery: Allestimento e validazione della versione italiana [Validation on the Italian version of the Severe Impairment Battery]. *Archivio di Psicologia, Neurologia, e Psichiatria, 53,* 371–385.

Pattie, A. H., & Gilleard, C. J. (1979). *Manual of the Clifton Assessment Procedures for the Elderly (CAPE).* Sevenoaks, England: Hodder & Stoughton.

Peavy, G. M., Salmon, D. P., Rice, V. A., & Butters, N. (1995). Assessment of severely demented elderly. *Journal of the International Neuropsychological Society, 1,* 185.

Pfeffer, R. I., Kuroski, T. T., Harrah, C. H., Chance, J. M., Bates, D., Detels, R., Filos, S., & Butzke, C. (1981). A survey diagnostic tool for senile dementia. *American Journal of Epidemiology, 114,* 515–527.

Pfeiffer, E. (1975). Short Portable Mental Status Questionnaire for the assessment of organic brain deficit in elderly patients. *Journal of the American Geriatrics Society, 23,* 433–441.

Plutchik, R., Conte, H., Lieberman, M., Bakur, M., Grossman, J., & Lehrman, N. (1970). Reliability and validity of a scale for the assessment of functioning of geriatric patients. *Journal of the American Geriatrics Society, 18,* 491–500.

Powell, T., Brooker, D. J. R., & Papadopolous, A. (1993). Test–retest reliability of the Middlesex Assessment of Mental State (MEAMS): A preliminary investigation in people with probable dementia. *British Journal of Clinical Psychology, 32,* 224–226.

Proctor, A. W., Francis, P. T., Strattman, G. C., & Bowen, D. M. (1992). Rapid autopsy brains for biochemical research: Experiences in establishing a program. *Neurochemical Research, 17,* 917–922.

Reglà, J. L., Gallego, M. L., Lòpez, O. L., Portabella, M. G., Lòpez-Pousa, S., Franch, J. V., & Saxton, J. (in press). Validaciòn de la adaptaciòn española de la "Severe Impairment Battery" (SIB) [Validation of the Spanish Adaptation of the "Severe Impairment Battery"]. *Neurologia,*

Reid, D. W., Tierney, M. C., Zorzitto, M. L., Snow, G., & Fisher, R. H. (1991). On the clinical value of the London Psychogeriatric Rating Scale. *Journal of the American Geriatrics Society, 39,* 368–371.

Reisberg, B. (1988). Functional Assessment Staging (FAST). *Psychopharmacology Bulletin, 24,* 653–659.

Reisberg, B., Ferris, S. H., de Leon, M. J., & Crook, T. (1982). The Global Deterioration Scale for the assessment of primary degenerative dementia. *American Journal of Psychiatry, 139,* 1136–1139.

Reisberg, B., Ferris, S. H., de Leon, M. J., & Crook, T. (1988). The Global Deterioration Scale (GDS). *Psychopharmacology Bulletin, 24,* 661–663.

Reisberg, B., Ferris, S. H., Kluger, A., Franssenm, E., de Leon, M. J., Mittelman, M., Borenstein, J., Rameshwar, K., & Alba, R. (1989). Symptomatic changes in CNS aging and dementia of the Alzheimer's type: Cross-sectional, temporal, and remediable concomitants. In M. Bergener & B. Reisberg (Eds.), *Diagnosis and treatment of senile dementia* (pp. 193–223). Berlin: Springer-Verlag.

Rey, A. (1964). *L'Examen Clinique en Psychologie* [The clinical tests of psychology]. Paris: Press Universitaire de France.

Ritchie, K., & Ledesert, B. (1991). The measurement of incapacity in the severely demented elderly: The validation of a behavioral assessment scale. *International Journal of Geriatric Psychiatry, 6,* 217–226.

Roccaforte, W. H., Burke, W. J., Bayer, B. L., & Wengel, S. P. (1994). Reliability and validity of the Short Portable Mental Status Questionnaire administered by telephone. *Journal of Geriatric Psychiatry and Neurology, 7,* 33–38.

Rozenbilds, U., Goldney, R. D., Gilchrist, P. N., Martin, E., & Connelly, H. (1986). Assessment by relatives of elderly patients with psychiatric illness. *Psychological Report, 58,* 795–801.

Salmon, D. P., Thal, L. J., Butters, N., & Heindel, W. C. (1990). Longitudinal evaluation of dementia of the Alzheimer type: A comparison of 3 standardized mental status examinations. *Neurology, 40,* 1225–1230.

Saxton, J., McGonigle-Gibson, K., Swihart, A., & Boller, F. (1993). *The Severe Impairment Battery (SIB) manual.* Suffolk, England: Thames Valley Test Company.

Saxton, J., McGonigle-Gibson, K., Swihart, A., Miller, M., & Boller, F. (1990). Assessment of the severely impaired patient: Description and validation of a new neuropsychological test battery. *Psychological Assessment, 2,* 298–303.

Schmage, N., Boehme, K., Dycka, J., & Schmitz, H. (1989). Nimodipine for psychogeriatric use: Methods, strategies, and considerations based on experience with clinical trials. In M. Bergener & B. Reisberg (Eds.), *Diagnosis and treatment of senile dementia* (pp. 374–381). Berlin: Springer-Verlag.

Sclan, S. G., Foster, J. R., Reisberg, B., Franssen, E., & Welkowitz, J. (1990). Application of Piagetian measures of cognition in severe Alzheimer's disease. *Psychiatric Journal of the University of Ottawa, 15,* 221–226.

Shiel, A., & Wilson, B. A. (1992). Performance of stroke patients on the Middlesex Elderly Assessment of Mental State. *Clinical Rehabilitation, 6,* 283–289.

Smith, A. (1982). *Symbol Digit Modalities Test: Manual.* Los Angeles: Western Psychological Services.

Smith, G. E., Ivnik, R. J., Malec, J. F., Petersen, R. C., Kokmen, E., & Tangalos, E. G. (1994). Mayo cognitive factor scales: Derivation of a short battery and norms for factor scores. *Neuropsychology, 8,* 194–202.

Social Psychiatry Research Unit. (1992). The Canberra Interview for the Elderly: A new field instrument for the diagnosis of dementia and depression by the ICD-10 and DSM-III-R. *Acta Psychiatric Scandinavica, 85,* 105–113.

Spiegel, R., Bruner, C., Ermini-Fünfschilling, D., Monsch, A., Notter, M., Puxty, J., & Tremmel, L. (1991). A new behavioral assessment scale for geriatric out- and inpatients: The NOSGER (Nurses' Observation Scale for Geriatric Patients). *Journal of the American Geriatrics Society, 39,* 339–347.

Stern, R. G., Mohs, R. C., Bierer, L. M., Silverman, J. M., Schmeidler, J., Davidson, M., & Davis, K. L. (1992). Deterioration on the Blessed test in Alzheimer's disease: Longitudinal data and their implications for clinical trials and identifications of subtypes. *Psychiatry Research, 42,* 101–110.

Storandt, M. (1994). General principles of assessment of older adults. In M. Storandt & G. R. Van den Bos (Eds.), *Neuropsychological assessment of depression and dementia in older adults: A clinician's guide* (pp. 7–32). Washington, DC: American Psychological Association.

Sultzer, D. L., Levin, H. S., Mahler, M. E., High, W. M., & Cumings, J. L. (1992). Assessment of cognitive, psychiatric, and behavioral disturbances in patients with dementia: The Neurobehavioral Rating Scale. *Journal of the American Geriatrics Society, 40,* 549–555.

Sultzer, D. L., Levin, H. S., Mahler, M. E., High, W. M., & Cumings, J. L. (1993). A comparison of psychiatric symptoms in vascular dementia and Alzheimer's disease. *American Journal of Psychiatry, 150,* 1806–1812.

Teasdale, G., Knill-Jones, R., & Van der Sande, J. (1978). Observer variability in assessing impaired consciousness and coma. *Journal of Neurology, Neurosurgery and Psychiatry, 41,* 603–610.

Teng, E. L., Chiu, H. C., Schneider, L. S., & Erickson-Metzger, L. (1987). Alzheimer's dementia: Performance on the Mini-Mental State Exam. *Journal of Consulting and Clinical Psychology, 55,* 96–100.

Teri, L., Larson, E. B., & Reifler, B. V. (1988). Behavioral disturbance in dementia of the Alzheimer type. *Journal of the American Geriatrics Society, 36,* 1–6.

Thal, L. J., Grundman, M., & Golden, R. (1986). Alzheimer's disease: A correlational analysis of the Blessed Information-Memory-Concentration Test and the Mini-Mental State Exam. *Neurology, 36,* 262–264.

Tombaugh, T. N., & McIntyre, N. J. (1992). The Mini-Mental State Examination: A comprehensive review. *Journal of the American Geriatrics Society, 40,* 922–935.

Tremmel, L., & Spiegel, R. (1993). Clinical experience with the NOSGER (Nurses' Observation Scale for Geriatric Patients): Tentative normative data and sensitivity to change. *International Journal of Geriatric Psychiatry, 8,* 311–317.

Uzgiris, I., & Hunt, J. M. (1975). *Assessment in infancy: Ordinal Scales of Psychological Development.* Urbana: University of Illinois.

Vilkki, J., Ahola, K., Holst, P., Öhman, J., Servo, A., & Heiskanen, O. (1994). Prediction of psychosocial recovery after head injury with cognitive tests and neurobehavioral ratings. *Journal of Clinical and Experimental Neuropsychology, 16,* 325–338.

Vitaliano, P. P., Breen, A. R., Albert, M. S., Russo, J., & Prinz, P. N. (1984a). Memory, attention, and functional status in community-residing Alzheimer-type dementia patients and optimally healthy aged individuals. *Journal of Gerontology, 39,* 58–64.

Vitaliano, P. P., Breen, A. R., Russo, J., Alberg, M. S., Vitiello, M., & Prinz, P. N. (1984b). The clinical utility of the Dementia Rating Scale for assessing Alzheimer's patients. *Journal of Chronic Disabilities, 37,*743–753.

Ward, T., Dawe, B., Proctor, A., Murphy, E., & Weinman, J. (1993). Assessment in severe dementia: The Guy's Advanced Dementia Schedule. *Age and Ageing, 22,* 183–189.

Ward, T., Murphy, E., & Proctor, A. (1991). Functional assessment in severely demented patients. *Age and Ageing, 20,* 189–198.

Wechsler, D. (1945). *Wechsler Memory Scale.* New York: Psychological Corporation.

Wechsler, D. (1955). *Wechsler Adult Intelligence Scale manual.* New York: Psychological Corporation.

Wechsler, D. (1981). *Manual for the Wechsler Adult Intelligence Scale—Revised.* New York: Psychological Corporation.

Weiler, P. G., Chiriboga, D. A., & Black, S. A. (1994). Comparison of mental status tests: Implications for Alzheimer's patients and their caregivers. *Journal of Gerontology, 49,* S44–S51.

Wild, K., Lear, J., & Kaye, J. (1995, February). *The severely impaired Alzheimer's disease patient: Can rates of cognitive change be assessed?* Poster presented at the annual meeting of the International Neuropsychological Society, Seattle, WA.

Wilson, B., Cockburn, J., & Baddeley, A. (1991). *The Rivermead Behavioural Memory Test manual.* Suffolk, England: Thames Valley Test Company.

Wilson, R., & Kaszniak, A. (1986). Longitudinal changes: Progressive idiopathic dementia. In L. Poon (Ed.), *Handbook for clinical memory assessment* (pp. 285–293). Washington, DC: American Psychological Association.

World Health Organization. (1980). *International classifications of impairments, disabilities and handicaps.* Geneva: Author.

Yesavage, J. A., Brink, T. L., Rose, T. L., Lum, O., Huang, O., Adey, V., & Leirer, V. (1983). Development and validation of a geriatric depression screening scale: A preliminary report. *Journal of Psychiatric Research, 17,* 37–49.

Yue, M., Fainsinger, R. L., & Bruera, E. (1994). Cognitive impairment in a patient with a normal Mini-Mental State Examination (MMSE). *Journal of Pain and Symptom Management, 9,* 51–53.

Zarit, S. H., Eiler, J., & Hassinger, M. (1985). Clinical assessment. In J. E. Birren & K. W. Schaie (Eds.), *Handbook of the psychology of aging* (pp. 725–754). New York: Van Nostrand Reinhold.

10

Psychopathology and Neuropsychological Assessment

JERRY J. SWEET AND CYNTHIA WESTERGAARD

INTRODUCTION

Vast changes in the knowledge and conceptualization of psychopathology have occurred in the last century. Today, the inextricable involvement of the central nervous system in severe psychopathology is no longer a debatable subject. Indeed, the body of knowledge pertaining to the interface of psychopathology and neuropsychology is now reaching a daunting size; much of it is relevant to clinical neuropsychologists.

Simultaneous with the rapid growth and evolution of clinical neuropsychology, including its assessment instrumentation, there have been complementary advances in: (1) structural and functional neurodiagnostic procedures of the brain; (2) neurobiology and neuroanatomy of mental disorders and psychopathology; (3) psychological methods of measuring psychopathology, including mood, affect, and personality characteristics; and (4) the effects of various psychopathological states on neuropsychological test performance. These simultaneous advances have strong implications for the practicing clinical neuropsychologist. Within this chapter one of our goals is to impart pertinent information regarding the current cross-disciplinary understanding of brain function and psychopathology, in order to go beyond the long-outdated, traditional "functional versus organic" distinction. In so doing, our use of the term *psychopathology* encompasses severe mental disorders (e.g., schizophrenia and psychotic spectrum disorders), unipolar and bipolar mood disorders, anxiety disorders, personality disorders, as well as mental disorders (e.g., delirium, dementia, amnesia) due to a general medical condition (e.g., infection, tumor, stroke, cardiovascular disease, Parkinson's disease).

JERRY J. SWEET and CYNTHIA WESTERGAARD • Evanston Hospital, Evanston, Illinois 60201

Additionally, this chapter will describe and briefly review current psychological methods used by clinical neuropsychologists to evaluate psychopathology. Along with information concerning increasingly sophisticated interpretation of neuropsychological measures in psychopathological states, we believe that such background knowledge can be quite useful and relevant for the practicing clinical neuropsychologist.

The inclusion of a chapter on psychopathology within this volume on the neuropsychology is based, in part, on the relatively high frequency of instances in which many neuropsychologists will have to address issues of psychopathology. Given that the top two referral sources of neuropsychologists have consistently been neurologists and psychiatrists (Sweet, Moberg, & Westergaard, 1996), it is not surprising that many patients have either known or diagnosable primary or secondary psychopathology when seen by the consulting neuropsychologist. The interested reader should see Sweet (1991) for a listing of common referral questions by medical specialty. Regardless of referral source, among the most common referral questions are: (1) to what extent does psychological condition X account for the overall clinical presentation; (2) beyond the presence and effect of psychological condition X, is brain dysfunction present; and (3) is the patient's current presentation the result of psychological condition X or brain dysfunction, or some combination of both? It follows, then, that neuropsychologists need an understanding of: (1) the neurobehavioral presentations of psychopathology; (2) the neuropathological dysfunction associated with major types of psychopathology; and (3) relevant assessment procedures.

From the practical standpoint of differential diagnosis, there can be legitimate confusion with patients whose reported symptoms, by their very nature, could be either psychiatric or neurological. Among the many symptoms that can be reported by patients in both diagnostic groups are: decreased attention and/or concentration, decreased learning and memory, work-finding difficulties, changes in judgment, reduced awareness of one's own behavior, impulsivity, affective disturbance, social withdrawal, difficulty expressing ideas, inefficiency of cognitive operations, and poor awareness of, or little benefit derived from, social feedback indicating inappropriateness of behavior. This partial listing is not intended to suggest that patients be placed in one particular diagnostic group that excludes other diagnoses (i.e., patients can, and do, have both psychological and neuropsychological disorders concurrently, either as primary sequelae to neurological events, or secondarily).

Further, as a part of everyday practice, almost regardless of the particular population being studied, there is a need for clinicians to consider alternative hypotheses to the conclusion that poor performance on neuropsychological tests represents brain dysfunction. Among the alternative hypotheses are a number of moderator variables relevant to the present chapter, as can be see from the listing found in Table 1 (Sweet, 1997). Psychopathology-related factors such as emotional states, significant psychiatric disorder, substance abuse, and feigning of

TABLE 1. Partial Listing of Moderator Variables or Alternative Hypotheses Commonly Considered in the Neuropsychological Interpretive Process[a]

Age
Gender
Handedness
Emotional state (e.g., depression, anxiety)
Suboptimal motivation and effort on part of patient
Poor physical stamina or fatigue
Low education
Congenital learning disorder
Premorbid or congenital cognitive or intellectual deficiency
Significant psychiatric disorder (e.g., bipolar disorder, schizophrenia)
Peripheral injury or non-CNS medical disorder that impairs task performance
Acute effects of substances (recreational, prescription or nonprescription)
External distraction in the testing environment
Internal distractions (e.g., pain, tingling, or other internal bodily discomforts)
English as a second language
Sociocultural background
Nonneurological medical disorders that may affect the central nervous system (e.g., liver disease causing hepatic encephalopathy)
Deliberate attempts to feign deficit (i.e., malingering)

[a]From Rozensky, Sweet, & Tovian (1997), with permission.

symptoms need to be considered as alternative causes of poor performance on formal neuropsychological tests in many clinical cases. Most importantly, it is the obligation of clinical practitioners to understand the psychometric properties of their assessment tools (e.g., discriminability of tests A and B), in order to determine whether differential task performance is due to variable specificity/ability of the test(s) to correctly identify pathology, or is due to true differences in abilities across tasks and groups (see Chapman & Chapman, 1975, 1987; Miller, Chapman, Chapman, & Collins, 1995).

Our discussion will now focus on select psychopathological disorders, relevant to the goal of understanding the basic nature of brain function and dysfunction within each. At the very least, the discussion to follow should give pause when confronted with the outdated, but still commonplace, referral question asking for a distinction between functional versus organic (i.e., psychological vs. brain-based) etiology.

NEUROPSYCHOLOGY OF SPECIFIC DISORDERS

Space limitations require that the present discussion be limited to a few of the more common, well-known psychopathologies that, from a neuropsychological standpoint, have been at least preliminarily investigated at present. While we had expected to summarize a broader variety of psychopathological conditions, our literature review suggests that many psychopathological disorders have undergone scant empirical neuropsychological investigation. The interested reader may wish to track down some of the infrequent studies in a particular area, such as sociopathy (e.g., Dolan, 1994; Malloy, Noel, Longabough, & Beattie, 1990), impulsive personality disorders (Stein, et al., 1993), dramatic personality disorders (Burgess, 1992), panic disorder (e.g., Lucas, Telch, & Bigler, 1991), and eating disorders (e.g., Hamsher, Halmi, & Benton, 1981; Kowalski, 1986; Strauss & Ryan, 1988; Touyz, Beumont, & Johnstone, 1986). However, we do not believe that enough empirical research exists at present to warrant summarizing here. Within this chapter, much more detailed attention will be given to schizophrenia because of the enormous, diverse literature on this subject.

Schizophrenia

Neuropathology

Kraepelin (1971, 1987) provided the first attempt to describe dementia praecox, the psychiatric disorder we now call schizophrenia. Dementia praecox was originally named after a "praecocious" child who presented with psychotic symptoms and a progressively deteriorating course to dementia. While Kraepelin and Alzheimer considered dementia praecox to be a progressively dementing brain-based disease (Kraepelin, 1987; Southard, 1919; Sweeney, Haas, & Clementz, 1993), Bleuler and other members of the psychiatric community argued that, since not all patients with dementia praecox became demented, and since not all postmortem schizophrenics showed signs of degenerative brain disease, dementia praecox would have to be reconceptualized. The psychiatric community, led by Bleuler, renamed the disorder "schizophrenia," and allowed a widely varying course of illness across patients (Bleuler, 1950; Marquart, 1935; White, 1921).

Today, the *Diagnostic and Statistical Manual of Mental Disorders,* 4th edition (DSM-IV) (American Psychiatric Association, 1994) conceptualizes schizophrenia (henceforth, SZ) as a syndrome of heterogenous symptoms, including at least 1 month of active-phase positive (delusions, hallucinations, disorganized speech, grossly disorganized or catatonic behavior) or negative symptoms (affective flattening, alogia, or avolition), with persisting symptoms and a disturbance in occupational, interpersonal, or cognitive functioning for at least 6 months. Whereas Kraepelin (1971, 1987) conceived of subtypes of dementia praecox as stable and unique, the DSM-IV recognizes five distinct subtypes of SZ, contingent on current symptomatology. As such, the nosology of SZ is clinically heterogeneous. For example, the same patient may meet subtype criterion such as catatonic at one time in their illness and later be diagnosed as disorganized, as their clinical features change.

Obstetrical complications, fetal and neonatal development, and low birth weight (Cannon, Barr, & Mednick, 1991; Kinney, Yurgelun-Todd, Waternaux, & Matthysse, 1994; Murray, O'Callaghan, Castle, & Lewis, 1992), abnormal brain and/or neuromotor development (Auerbach, Hans, & Marcus, 1993; Crow, 1990; Fish, 1977; McNeil, Harty, Blennow, & Cantor-Graae, 1993; Meehl, 1990; Nuechterlein & Dawson, 1984; Walker, 1994; Walker, Savoie, & Davis, 1994; Weinberger, 1987), chaotic family like and/or deviant communication styles (Bateson, Jackson, Haley, & Weakland, 1956; Docherty, 1994; Fromm-Reichman, 1948) or little expressed emotion (Vaughn & Leff, 1976), adult neuroanatomic and functional or metabolic brain abnormalities (e.g., Andreasen, 1994; Neuchterlein, 1987; Raz & Raz, 1990), abnormal neurotransmitter systems (Cross, Crow, & Owen, 1981; Seeman & Niznik, 1990), and genetic vulnerability (Baron, 1986a,b; Clementz & Sweeney, 1990, 1992; Faraone et al., 1995; Gottesman, 1991; Kaufmann & Malaspina, 1993; Kendler & Diehl, 1993; Kessler, 1980; Kremen, Tsuang, Faraone, & Lyons, 1992; Kremen et al., 1994; Meehl, 1990; Nasrallah, 1993; Prescott & Gottesman, 1993; Sweeney et al., 1993; Zubin, 1988) have all been hypothesized etiological factors of SZ. Yet, no single etiological factor is present in all persons with SZ. With SZ being the area of severe psychopathology that has amassed the greatest research knowledge base, the importance of understanding the union of what are sometimes viewed as independent neural and behavioral systems seems clear. It is this point of union that is particularly relevant to neuropsychologists, as they collaborate with other health specialists in attempting to delineate etiologies and treatments of psychopathology.

SZ is considered to be a heterogeneous neurobehavioral disorder with associated structural and physiological brain abnormalities. Contemporary postmortem examination, computer-assisted tomography (CT) studies, and magnetic resonance imaging (MRI) studies have shown that some SZs have reduced corpus callosum size, mild to severe atrophy of the prefrontal cortex, reduced volume of temporal–limbic–hippocampal structures, and reduced brain densities (Breier et al., 1992; Golden, 1981; Golden, Graber, et al., 1980; Gur et al., 1994; Hoff, Neal, Kushner, & DeLisi, 1994).

Enlargement of the third and the lateral ventricles (ventriculomegaly) has consistently been found to be a reliable phenomenon and possible indication of cerebral damage in SZ, resulting in measures of increased ventricular–brain ratios (VBR) (Cannon & Marco, 1994; Daniel, Goldbery, Gibbons, & Weinberger, 1991; DeQuardo et al., 1994; Gur et al., 1994; Raz, 1994; Raz & Raz, 1990). Andreasen et al. (1990) found that SZs with greater negative symptoms had significantly larger ventricular size than those with mixed or positive clinical features. Raz (1993, 1994) provides data that suggest that the cerebral atrophy of SZ may not only include the frontotemporal region and cerebrospinal fluid (CSF) cavities adjacent to the basal ganglia, but may also include the CSF-filled spaces neighboring the diencephalon and cerebellum; hence, abnormal brain morphology of SZ may include both cortical and subcortical structures, as well as their neural interconnections (see also Freeman & Karson, 1993). However, while perhaps the most prevalent CT finding in SZ, many SZs fail to show increased VBR–cortical atrophy (Bachneff, 1991).

Studies of regional cerebral blood flow ($_r$CBF) using functional brain-imaging techniques [e.g., positron emission tomography (PET), or single photon emission tomography (SPECT)], have shown that reduced metabolic activity (hypometabolism) of the brain is highly related to locally reduced cerebral blood flow (Bachneff, 1991; Sharif, Gewirtz, & Iqbal, 1993). Reduced metabolism and $_r$CBF have been found in the prefrontal brain of both chronic and neuroleptic naive SZs, with greater hypofrontality in negative symptoms SZs (Andreasen et al., 1992; Bachneff, 1991; Berman, Torrey, Daniel & Weinberger, 1992; Weinberger, Berman, & Illowsky, 1988; Weinberger, Berman, & Zec, 1986; Wolkin et al., 1992). Buchsbaum et al. (1992) replicated hypofrontality in neuroleptic naive SZs, and also discovered diminished metabolism in the basal ganglia and occipital cortex. Buchsbaum et al. concluded that they had discovered evidence of a combined frontostriatal dysfunction in SZ. While research had not produced consistent results regarding frontal lobe functioning in SZs (Andreasen, 1994; Heinrichs, 1993), sampling and other methodological differences may account for conflicting findings (Bachneff, 1991; Berman et al., 1992; Buchsbaum et al., 1992).

Abnormal auditory event related potentials, i.e., reductions in the P300 amplitude, also have been associated with abnormal frontal lobe functioning in neuroleptic naive and chronic SZ (Wolkin et al., 1992), as well as in their unaffected first-degree relatives (Roxborough, Muir, Blackwood, Walker, & Blackburn, 1993). These findings appear to be independent of medication effects, clinical state, and subtype.

Finally, electrophysiological studies have shown greater diffuse electroencephalographic (EEG) abnormalities in SZs than in other psychiatric patients or controls. These nonspecific EEG abnormalities are present in 20–40% of SZs, and have been reported to be independent of chronicity or severity of illness, subtyping, or medication status (Seidman, Cassens, Kremen, & Pepple, 1992). Numerous studies have replicated abnormally slow P300 wave phenomena in chronic SZs while they were performing frontal lobe, attentional tasks, such as the Wisconsin Card Sorting Task (Berman et al., 1992; Seidman et al., 1992, 1994; Weinberger et al., 1986, 1988).

A biochemical approach to the study of SZ proposes that the psychopathology of SZ is related to hyperdopamine activity (Wyatt, 1986, 1991) and elevated densities of dopamine D2 (but not D1) receptors in the basal ganglia, (e.g., striatal tissue), even in neuroleptic naive SZs. Pharmacological studies have shown that blockage of dopamine D2 receptors by neuroleptics results in the reduction in positive symptoms of delusions and hallucinations. Conversely, increased dopamine uptake can increase psychotic symptoms (Andreasen 1994; Cross et al., 1981; Farde et al., 1990; Gur & Pearlson, 1993; Seeman et al., 1984; Seeman & Niznik, 1990). However, the hyperdopamine hypothesis cannot explain many aspects of

SZ psychopathology. For example, neuroleptics often do not significantly affect negative symptoms, and some SZ's are treatment resistent to neuroleptics. Also, change in positive symptoms does not neatly coincide with dopamine blockage, i.e., it can take weeks or months to lower positive symptoms on neuroleptics (Heinrichs, 1993). Additional difficulties include the fact that non-SZ psychiatric groups also present with abnormal dopamine activity (i.e., not specific to SZ), and further, abnormal dopamine activity is not found in all SZs (Kay & Sandyk, 1991).

Bachneff (1991) argues that SZ research should shift its attention from studies of quantitative focal neuronal deficits (e.g., reduced dopamine neuronal densities in the prefrontal cortex) to the neural systems that are modulated by dopamine [e.g., local circuit neurons (LCNs)], formerly known as interneurons or Golgi type II neurons (see Bachneff, 1991, pp. 873–877). For example, Bachneff cites evidence that LCNs provide empirical support for "an admittedly speculative" theoretical model of distributed "basic operational units" essential for "higher brain functions" associated with an intact prefrontal lobe, as well as functions related to the temporolimbic areas (p. 874). Interestingly, LCNs do not become mature in humans before the second or third decade, concomitant with the typical age of onset of SZ.

In sum, the etiology, onset, course, and subtype of SZ are each highly variable, causing some researchers to question whether SZ is a unitary construct or a heterogenous group of unrelated or partially related disorders with multiple etiologies. At present, the construct of SZ remains polythetic (Andreasen, 1994; Andreasen & Carpenter, 1993; Andreasen & Flaum, 1991; Bellack & Blanchard, 1993; Heinrichs, 1993; Sweeney et al., 1993).

Neuropsychological Presentation

Clearly heterogeneous in its clinical presentation within and across individuals, heterogeneity further confounds generalized conclusions in neuropsychological test performance (Gold & Harvey, 1993; Gray, Feldon, Rawlins, Hemsley, & Smith, 1991; Strauss, 1993). For example, some SZs perform poorly across a variety of tests (Heaton, Baade, & Johnson, 1978; Saykin et al., 1991, 1994), some perform poorly on a few specific tasks while other neurocognitive functions are relatively preserved (Goldstein, 1986; Heinrichs & Awad, 1993), and a minority perform within normal limits on neuropsychological tasks (Bellack & Blanchard, 1993; Heinrichs & Awad, 1993; Moses & Maruish, 1988). Although neuropsychological testing has not produced a consistent pattern of findings across all persons with SZ or a universal schizophrenic profile, some generalizations can be made, at least with respect to neuropsychological subsets of SZs (Heinrichs & Awad, 1993).

Some SZs present with diffuse, global, or generalized cognitive impairments, as has been demonstrated by a variety of researchers (Buchsbaum et al., 1992; Gold & Harvey, 1993). For example, age- and education-controlled studies have shown that the Pathognomonic scale of the Luria–Nebraska Neuropsychological

Battery (LNNB) provides a quick measure of gross brain dysfunction that discriminates chronic SZs from psychiatric and neurologically normal controls (Moses & Maruish, 1988; Purish, Golden, & Hammeke, 1987). Using the full LNNB, Bellini, Gambini, Palladino, & Scarone (1988) demonstrated bilateral neurofunctional impairment in SZ and affective patients. More importantly, they showed that affective patient were clearly separable from SZs given their greater impairment on two subscales (Rhythm and Intelligence). Dickerson, Ringel, and Boronow (1991) examined a group of chronic inpatient SZ and found that positive symptoms of thought disorder and hallucinations were predictors of LNNB performance: specifically, the Left Frontal and the Memory scales of the LNNB showed the strongest positive relationship. Saykin et al. (1991) demonstrated that SZs perform at least one standard deviation below normal controls on ten cognitive factor scores derived from a large battery of neuropsychological tests, suggestive of cognitive dysfunctions instantiated by diverse anatomical systems (Gold & Harvey, 1993).

Golden, Moses, et al. (1980) demonstrated that neuropsychological impairment on the LNNB was related to brain atrophy in younger chronic SZs, as well as a subgroup of "organic schizophrenics," which was separable from other young chronic SZs on neuropsychological measures. Golden (1981) described a group of SZ with diffuse deficits as seriously impaired on tasks of sustained attention and concentration, and on tasks that are complex or involve "higher cognitive functioning," but with generally intact basic motor and sensory skills. Puente, Rodenbough, and Orrell (1993) showed that chronic brain-damaged SZs scored significantly higher than chronic non-brain-damaged SZs on the Profile Elevation scale of the LNNB, but more importantly, they showed that LNNB scores were unrelated to medication (namely, chlorpromazine equivalents). Rossi et al. (1990) grouped SZs according to LNNB performance and discovered a distinct subgroup of patients with enlarged lateral ventricles, higher negative symptoms, and difficulty understanding task instructions. They concluded that they had found a subset of SZs that met criteria for Kraepelin's dementia praecox.

In an excellent review of intellectual functioning in SZ, Seidman et al. (1992) point out that 5- to 10-point lower IQ scores exist premorbidly or during early phases of SZ (also Heaton et al., 1994). The range of SZ IQ scores show the same type of variation in the general population, such that higher mean IQs are obtained in higher socioeconomic status groups. These significant IQ deficits have been associated with early onset, male gender, attentional dysfunction, poor childhood academic performance, and marked childhood behavior disorder. Finally, Seidman et al. point out that Verbal IQ scores tend to be greater than Performance IQ scores in SZs versus controls, but that this finding is not specific to SZ and is found in other psychotic and brain-injured groups as well.

Some Szs perform poorly on tests of prefrontal lobe functioning, with deficits in sustained attention/vigilance, ability to inhibit interference or perseverative responses, ability to formulate and reason deductively with abstract concepts, ability to filter out irrelevant or distracting information, ability to integrate different sources or types of information, poor cognitive flexibility or ability to shift mental sets, poor word and design fluency, poor planning abilities, impaired social judgment and insight, organization, and mental tracking (Cornblatt & Erlenmeyer-Kimlint, 1985; Cornblatt & Keilp, 1994; Gjerde, 1983; Randolph, Goldberg, & Weinberger, 1993; Young, Davila, & Scher, 1993). Levin, Yurgelun-Todd, & Craft (1989) argue that this group of frontal lobe SZ's can be further subdivided, with negative symptom SZ's evidencing inattention or distractibility primarily by errors of omission (e.g., failure to respond), while positive symptoms SZ's evidence inattention primarily with errors of commission (i.e., impulsively overresponding). Overall, studies have shown that impairment of selective attention is characteristic of some SZs, but is not characteristic of SZs in general (Goldsampt, Barros, Schwartz, Weinstein, & Iqbal, 1993). Gureje, Acha, and Osuntokun (1994) demonstrated that SZ and manic subjects performed worse on a neuropsychological battery than normal controls and that SZ performed worse than manic patients on some measures. They concluded that, unrelated to age, chronicity, or years of institutionalization, general cognitive deficits are a feature of SZs and manics, but that frontal lobe dysfunction may be more specific to SZ.

Morrison-Stewart et al. (1992) demonstrated that SZs performed worse than controls on putative tests of frontal lobe dysfunction [Wisconsin Card Sorting Test (WCST)], and, surprisingly, that nonmedicated SZs performed better than age-, education-, and IQ-matched medicated SZs. Their combined group of SZs were not significantly different on non-frontal lobe tasks [e.g., Wechsler Memory Scale (WMS)]. Goldsampt et al. (1993) describe a study in which the WCST was administered to SZ, bipolar, and normal control groups. As expected, the SZ and bipolar groups performed worse than normal controls, and SZs worse than bipolars. However, the SZs performed worse because of cognitive flexibility and perserverative responses, while bipolar performance was characterized by a failure to inhibit impulsive responses, resulting in a failure to maintain an appropriate semantic category or set. The difference in performance was, therefore, based on differential impairments in cognitive or "executive" functions (Goldsampt et al., 1993, p. 153).

Gold and Harvey (1993) correctly remind us that it is not pathognomonic for SZs to perform poorly on the WCST, and patients with other psychiatric diagnoses may also perform poorly on the task. Hence, while overall performance on the WCST is neither sensitive nor specific to SZ, specific types of errors may contribute to task errors that differentiate psychiatric groups (Morrison-Stewart et al., 1992).

Summarizing a decade of research on memory impairments in SZ, Randolph et al. (1993) concluded that "the bulk of recent data suggest that memory deficits are a core feature of the neuropsychological profile of SZs, strongly suggesting bilateral dysfunction of medial temporal lobe systems in SZ: (p. 508). Some SZs perform poorly on test of semantic memory (WMS-R, Warrington Word Recognition) and verbal learning (California Verbal Learning Test). These memory functions have been implicated with the left temporal–hippocampal system (Saykin et al., 1994), hippocampal–diencephalic neuronal loss (Benes, Sorensen, & Bird, 1991), and impaired temporal–hippocampal and frontal–hippocampal functions. These temporal lobe–hippocampal SZs exhibit impaired verbal memory and verbal learning, with rapid forgetting of new information and significant free recall intrusions (Heinrichs & Awad, 1993; Jeste & Lohr, 1989; Saykin et al., 1991; Young et al., 1993). While memory disturbance may appear commonplace in SZ, a true amnestic disorder is rare (Heinrichs & Awad, 1993). First episode, neuroleptic-naive SZs have been shown to perform as poorly as chronic, unmedicated but previously neruoleptically exposed SZ on verbal memory and learning tasks, suggesting that verbal memory may be "a primary neuropsychological deficit early in the course of SZ" (Saykin et al., 1994, p. 124).

Similarly, some SZs exhibit language and speech dysfunction associated with dysfunction in Broca's area in the left frontal lobe (Young et al., 1993). These frontal lobe SZs exhibit neologisms, paraphasias, confabulation, clanging or echolalic speech, incomprehensible speech constructed out of meaningful words ("word salad"), and derailment; other deficits such as impaired confrontation naming and verbal fluency have also been observed.

Another subset of SZs show abnormalities in gait, posture, balance, coordination, and reaction time, possible secondary to sensory or neuromotor dysfunction. For example, some SZ show diminished ability in initiate, execute, sustain, and complete simple to complex motor tasks, suggestive of possible frontal/sensorimotor, basal ganglia, or cerebellar dysfunction (Bigler, 1988; Heinrichs & Awad, 1993; Marsden, 1982; Weinberger et al., 1986), and these clinical observations have been observed well before the neuroleptic medication era (Bleuler, 1950; Diefendorf & Dodge, 1908; Kraepelin, 1971). Motor anomalies evidenced in today's SZs include stereotypies, slowed reaction times, spasmodic jerkiness, reduced efficiency of fine movements, dystonias, generalized loss of smooth muscular coordination, and abnormalities in manual control and tracking (Asarnow, Marder, Mintz, Van Putten, & Zimmerman, 1988; Caligiuri & Lohr, 1990: Caligiuri, Lohr, Panton, & Harris, 1993; DeAmicis, & Cromwell, 1979; Goode, Meltzer, Crayton, & Mazura, 1977; Holzman & Levy, 1977; King, 1965; Lipton, Levy, Holzman, & Levin, 1983; Manschreck, 1986; Manschreck et al., 1990; Mather & Putchat, 1984; Meltzer, 1976; Rosofsky, Levin, & Holzman, 1982; Schwartz et al., 1989, 1990; Vrtunski, Simpson, & Meltzer, 1989).

Some SZs have structural abnormalities of their neuromuscular system. Specifically, irregular atrophy of individual muscle fibers and an increase in intramuscular nerve branching have been consistent findings (Crayton, Stalberg, & Hilton-Brown, 1977; Meltzer, 1976, 1987; Schneider & Grossi, 1979; Stevens, 1992). However, neuronal atrophy, abnormal innervation, and increased neuromuscular jitter are not specific to SZ, but can be found in other severe psychiatric patients, as well as in persons with Parkinson's disease (Crayton et al., 1977; Stevens, 1992). Hence, it is unclear whether neuromuscular abnormalities are related to exposure to neuroleptics or chronicity of severe mental illness, or whether they constitute true neuromotor disease related to SZ.

Holzman, Proctor, and Hughes (1973), followed by Holzman and Levy (1977), reported abnormal eye tracking in SZ by assessing the congruence of a subject's eye tracking behavior with a sinusoidal wave target. Levy, Holzman, Matthysse, and Mendell (1994) present an impressive list of studies from 1908 to the present in which there has not been a single failure to replicate eye tracking dysfunction in SZ. Eye tracking dysfunction does not appear to be an artifact of neuroleptic exposure, acute psychotic state, poor motivation, or inattention, and is not specific to SZ (Altman et al., 1990; Levy et al., 1994).

On a task sustaining isometric force on a hand dynamometer with auditory feedback, Rosen, Lockhart, Gants, and Westergaard (1991) reported that SZs and their non-SZ first-degree relatives consistently performed worse than affective disordered patients and normal controls. Grip strength, age, gender, education, work status, medication level, neuroleptic exposure, hospitalization status, chronicity, and clinical symptomatology were each unrelated to dynamometer performance. Rosen et al. (1991) concluded that the dynamometer task provided a sensitive and reliable behavioral and vulnerability marker of SZ.

Westergaard (1994) examined a diverse set of quantified measures of abnormal neuromotor behaviors in time series data of force exerted during the dynamometer task. Comparing SZ and bipolar patients with psychiatrically normal controls, Westergaard found that SZs had a disturbance in their ability to appropriately activate and sustain muscle force. Specifically, SZ showed slower response and recovery times, more time off target, poor motor steadiness, negativism, and disorganized, erratic, idiopathic motor behaviors. Bipolar patients were also less "motor steady" than controls. None of the above findings were related to demographic or clinical variables. Clinical decision rules incorporating abnormal motor behaviors correctly distinguished patients from controls (91–100% sensitivity) and bipolar patients from SZ (100% specificity). While it is true that abnormal psychomotor performance may be iatrogenic in studies that use chronic neuroleptic-exposed SZs (Blanchard & Neale, 1992; Heaton & Crowley, 1981; Manschreck et al., 1990), there is also substantial evidence from archival reports (Owens, Johnstone, & Frith, 1982; Reiter, 1925; Turner, 1989; Waddington & Crow, 1988), developmental studies (Fish, 1977; Walker, 1994; Walker, Savoie, & Davis, 1994; Walker & Shaye, 1982), and current research using neuroleptic-naive SZs (Caligiuri, Lohr, & Jeste, 1993; Crow, Owens, Johnstone, Cross, & Owen, 1983; Farde et al., 1990; Khot & Wyatt, 1991; Moses, 1984; Moses & Maruish, 1989; Owens et al., 1982; Verdoux, Magnin, & Bourgeois, 1995; Waddington & Youssef, 1990) to demonstrate that not all dyskinesia (or poor neuromotor performance) can be explained away as secondary to tardive dyskinesia.

Relating neuropsychological functioning to structural and functional brain abnormalities, Seidman et al. (1992) tentatively propose two distinct syndromes of SZ defined by unique frontolimbic dysfunction. Syndrome I SZ (orbitofrontal, temporal–limbic) is characterized by "paranoid, positive symptom, good premorbid status relatively preserved intellectual ability, adequate premorbid achievement, good visuospatial, motor and executive functions. At the same time there are impairments in attention (hypervigilance, commission errors), language, reasoning and abstraction, verbal learning and memory." Syndrome II SZ (dorsolateral, limbic–prefrontal) is characterized by "nonparanoid, negative symptom, poor premorbid status, limited intellectual and academic achievement, attention dysfunction (omission errors and response slowing), poor working memory, significant executive dysfunctions, concrete thinking, verbal deficits, pronounced motor slowing, lack of the usual cerebral dominance on motor tasks, and bilateral impairment" (p. 428). Later, Seidman et al. (1994) reported that poor performance on neuropsychological measures testing frontal and left temporal lobe functions (i.e., attentional, and "executive" and memory, respectively) were highly associated with MRI area or volume measures of dorsolateral prefrontal cortex in SZ. In particular, left dorsal lateral prefrontal cortex reduction showed worse performance on the following: WCST, Wechsler Adult Intelligence Scale—Revised (WAIS-R) Similarities, lower IQ, and WMS-R verbal and visual memory. Smaller right dorsal lateral prefrontal cortex was associated with impairment in attention and vigilance.

Just as memory function was unrelated to temporal lobe volume, Seidman et al. (1994) concluded that "in schizophrenia, recall memory may be associated as much with prefrontal contributions of attention, organization, and encoding as with temporal–limbic contributions of retrieval" (p. 242). Similarly, Gold et al. (1994) compared 66 SZs with 48 medically intractable focal left temporal and 53 right temporal lobe epilepsy patients on a comprehensive neuropsychological battery. While all three patient groups demonstrated memory impairments compared to national norms, semantic knowledge and verbal memory in SZs was significantly better than the left temporal lobe epilepsy group. Also, SZs showed the greatest attentional impairment and motor slowing than the epilepsy groups on tasks thought to reflect frontal lobe or executive functioning (e.g., Trails, Tapping, WCST Categories learned/completed). Gold et al. (1994) concluded that lateralized medial–temporal lobe dysfunction is not a sufficient explanation of the cognitive impairments in SZ, and that compromised frontal–executive functioning may play a greater role in task performance than widely believed. Goldberg and Weinberger (1994) caution that WCST scores may best be understood as the combined result of diverse psychological–semantic, physiological, and neuroanatomic mechanisms.

Unipolar Depression

Neuropathology

Epidemiological studies have reported lifetime major depression prevalence estimates as high as 17% (Blazer, Kessler, MacGonagle, & Swartz, 1994), making this disorder a major public health problem. Reviews of relevant literature have suggested fairly consistently that patients with major depression have associated dysfunction within the right hemisphere, particularly within the right frontal lobe, or anteriorly within the right hemisphere (e.g., Cassens, Wolfe, & Zola, 1990; Flor-Henry, 1983; Newman & Sweet, 1992).

Based on studies of psychiatric surgery, unilateral lesions, hemispheric activation, EEG, evoked potentials, epilepsy, and PET scans, Flor-Henry (1983) suggested that rather than a simple localized dysfunction, the regulation of emotion results from interaction of the two hemispheres through transcallosal neural inhibition. That is, while right hemisphere dysfunction has been related to depression, it is the failure of the left hemisphere to adequately control (i.e., inhibit) the expression of symptoms of depression. Similarly, failure of the right hemisphere to inhibit the left hemisphere can result in anger, paranoia, or euphoria. According to Flor-Henry (1983), the "release of emotion" may be due to the loss of contralateral inhibition with subsequent ipsilateral activation to an "abnormal emotional state" (see pp. 282–283).

Building on Flor-Henry's theoretical model of emotion, Tucker (1988) posited that intrahemispheric cortical activation and regulation between anterior and posterior regions of the brain were also involved in the expression of emotion. Accordingly, within each hemisphere, anterior regions were viewed as providing a regulatory function, such that increased frontal activation presumably would lead to decreased activation in posterior regions, and posterior regions were hypothesized to be representational, or contain contextual information about a given emotional state. Hence, increased frontal activation would presumably inhibit (i.e., decease activation of) posterior regions. This notion has, in fact, received some support in the literature in terms of increased right frontal lobe EEG activation in depressives (e.g., Schaffer, Davidson, & Saron, 1983), or alternatively, that decreased activation of the left, relative to the right, anterior region is a marker of vulnerability to depression (see review by Davidson, 1992).

Supporting evidence for the contributions of interhemispheric and intrahemispheric mechanisms in depression can be found within the stroke literature, most notably in the work of Robinson and colleagues (e.g., Starkstein & Robinson, 1988). Generally supported by the literature, although not without opponents (e.g., House, Dennis, Warlow, Hawton, & Molyneux, 1990), there seems to be a strong relationship between lesion location and affective disturbance (see Sweet, Newman, & Bell, 1992, for review). Within the left hemisphere, more anterior lesions are associated with a greater frequency of major depression, while to a much smaller degree, within the right hemisphere, posterior lesions are more likely to produce depression. Overall, the greater number of poststroke major depressions occur with lesions in the left hemisphere (Robinson & Starkstein, 1990).

Neuropsychological Presentation

In reviewing the literature, Sweet et al. (1992) concluded that deficits in clinically depressed individuals appeared to cluster around three major areas of impairment: psychomotor speed, motivation and attention (including difficulty with sustained, effortful tasks requiring concentration), and memory and learning. With regard to memory and learning, incidental (versus intentional) memory may be relatively intact, as is recognition memory (versus free recall), and memory for related (versus unrelated) words. Newman and Sweet (1992) also note preliminary research suggesting that productive naming may be decreased in depressives. Cassens et al. (1990), in their review, describe unipolar depression deficits as including mild to moderate dysnomia, motor slowing and slowed performance on nonverbal visual–spatial tasks (e.g., Block Design, Objects Assembly), and greater memory impairment for nonverbal than verbal stimuli. Given that "slowing" or psychomotor retardation seems to affect timed tests (e.g., Newman & Sweet, 1986), such as Block Design and Object Assembly, one must be careful about using such tests to support a conclusion of right hemisphere dysfunction. Nonverbal memory impairment in untimed memory tests (such as those cited by Abas, Sahakian, & Levy, 1990; Cassens et al., 1990; Goulet-Fisher, Sweet, & Pfaelzer-Smith, 1986) may provide stronger evidence of right hemisphere dysfunction, consistent with the areas of neuropathology noted earlier.

Lachner and Engel (1994) performed a meta-analysis on studies that attempted to differentiate depression and dementia using various tests of memory. Results showed greater effect sizes for memory test that contained the following characteristics: delayed rather than immediate retrieval, distraction prior to recall, and "high-capacity demand" (greater cognitive demand and effort).

Based on their review of the literature, Sweet et al. (1992) recommended that clinicians consider a number of points when evaluating patients who are depressed:

1. Administer neuropsychological measures that evaluate domains suggested by the literature to differentiate depression from brain dysfunction (e.g., incidental versus intentional learning, recognition versus recall memory, initial learning versus delayed recall).
2. Avoid isolated test score interpretation; seek collateral information of patient's behaviors and capabilities; be familiar with common behavioral characteristics of pseudodementia.
3. Do not use customary "cutoffs" to determine impairment for tests known to be sensitive to depression effects (e.g., Trail Making, WAIS-R Digit Symbol).
4. Avoid diagnosing brain dysfunction in depressed patients, if only based on poor findings in decreased cognitive efficiency or mild attentional or mild memory problems. In other words, look for patterns of impairment not associated with depression (e.g., impaired recall *and* recognition, a true "Stroop effect").

5. If questions concerning effort, inattention, or other depression-related variables cannot be addressed satisfactorily within the testing session, readminister at least a portion of the testing on another day, perhaps after a period of pharmacological or psychotherapeutic intervention.

The above discussion is not intended to suggest that the effect of depression on neuropsychological function must be limited inherently to only certain domains. In fact, the effects of depression in some individual cases of depressive pseudodementia can include nearly all possible neuropsychological functions, even those that are purportedly pathognomonic of brain dysfunction (see case discussions in Newman & Sweet, 1992).

Obsessive–Compulsive Disorder

Neuropathology

Epidemiological studies have indicated that obsessive–compulsive disorder (OCD) may be twice as common as SZ and panic disorder, with perhaps 1 to 2 million Americans suffering from OCD (Rasmussen & Eisen, 1990). OCD has been associated with head trauma, encephalitis, premorbid neurological illness, birth trauma, abnormal EEGs and evoked-potentials, abnormal CT and PET of the brain, and abnormalities of neuropsychological testing (Hollander et al., 1990). Although not all evidence of nervous system integrity in OCD patients is consistent, Hollander et al. (1990) found that OCD patients had significantly more neurological soft signs in both initial and replication groups than did controls. Further, the more severe the obsessions, the more soft signs present. A number of fine motor coordination problems were evident, with worse performance in the left hand, and on cube drawings, thought to suggest right frontal dysfunction. OCD has been compared to disorders of movement, such as Parkinson's disease, Tourette's syndrome, Sydenham's chorea, and chronic motor tics, with the results suggestive of similar loci of striatal dysfunction, particularly the caudate nucleus in the case of OCD (Baxter, 1990; Schwartz, Martin, & Baxter, 1992).

Neuropsychological Presentation

Among neuropsychological studies, fairly consistent evidence has been found of visuospatial or visuoconstructional deficit (viewed as indication of right hemisphere dysfunction) (Boone, Ananth, Philpott, Kaur, & Djenderedjian, 1991; Hollander et al., 1993; reviews by Alarcon, Libb, & Boll, 1994; Otto, 1992), nonverbal memory deficit (Boone et al., 1991; Christensen, Kim, Dysken, & Hoover, 1992; Zielinski, Taylor, & Juzwin, 1991), and intact verbal functions, including intact verbal memory (Boone et al., 1991; Christensen et al., 1992; Zielinski et al., 1991). Given the frequent mention in the literature of frontal pathophysiology in

OCD, the lack of strong evidence of deficiencies in executive functions and attention in the neuropsychological findings is noteworthy (Boone et al., 1991; Zielinski et al., 1991) and difficult to explain.

The Special Case of Malingering

Clearly, malingering is not representative of a specific psychopathology. Further, malingering is not a legitimate disorder, but, to paraphrase the DSM-IV, is instead the deliberate production of false or greatly exaggerated symptoms motivated by external incentives (American Psychiatric Association, 1994). Malingers may present to neuropsychologists with fraudulent cognitive or emotional complaints. Given the now commonplace involvement of neuropsychologists with forensic cases, the issue of identifying malingerers and not confusing them with genuine cases of cognitive or emotional disturbance is increasingly important. The vast majority of the literature on this subject has been published within the last 5–8 years, with numerous articles continuing to be published on an annual basis. Nies and Sweet (1994) have reviewed the literature pertaining to neuropsychological assessment and malingering, and have concluded that while difficult, it is possible to identify at least some malingerers, if looked for deliberately. Multiple measures and methods are necessary, since no single measure or methodology has proven sufficient to date. Nies and Sweet recommend consideration of the following:

1. The use of specific tests of malingering.
2. Evaluation of patterns of performance on common neuropsychological measures that are "forced choice" in structure and for which below-chance-level performances can be computed. However, while typically performing worse than real patients, it is important to note that not all malingerers will perform below chance levels.
3. Evaluation of nonsensical test patterns that have not been found to occur in real psychiatric or neurological patients (e.g., Rawling & Brooks, 1990; Mittenberg, Azrin, Millsaps, & Heilbronner, 1993; Tenhula & Sweet, 1996).
4. Examination of excessive inconsistency of test scores within and across test sessions.
5. Confirmation of test behaviors by comparison with independently obtained information pertaining to everyday life and work-related activities.
6. Detailed clinical history taking that allows determination of whether the patient has suffered significant and lasting real life losses (e.g., divorce from previously contented spouse, loss of property due to bankruptcy, loss of secure and rewarding long-time vocation) attributable to the claimed disorder.

Consideration of malingering by clinical neuropsychologists has become extremely important, as other disciplines may not have the methods and instrumentation available to accurately distinguish between genuine psychopathology and fraudulent behavior. No doubt, most senior clinicians have a variety of case anecdotes ranging from patients who clearly malingered all their symptoms to those who may have an area of legitimate injury (i.e. herniated disk requiring spinal fusion) and who nevertheless malinger cognitive symptoms. Often, malingerers have already been seen and have validated as legitimately injured by physicians or other psychologists, who then have difficulty with their own cognitive dissonance in changing their original diagnosis. Conversely, neuropsychologists must be familiar with a wide range of medical conditions in order not to rule out genuine brain dysfunction in patients whose presentation may initially appear odd or unusual (e.g., some presentations of aphasia or apraxia, and some presentations of acute medical diseases, such as encephalitis, epilepsy, endocrine disorders or pseudotumor cerebri).

AVAILABLE PROCEDURES/TESTS FOR EVALUATING PSYCHOPATHOLOGY

The number of formal tests and procedures available today is substantially larger than in the recent past of even 10 years ago. Before discussing these choices, it may be helpful to first consider the broader question of what types of psychopathology measures clinical neuropsychologists currently employ. In a recent survey of 279 neuropsychologists, Sweet, Moberg, and Westergaard (1996) found that 74% used objective personality tests either "often" or "always." This high degree of frequency of usage is in striking contrast to the 85% who stated that they "never" or only "occasionally" used projective personality tests. Comparison to earlier data gathered for objective personality tests by Sweet and Moberg (1990) indicates similar and therefore stable usage 5 years earlier. However, the projective personality tests had been used at a somewhat higher rate 5 years earlier (77% indicated "never" or "occasionally," and 5 years ago, 16% indicated "often" compared to only 10% in the most recent survey), and thus seems to be in declining usage by neuropsychologists.

Dies (1994) argues that the Rorschach should not be used as a "diagnostic instrument," but should rather be used descriptively to assess present clinical state, presumably for psychiatric patients. While not possible to determine with certainty, there appear to be several possible reasons that projective techniques are specifically in low favor and decreasing usage by neuropsychologists. First, reliance of some of the more popular projective techniques, such as the Rorschach, on visual perception of vague, ambiguous stimuli introduces a confound for many brain-impaired patients who have visual field cuts, diplopia, visual attention, visual discrimination, visual–spatial, or other visual disturbances. Memory disturbances may obfuscate the Rorschach's formal inquiry, which asks the patient to explain their previous answers. Language disturbances may also impair the patient's ability to accurately report characteristics of the inkblots. Clearly, there is no objective method for identifying the degree to which the normal process of reporting visual percepts of the inkblots will be altered and therefore invalidated in any individual case of brain dysfunction. Second, Exner's system for scoring and interpreting the Rorschach has empirically derived construct validity and test–retest and interrater reliability, but norms are not available for populations whose cognitive and emotional disturbances from neurological disorder's may be static or likely to change dramatically over time (e.g., traumatic brain injury or cerebral vascular disease).

Other popular projective techniques, such as the Thematic Apperception Test or any of the incomplete sentences procedures, may also suffer from a degree of invalidity because of the impairment of neuropsychological abilities required to complete the tasks accurately. Further, neuropsychologists tend to prefer measures with well-documented, reliable scoring procedures, something lacking with the Thematic Apperception Test and most incomplete sentence tasks. In fact, to many psychologists, such assessment procedures are not deemed to be psychological tests at all, in that they fail to meet the definitional criteria (i.e., objective, standardized, quantifiable, with the ability to establish degree of reliability, validity, and utility) (see Anastasi, 1988; Murphy & Davidshofer, 1994; Walsh & Betz, 1990), and are therefore referred to as psychological techniques. Given these distinctions and concerns, the discussion that follows will focus on objective measures of personality and emotion because of their greater relevance to neuropsychologists. An important caveat is warranted regarding the general inappropriateness and ineffectiveness of using any projective or objective personality measure expressly to diagnose the presence or absence of brain dysfunction, since the research literature has convincingly failed to provide empirical support for doing so (Chelune, Ferguson, & Moehle, 1986).

Objective Personality Measures

Minnesota Multiphasic Personality Inventory

The Minnesota Multiphasic Personality Inventory (MMPI) and Minnesota Multiphasic Personality Inventory—2 (MMPI-2) are well known to all clinical psychologists and therefore do not require general description. There are several reasons that the MMPI-2, following on the heels of its predecessor, has remained the most frequently used objective personality test. These reasons include: (1) the vast, and for the most part still relevant, MMPI literature established over decades of use (allowing clinicians to be very familiar with the appropriate uses and limitations of the instrument); (2) the effectiveness of the MMPI and MMPI-2 validity scales; (3) the empirical basis for item selection (leading to a substantial number of items having low face validity, and thus decreasing "impression management" by patients); and (4) the adaptability of the test format for computerized scoring (allowing for very efficient use of clinician time, while obtaining extensive breakdowns and analyses of the many available scales and items). As alluded to earlier, since the MMPI and MMPI-2 have significant limitations in the diagnosis of brain dysfunction (e.g., Golden, Sweet, & Osmon, 1979), the popularity of the instrument with clinical neuropsychologists has been to elucidate an individual's coping styles, emotional distress, adjustment to medical conditions, and general psychological function (cf. Graham, 1993; Greene, 1991; Keller & Butcher, 1991). Additionally, the MMPI and MMPI-2 can help indicate substance abuse potential and other specific disorders that may affect diagnosis and treatment planning of patients with brain dysfunction who either have independent psychological disturbance or for whom such disturbance is a primary or secondary effect of the brain dysfunction itself. Importantly, readers should appreciate that, as paper-and-pencil self-report measures, the MMPI and MMPI-2 cannot discriminate between medical and psychological conditions. Given that an absence of abnormal medical findings does not automatically mean that the condition is psychological, and vice versa, this latter goal is best achieved through the active collaboration of physicians and psychologists. Attempting to address these issues, neuropsychologists have begun to elucidate more appropriate normative data for head-injured, cerebrovascular, and neurologically disordered patients (Alfano, Finlayson, Stearns, & Nellson, 1990; Gass, 1991, 1992; Gass & Russell, 1991; Rothke et al., 1994).

Last, it may be very important to evaluate reading (comprehension, rather than simple work recognition) ability, if a current eighth grade reading comprehension level is not assured. Unfortunately, for some patients seen by neuropsychologists, this required level of reading ability will preclude use of the MMPI-2.

Personality Assessment Inventory

The Personality Assessment Inventory (PAI) (Morey, 1991) is a recently developed test that appears to have substantial potential for use by clinical neuropsychologists. Rather than the true–false format of the MMPI-2, the PAI uses a four-item response set of false, slightly true, mainly true, and very true. The inventory has 344 items that form 22 nonoverlapping scales. These scales include four validity scales (Inconsistency, Infrequency, Negative Impression, Positive Impression), 11 clinical scales (Somatic Complaints, Anxiety, Anxiety-related Disorders, Depression, Mania, Paranoia, Schizophrenia, Borderline Features, Antisocial Features, Alcohol Problems, Drug Problems), five treatment scales (Aggression, Suicidal Ideation, Stress, Nonsupport, Treatment Rejection), and two interpersonal scales (Dominance, Warmth). Ten of the scales have conceptually derived subscales. Linear T scores are used for normative comparisons, with the manual presenting extensive data based on over 3000 normal and clinical subjects.

Importantly, there are two features of the PAI that have special promise, in the event that future research supports the diagnostic validity and utility of the instrument. Specifically, the PAI requires a lower reading level than the MMPI-2 (i.e., fourth grade instead of eighth grade), and because it is briefer, it does not require as much time to complete as the MMPI-2. Because it has only recently become available to clinicians, we may not know for some time whether the PAI will merit regular consideration by neuropsychologists. The history of the MMPI suggests that, similarly, appropriate applications and limitations of the PAI will require extensive investigation and time to identify. Similar to the MMPI, a recent study by Rogers, Ornduff, and Sewell (1993) found that the PAI is highly effective in identifying individuals feigning SZ, but only marginally effective in identifying individuals feigning depression and ineffective in identifying individuals feigning anxiety disorder.

Millon Clinical Multiaxial Inventory—III

The Millon Clinical Multiaxial Inventory—III (MCMI-III) (Millon, Millon, & Davis, 1994) has recently been released for use. This latest version has 175 items (95 new items) at the eighth grade reading level. Scales are divided into personality pattern scales (Schizoid, Avoidant, Depressive, Dependent, Histrionic, Narcissistic, Antisocial, Aggressive, Compulsive, Passive–Aggressive, Self-defeating, Schizotypal, Borderline, Paranoid), clinical syndromes (Anxiety, Somatoform, Bipolar Mania, Dysthmia, Alcohol Dependence, Drug Dependence, Posttraumatic Stress Disorder, Thought Disorder, Major Depression, Delusional Disorder), modifying indices (Disclosure, Desirability, Debasement), and a validity index.

Given that the MCMI-III has just been released, there is as yet no published independent research in the professional literature. The literature on the predecessor instrument, the MCMI-II, is of reasonable size. Among other topics, the MCMI-II literature has addressed detection of spurious posttraumatic stress disorder claims (Lees-Haley, 1992), detection of random responding (Bagby, Gillis, & Rogers, 1991), hits and misses in detection of response bias (Retzlaff, Sheehan & Fiel, 1992), diagnostic accuracy with psychopathy, personality disorder, and psychotic disorders (Hart, Forth, & Hare, 1991; Inch & Crossley, 1993; McCann, Flynn, & Gersh, 1992; Retzlaff, Ofman, Hyer, & Matheson, 1994; Soldz, Budman, Demby, & Merry, 1993; Strack, Lorr, Campbell, & Lamnin, 1992), correspondence of factor structure to personality dimensions (Retzlaff, Lorr, Hyer, & Ofman, 1991; Strack, 1991), and comparison with the MMPI (Libb, Murray, Thurstin, & Alarcon, 1992; McCann, 1991). As one can imagine with any published test, not all of these studies are favorable to the MCMI-II, such as that of Inch and Crossley (1993), which found that both the MCMI-I and MCMI-II underestimated the incidence of psychotic disorders and overestimated the incidence of nonpsychotic disorders and personality disorders. Similarly, Piersma (1991) found the MCMI-II depression scales to underdiagnose major depression. More fundamentally difficult are the empirical findings (Miller, Goldberg, & Streiner, 1993; Streiner & Miller, 1989; Streiner, Goldberg, & Miller, 1993) that demonstrate that the method of assigning item weights or applying modifier and correction indices, all of which requires use of the computerized resources of the test publisher at a cost, provides no psychometric advantage, no appreciable advantage to the clinician, and may inhibit use of the instrument.

We should note that the above summary of a portion of the MCMI-II literature is by no means guaranteed to reflect the capabilities or limitations of the MCMI-III. As we have stated, it will take time for independent researchers to develop a substantive literature on the MCMI-III.

Millon Behavioral Health Inventory

The Millon Behavioral Health Inventory (MBHI) (Millon, Green, & Meagher, 1979, 1982) was conceptualized specifically for use by psychologists who work with medical patients. The MBHI is relatively brief to administer, with 150 items at the eighth grade reading level. Items break down into eight basic coping styles (Introversive, Inhibited, Cooperative, Sociable, Confident, Forceful, Respectful, Sensitive), six psychogenic attitudes scales (Chronic Tension, Recent Stress, Premorbid Pessimism, Future Despair, Social Alienation, Somatic Anxiety), three psychosomatic correlates (Allergic Inclination, Gastrointestinal Susceptibility, Cardiovascular Tendency), three prognostic indices scales (Pain Treatment Responsivity, Life Threat Reactivity, Emotional Vulnerability), and a three-item validity index. Neuropsychologists often see patients who have acute and chronic medical conditions, sometimes extending beyond the central nervous system, as in the case of the co-occurrence of pain from motor vehicle accidents, falls, and assaults. This being the case, an inventory designed to assess health attitudes and coping styles would seem to have particular relevance and therefore potential usefulness for the neuropsychologist whose job it is to fully appreciate brain function and dysfunction within the context of overall psychological, social, and physical function.

Unfortunately, given the length of time it has been available, the MBHI has received little attention from clinical researchers, and therefore numerous questions remain regarding its usefulness (Allen, 1985; Lanyon, 1985). For example, within the research pertaining to chronic pain patients, there have been concerns regarding the following: high degree of scale correlations within the MBHI (Lee-Riordan & Sweet, 1995), lack of specificity of the Pain Treatment Responsivity scale to chronic pain in general or to subtypes of pain (Gatchel, Deckel, Weinberg, & Smith, 1985; Wilcoxson, Zook, & Zarski, 1988), lack of concurrent validity with other assessment instruments (Sweet, Breuer, Hazelwood, Toye, & Pawl, 1985; Wilcoxson et al., 1988), and the degree to which responses on the MBHI are affected by the respondent's tendency to deny psychopathology or to admit emotional distress, as well as the ineffectiveness of a three-item validity scale (Lee-Riordan & Sweet et al., 1985). Perhaps further research will lead to either revision or better delineation of the limitations and usefulness of the MBHI.

Self-Report Mood Inventories

The large number of available self-report measures of mood and emotion precludes presentation of an exhaustive list. These assessment tools tend to be brief and straightforward to complete, making them attractive to clinicians. In fact, approximately 77% of clinical neuropsychologists "often" or "always" include measures (most of which are self-report) of mood and affect in their evaluations (Sweet et al., 1996). Importantly, clinicians need to appreciate the typically face-valid nature of these measures. In other words, it is certainly possible and relatively easy for a patient to engage in "impression management." For example, a hospitalized patient who meets criteria for major depression following a suicide attempt may in fact attain a score within the normal range on a self-report depression inventory, and conversely a patient who is not depressed may attain a very abnormal score, if he or she desires to do so. Nevertheless, the popularity of this type of test stems from the fact that most patients will endeavor to accurately describe their status. Among the available self-report mood inventories are the following: Beck Depression Inventory (Beck & Steer, 1987), Beck Hopelessness Scale (Beck & Steer, 1988), Beck Anxiety Inventory (Beck & Steer, 1990), Beck Scale for Suicide Ideation (Beck & Steer, 1991), State–Trait Anxiety Inventory (Spielberger, 1983), Multiple Affect Adjective Check List—Revised (Zuckerman & Lubin, 1985), State–Trait Anger Expression Inventory (Spielberger, 1988), and the Penn Inventory of Posttraumatic Stress Disorder (Hammerberg, 1992).

Rating Scales

As structured interviews become more and more popular, so does the use of formal rating scales that guide these interviews. Their use largely has grown out of large research projects that required standardization and verification of clinical diagnoses. From such projects, structured interviews are now available that relate to formal psychiatric diagnosis (Structured Clinical Interview for DSM-III-R, Spitzer, Williams, Gibbon, & First, 1990), posttraumatic stress disorder (Clinician Administered PTSD Scale—Form 1, Blake et al., 1990), malingering of psychiatric symptoms (Structured Interview of Reported Symptoms, Rogers, Bagby, & Dickens, 1992), and depression (Revised Hamilton Rating Scale for Depression, Warren, 1994) and other conditions.

The use of structured interviews is particularly well suited to specialty clinic practice because of the benefits of obtaining standardized information from all patients being seen for the same disorder. Clinicians seeing a broad spectrum of disorders would be well advised to learn a few relevant procedures, especially for those conditions that often lead to adversarial situations in which "proving" the condition definitively becomes important (e.g., litigated posttraumatic stress disorder).

THE CURRENT CHALLENGE

In recent years, much has changed in the understanding of the etiology, central nervous system involvement, assessment, and treatment of psychopathology. This is perhaps best exemplified in the SZ literature reviewed in this chapter. Even though especially knowledgeable regarding diagnostic and treatment issues pertaining to disorders of the brain, clinical neuropsychologists are also intimately involved in diagnostic and treatment issues pertaining to psychopathology. Standards of practice have moved well beyond simplistic notions of organic versus functional etiologies and similarly narrow treatment approaches. With the burgeoning knowledge of such exciting areas as functional neuroimaging techniques, neurochemistry, neurobiology, and psychopharmacology comes a growing body of knowledge that is more sharply and clearly delineating the basic nature and neuropsychological concomitants of psychopathological disorders. Keeping abreast of the rapid growth of relevant neuroscience information is a challenging, but requisite, task. Similarly, the proliferation of assessment techniques pertaining, not only to neuropsychological functioning, but also to psychopathology demands copious attention and effort, if we are to accomplish effectively our labyrinthine diagnostic and treatment tasks.

How can one identify an effective clinical neuropsychologist? We propose that one of the more palatable answers is that he or she does not simply focus on neuropsychological test data, but rather successfully integrates the often broad, disparate data available (including psychosocial, medical, neurological and personality/emotional) into the fullest possible understanding of the patient, and then, when appropriate, endeavors toward effective therapeutic intervention.

REFERENCES

Abas, M., Sahakian, B., & Levy, R. (1990). Neuropsychological deficits and CT scan changes in elderly depressives. *Psychological Medicine, 20,* 507–520.

Alarcon, R., Libb, J., & Boll, T. (1994). Neuropsychological testing in obsessive compulsive disorder: A clinical review. *Journal of Neuropsychiatry, 6,* 217–228.

Alfano, D., Finlayson, A., Stearns, G., & Nellson P. (1990). The MMPI and neurologic dysfunction: Profile configuration and analyses. *The Clinical Neuropsychologist, 4,* 69–79.

Allen, M. (1985). Review of Millon Behavioral Health Inventory. In J. V. Mitchell, Jr. (Ed.), *The ninth mental measurements yearbook* (Vol. 1). Lincoln: University of Nebraska Press.

Altman, E., Hedeker, D., Davis, J., Comaty, J., Jobe, T., & Levy, D. (1990). Neuropsychological test deficits are associated with smooth pursuit eye movement impairment in affective disorders but in schizophrenia. *International Journal of Clinical Neuropsychology, 12,* 49–59.

American Psychiatric Association. (1994). *Diagnostic and statistical manual of mental disorders* (4th ed.). Washington, DC: Author.

Anastasi, A. (1988). *Psychological testing* (6th ed.). New York: Macmillan.

Andreasen, N. (Ed.). (1994). *Schizophrenia: From mind to molecule.* Washington DC: American Psychiatric Press.

Andreasen, N., & Carpenter, W. (1993). Diagnosis and classification of schizophrenia. *Schizophrenia Bulletin, 2,* 199–214.

Andreasen, N., Ehrhardt, J., Swayze, V. II, Aalliger, R., Yuh, W., Cohen, G., & Ziebell, S. (1990). Magnetic resonance imaging of the brain in schizophrenia. *Archives of General Psychiatry, 47,* 35–44.

Andreasen, N., & Flaum, M. (1991). Schizophrenia: The characteristic symptoms. *Schizophrenia Bulletin, 17,* 27–135.

Andreasen, N., & Olsen, S. (1982). Negative vs. positive schizophrenia. *Archives of General Psychiatry, 39,* 789–794.

Andreasen, N., Rezai, K., Alliger, R., Swayze, V., Flaum, M., Kirchner, P., Cohen, G., & O'Leary, D. (1992). Hypofrontality in neuroleptic-naive patients and in patients with chronic schizophrenia. *Archives of General Psychiatry, 49,* 943–958.

Asarnow, R. F., Marder, S. R., Mintz, J., Van Putten, T., & Zimmerman, K. E. (1988). Differential effect of low and conventional doses of fluphenazine on schizophrenic outpatients with good or poor information-processing abilities. *Archives of General Psychiatry, 45,* 822–826.

Auerbach, J., Hans, S., & Marcus, J. (1993). Neurobehavioral functioning and social behavior of children at risk for schizophrenia. *Israel Journal of Psychiatry and Related Sciences, 30,* 40–49.

Bachneff, S. (1991). Positron emission tomography and magnetic resonance imaging: A review of local circuit neurons hypo(dys)function hypothesis of schizophrenia. *Biological Psychiatry, 30,* 857–886.

Bagby, R., Gillis, J., & Rogers, R. (1991). Effectiveness of the Millon Clinical Multiaxial Inventory Validity Index in the detection of random responding. *Psychological Assessment: A Journal of Consulting and Clinical Psychology, 3,* 285–287.

Baron, M. (1986a). Genetics of schizophrenia: I. Familial patterns and mode of inheritance. *Biological Psychiatry, 21,* 1051–1066.

Baron, M. (1986b). Genetics of schizophrenia: II. Vulnerability traits and gene markers. *Biological Psychiatry, 21,* 1189–1211.

Bateson, G., Jackson, D., Haley, J., & Weakland, J. (1956). Toward a theory of schizophrenia. *Behavioral Science, 1,* 251–264.

Baxter, L. (1990). Brain imaging as a tool in establishing a theory of brain pathology in obsessive compulsive disorder. *Journal of Clinical Psychiatry, 51,* 22–25.

Beck, A., & Steer, R. (1987). *Beck Depression Inventory manual.* San Antonio, TX: Psychological Corporation.

Beck, A., & Steer, R. (1988). *Beck Hopelessness Scale manual.* San Antonio, TX: Psychological Corporation.

Beck, A., & Steer, R. (1990). *Beck Anxiety Inventory manual.* San Antonio, TX: Psychological Corporation.

Beck, A., & Steer, R. (1991). *Beck Scale for Suicide Ideation manual.* San Antonio, TX: Psychological Corporation.

Bellack, A., & Blanchard, J. (1993). Schizophrenia: Psychopathology. In A. Bellack & M. Hersen (Eds.), *Psychopathology in adulthood* (pp. 216–233). Boston: Allyn and Bacon.

Bellini, L., Gambini, O., Palladino, F., & Scarone, S. (1988). Neuropsychological assessment of functional central nervous system disorders: I. Hemispheric functioning characteristics in schizophrenia and affective illness. *Acta Psychiatry Scandinavia, 78,* 242–246.

Benes, F., Sorensen, I., & Bird, E. (1991). Reduced neuronal size in the posterior hippocampus of schizophrenic patients. *Schizophrenia Bulletin, 17,* 597–608.

Berman, K., Torrey, E., Daniel, D., & Weinberger, D., (1992). Regional cerebral bloodflow in monozygotic twins discordant and concordant for schizophrenia. *Archives of General Psychiatry, 49,* 927–934.

Bigler, E. (1988). *Diagnostic clinical neuropsychology* (rev. ed.). Austin: University of Texas Press.

Blake, D., Weathers, F., Nagy, L., Kaloupek, D., Klauminzer, G., Charney, D., & Keane, T. (1990). A clinician rating scale for assessing current and lifetime PTSD: The CAPS-1. *Behavior Therapist, 13,* 187–188.

Blanchard, J., & Neale, J. (1992). Medication effects: Conceptual and methodological issues in schizophrenia research. *Clinical Psychology Review, 12,* 345–361.

Blazer, D., Kessler, R., MacGonagle, K., & Swartz, M. (1994). The prevalence and distribution of major depression in a national community sample: The national comorbidity survey. *American Journal of Psychiatry, 151,* 979–986.

Bleuler, E. (1950). *Dementia praecox or the group of schizophrenias* (J. Zinkin, trans). New York: International Universities Press (original work published 1911).

Boone, K., Ananth, J., Philpott, L., Kaur, A., & Djenderedjian, A. (1991). Neuropsychological characteristics of nondepressed adults with obsessive compulsive disorder. *Neuropsychiatry, Neuropsychology, and Behavioral Neurology, 4,* 96–109.

Breier, A., Buchanan, R., Elkashef, A., Munson, R., Kirkpatrick, B., & Gellad, F. (1992). Brian morphology and schizophrenia: A magnetic resonance imaging study of limbic, prefrontal cortex, and caudate structures. *Archives of General Psychiatry, 49,* 921–926.

Buchsbaum, M., Haier, R., Potkin, S., Nuechterlein, K., Bracha, H., Katz, M., Lohr, J., Wu, J., Lottenburg, S., Jerabek, P., Trenary, M., Tafalla, R., Reynolds, C., & Bunndy, W., Jr. (1992). Frontostriatal disorder of cerebral metabolism in never-medicated schizophrenics. *Archives of General Psychiatry, 49,* 935–942.

Burgess, J. (1992). Neurocognitive impairment in dramatic personalities: Histrionic, narcissistic, borderline, and antisocial disorders. *Psychiatry Research, 42,* 283–290.

Caligiuri, M. P., & Lohr, J. B. (1990). Fine force instability: A quantitative measure of neuroleptic-induced dyskinesia in the hand. *Journal of Neuropsychiatry, 2,* 395–398.

Caligiuri, M. P., Lohr, J. B., & Jeste, D. (1993). Parkinsonism in neuroleptic-naive schizophrenic patients. *American Journal of Psychiatry, 150,* 1343–1348.

Caligiuri, M. P., Lohr, J. B., Panton, D., & Harris, M. J. (1993). Extrapyramidal motor abnormalities associated with late-life psychosis. *Schizophrenia Bulletin, 19,* 747–754.

Cannon, T., Barr, C., & Mednick, S. (1991). Genetic and perinatal factors in the etiology of schizophrenia. In E. F. Walker (Ed.), *Schizophrenia: A life-course developmental perspective* (pp. 9–31). New York: Academic Press.

Cannon, T., & Marco, E. (1994). Structural brain abnormalities as indicators of vulnerability to schizophrenia. *Schizophrenia Bulletin, 20,* 89–102.

Cassens, G., Wolfe, L., & Zola, M. (1990). The neuropsychology of depressions. *Journal of Neuropsychiatry and Clinical Neurosciences, 2,* 202–213.

Chapman, L. J., & Chapman, J. P. (1975). Problems in the measurement of cognitive deficit. *Psychological Bulletin, 79,* 80–103.

Chapman, L. J., & Chapman, J. P. (1987). The search for symptoms predictive of schizophrenia. *Schizophrenia Bulletin, 13,* 497–503.

Chelune, G., Ferguson, W., & Moehle, K. (1986). The role of standard cognitive and personality tests in neuropsychological assessment. In T. Incagnoli, G. Goldstein, & C. Golden (Eds.), *Clinical application of neuropsychological test batteries* (pp. 75–119). New York: Plenum Press.

Christensen, K., Kim, S., Dysken, M., & Hoover, K. (1992). Neuropsychological performance in obsessive compulsive disorder. *Biological Psychiatry, 31,* 4–18.

Clementz, B., & Sweeney, J. (1990). Is eye movement dysfunction a biological marker for schizophrenia? A methodological review. *Psychological Bulletin, 108,* 77–92.

Clementz, B., & Sweeney, J. (1992). Smooth pursuit eye movement dysfunction and liability for schizophrenia: Implications for genetic modelling. *Journal of Abnormal Psychology, 101,* 117–129.

Cornblatt, B., & Erlenmeyer-Kimlint, L. (1985) Global attentional deviance as a marker of risk for schizophrenia: Specificity and predictive ability. *Journal of Abnormal Psychology, 94,* 470–486.

Cornblatt, B., & Keilp. J. (1994). Impaired attention, genetics, and the pathophysiology of schizophrenia. *Schizophrenia Bulletin, 20,* 31–46.

Crayton, J., Stalberg, E., & Hilton-Brown, P. (1977). The motor unit in psychotic patients: A single fi-
bre EMG study. *Journal of Neurology, Neurosurgery, and Psychiatry, 40,* 455–463.

Cross, A., Crow, T., & Owen, F. (1981). Eh-flupenthixol binding in postmortem brains of schizophrenics: Evidence for a selective increase in dopamine D2 receptors. *Psychopharmacology,
74,* 122–124.

Crow, T. (1990). Schizophrenia as a genetic encephalopathy. *Recenti Progressi in Medicina, 81,*
738–745.

Crow, T., Owens, D., Johnstone, E., Cross, A., & Owens, F. (1983). Does tardive dyskinesia exist?
Modern Problems in Pharmacopsychiatry, 21, 206–219.

Daniel, D., Goldberg, T., Gibbons, R., & Weinberger, D. (1991). Lack of a bimodal distribution of ventricular size in schizophrenia: A gaussian mixture analysis of 1056 cases and controls. *Biological
Psychiatry, 30,* 887–903.

Davidson, R. (1992). Anterior cerebral asymmetry and the nature of emotion. *Brain and Cognition, 20,*
125–151.

DeAmicis, L., & Cromwell, R. (1979). Reaction time crossover in process schizophrenic patients, their
relatives, and control subjects. *Journal of Nervous and Mental Disease, 167,* 593–600.

DeQaurdo, J., Tandon, R., Goldman, R., Meador-Woodruff, J., McGrath-Giroux, M., Brunberg, J., &
Kim, L. (1994). Ventricular enlargement, neuropsychological status, and premorbid function in
schizophrenia. *Biological Psychiatry, 35,* 517–524.

Dickerson, F., Ringel, N., & Boronow, J. (1991). Neuropsychological deficits in chronic schizophrenics: Relationship with symptoms and behavior. *The Journal of Nervous and Mental Disease, 179,* 744–749.

Diefendorf, A., & Dodge, R. (1908). An experimental study of the ocular reactions of the insane from
photographic records. *Brain, 31,* 451–489.

Dies, R. (1994). The Rorschach Comprehensive System: Current status and clinical applications. *The
Independent Practitioner, Bulletin of Division 24 of the APA, 14,* 96–106.

Docherty, N. (1994). Cognitive characteristics of the parents of schizophrenic patients. *The Journal of
Nervous and Mental Disease, 182,* 443–451.

Dolan, M. (1994). Psychopathy—A neurobiological perspective. *British Journal of Psychiatry, 165,*
151–159.

Faraone, S., Seidman, L., Kremen, W., Pepple, J., Lyons, M., & Tsuang, M. (1995). Neuropsychological functioning among the nonpsychotic relatives of schizophrenic patients: A diagnostic efficiency analysis. *Journal of Abnormal Psychology, 104,* 286–304.

Farde, L., Wiesel, F., Stone-Elander, S., Halldin, C., Nordstrom, A. L., & Sedvall, G. (1990). D2
dopamine receptors in neuroleptic-naive schizophrenic patients. *Archives of General Psychiatry,
47,* 213–219.

Fish, B. (1977). Neurologic antecedents of schizophrenia in children: Evidence for an inherited, congenital neurointegrative defect. *Archives of General Psychiatry, 47,* 213–219.

Fish, B. (1977). Neurologic antecedents of schizophrenia in children: Evidence for an inherited, congenital neurointegrative defect. *Archives of General Psychiatry, 34,* 1297–1313.

Flor-Henry, P. (1983). *Cerebral basis of psychopathology.* Boston: Wright.

Flor-Henry, P. (1990). Neuropsychology and psychopathology: A progress report. *Neuropsychology
Review, 1,* 103–123.

Freeman, T., & Karson, C. (1993). The neuropathology of schizophrenia: A focus on the subcortex.
Psychiatric Clinics of North America, 16, 281–293.

Fromm-Reichman, F. (1948). Notes on the development of treatment of schizophrenia by psychoana-
lytic psychotherapy. *Psychiatry, 11,* 263–273.

Gass, C. (1991). MMPI-2 interpretation and closed head injury: A correction factor. *Psychological
Assessment, 3,* 27–31.

Gass, C. (1992). MMPI-2 interpretation of patients with cerebrovascular disease: A correction factor. *Archives of Clinical Neuropsychology, 7,* 17–27.

Gass, C., & Russell, E. (1991). MMPI profiles of closed head trauma patients: Impact of neurologic complaints. *Journal of Clinical Psychology, 47,* 253–260.

Gatchel, R., Deckel, A., Weinberg, N., & Smith, J. (1985). The utility of the Millon Behavioral Health Inventory in the study of chronic headaches. *Headache, 25,* 49–54.

Gjerde, P. (1983). Attentional capacity dysfunction and arousal in schizophrenia. *Psychological Bulletin, 93,* 57–72.

Gold, J., & Harvey, P. (1993). Cognitive deficits in schizophrenia. *Psychiatric Clinics of North America, 16,* 295–312.

Gold, J., Hermann, B., Randolph, C., Wyler, A., Goldberg, T., & Weinberger, D. (1994). Schizophrenia and temporal lobe epilepsy. *Archives of General Psychiatry, 51,* 265–272.

Goldberg, E., & Seidman, L. (1991). Higher cortical functions in normals and in schizophrenia: A selective review. In S. Steinhauer, J. Gruzelier, & J. Zubin (Eds.), *Handbook of schizophrenia: Vol 5. Neuropsychology, psychophysiology and information processing* (pp. 553–597). New York: Elsevier.

Goldberg, T., Weinberger, D. (1994). Schizophrenia, training paradigms, and the Wisconsin Card Sorting Test redux. *Schizophrenia research, 11,* 291–296.

Golden, C. (1981). *Diagnosis and rehabilitation in clinical neuropsychology* (2nd ed.). Springfield, IL: Charles C. Thomas.

Golden, C., Graber, B., Coffman, J., Berg, R., Bloch, S., & Brogan, D. (1980). Brain density deficits in chronic schizophrenia. *Psychiatry Research, 3,* 179–184.

Golden, C., Moses, J., Zelazowski, R., Graber, B., Zatz, L., Horvath, T., & Berger, P. (1980). Cerebral ventricular size and neuropsychological impairment in young chronic schizophrenics. *Archives of General Psychiatry, 37,* 619–623.

Golden, C., Sweet, J., & Osmon, D. (1979). The diagnosis of brain damage by the MMPI: A comprehensive evaluation. *Journal of Personality Assessment, 43,* 138–142.

Goldsampt, L., Barros, J., Schwartz, B., Weinstein, C., & Iqbal, N. (1993). Neuropsychological correlates of schizophrenia. *Psychiatric Annals, 23,* 151–157.

Goldstein, G. (1986). The neuropsychology of schizophrenia. In I. Grant & K. Adams (Eds.), *Neuropsychological assessment of neuropsychiatric disorders* (pp. 147–171). New York: Oxford University Press.

Goldstein, G. (1990). Neuropsychological heterogeneity in schizophrenia: A consideration of abstraction and problem-solving abilities. *Archives of Clinical Neuropsychology, 5,* 251–264.

Goode, D., Meltzer, H., Crayton, J., & Mazura, T. (1977). Physiological abnormalities of the neuromuscular system in schizophrenia. *Schizophrenia Bulletin, 3,* 121–138.

Gottesman, I. (1991). *Schizophrenia genesis: The origins of madness.* New York: Freeman.

Goulet-Fisher, D., Sweet, J., & Pfaelzer-Smith, E. (1986). Influence of depression on repeated neuropsychological testing. *International Journal of Clinical Neuropsychology, 8,* 14–18.

Graham, J. (1993). *MMPI-2: Assessing personality and psychopathology* (2nd ed.). New York: Oxford University Press.

Gray, J., Feldon, J., Rawlins, J., Hemsley, D., & Smith, A. (1991). The neuropsychology of schizophrenia. *Behavioral and Grain Sciences, 14,* 1–84.

Greene, R. (1991). *The MMPI-2/MMPI: An interpretive manual.* Boston: Allyn & Bacon.

Gur, R. E., Mozley, D., Shtasel, D., Cannon, T., Gallacher, F., Turetsky, B., Grossman, R., & Gur, R. C. (1994). Clinical subtypes of schizophrenia: Differences in brain and CSF volume. *American Journal of Psychiatry, 151,* 343–350.

Gur, R. E., & Pearlson, G. (1993). Neuroimaging in schizophrenia research. *Schizophrenia Bulletin, 19,* 337–353.

Gureje, O., Acha, R. A., & Osuntokun, B. O. (1994). Do young schizophrenics with recent onset of illness show evidence of hypofrontality? *Behavioral Neurology, 7,* 59–66.

Hammerberg, M. (1992). Penn Inventory of Posttraumatic Stress Disorder: Psychometric properties. *Psychological Assessment, 4,* 67–76.

Hamsher, K., Halmi, K., Benton, A. (1981). Prediction of outcome in anorexia nervosa from neuropsychological status. *Psychiatric Research, 4,* 79–88.

Hart, S., Forth, A., & Hare, R. (1991). The MCMI-II and psychopathy. *Journal of Personality Disorders, 5,* 318–327.

Heaton, R., Baade, L., & Johnson, K. (1978). Neuropsychological test results associated with psychiatric disorders in adults. *Psychological Bulletin, 85,* 141–162.

Heaton, R., & Crowley, T. (1981). Effects of psychiatric disorders and their somatic treatments on neuropsychological test results. In S. B. Filskov & T. J. Boll (Eds.), *Handbook of clinical neuropsychology* (pp. 481–525). New York: Wiley.

Heaton, R., Paulsen, J., McAdams, L., Kuck, J., Zisook, S., Braff, D., Harris, J., & Jeste, D. (1994). Neuropsychological deficits in schizophrenics: Relationship to age, chronicity, and dementia. *Archives of General Psychiatry, 51,* 469–476.

Heinrichs, W. (1993). Schizophrenia and the brain: Conditions for a neuropsychology of madness. *American Psychologist, 48,* 221–233.

Henrichs, W., & Awad, G. (1993). Neurocognitive subtypes of chronic schizophrenia. *Schizophrenia Research, 9,* 49–58.

Hoff, A., Neal, C., Kushner, M., & DeLisi, L. (1994). Gender differences in corpus callosum size in first-episode schizophrenics. *Biological Psychiatry, 35,* 913–919.

Hollander, E., Cohen, L., Richards, M., Mullen, L., DeCaria, C., & Stern, Y. (1993). A pilot study of the neuropsychology of obsessive compulsive disorder and Parkinson's disease: Basal ganglia disorders. *Journal of Neuropsychiatry, 5,* 104–107.

Hollander, E., Schiffman, E., Cohen, B., Rivera-Stein, M., Rosen, W., Gorman, J., Fyer, A., Papp, L., & Liebowitz, M. (1990). Signs of central nervous system dysfunction in obsessive compulsive disorder. *Archives of General Psychiatry, 47,* 27–32.

Holzman, P., & Levy, D. (1977). Smooth pursuit eye movements and functional psychoses: A review. *Schizophrenia Bulletin, 3,* 15–27.

Holzman, P., Proctor, L., & Hughes, D. (1973). Eye tracking patterns in schizophrenia. *Science, 181,* 179–181.

Holzman, P., Proctor, L., Levy, D., Yasillo, J., Meltzer, H., & Hurt, S. (1974). Eye tracking dysfunctions in schizophrenic patients and their relatives. *Archives of General Psychiatry, 31,* 143–151.

House, A., Dennis, M., Warlow, C., Hawton, K., & Molyneux, A. (1990). Mood disorders after stroke and their relation to lesion location: A CT scan study. *Brain, 113,* 1113–1129.

Inch, R., & Crossley, M. (1993). Diagnostic utility of the MCMI-I and MCMI-II with psychiatric outpatients. *Journal of Clinical Psychology, 49,* 358–366.

Jeste, D., & Lohr, J. (1989). Hippocampal pathologic findings in schizophrenia. *Archives of General Psychiatry, 46,* 1019–1024.

Kaufmann, C., & Malaspina, D. (1993). Molecular genetics of schizophrenia. *Psychiatric Annals, 23,* 111–122.

Kay, S., & Sandyk, R. (1991). Experimental models of schizophrenia. *International Journal of Neurosciences, 58,* 69–82.

Keller, L., & Butcher, J. (1991). *Assessment of chronic pain patients with the MMPI-2.* Minneapolis: University of Minnesota Press.

Kendler, K., Diehl, S. (1993). The genetics of schizophrenia: A current genetic–epidemiologic perspective. *Schizophrenia Bulletin, 19,* 261–285.

Kessler, S. (1980). The genetics of schizophrenia: A review. *Schizophrenia Bulletin, 6,* 404–416.

Khot, V., & Wyatt, R. J. (1991). Not all that moves is tardive dyskinesia. *American Journal of Psychiatry, 148,* 661–666.

King, H. (1965). Reaction time and speed of voluntary movement by normal and psychotic subjects. *The Journal of Psychology, 59,* 219–227.

Kinney, D., Woods, B., & Yergelun-Todd, D. (1986). Neurologic abnormalities in schizophrenic patients and their families. II: Neurologic and psychiatric findings in relatives. *Archives of General Psychiatry, 43,* 665–668.

Kinney, D., Yurgelun-Todd, D., Waternaux, C., & Matthysse, S. (1994). *Schizophrenia Research, 12,* 63–73.

Kowalski, P. (1986). Cognitive abilities of female adolescents with anorexia nervosa. *International Journal of Eating Disorders, 5,* 983–998.

Kraepelin, E. (1971). *Dementia praecox and paraphrenia* (R. M. Barclay, Trans, G. Robertson Ed.). New York: Krieger (original work published 1919).

Kraepelin, E. (1987). Senile and pre-senile dementias. In K. Bick, L. Amaducci, & G. Pepeu (Eds.), *The early story of Alzheimer's disease* (pp. 32–81). New York: Raven Press (original work published 1910).

Kremen, W., Seidman, J., Pepple, J., Lyons, J., Tsuang, M., & Faraone, S. (1994). Neuropsychological risk indicators for schizophrenia: A review of family studies. *Schizophrenia Bulletin, 20,* 103–119.

Kremen, W., Tsuang, M., Faraone, S., & Lyons, M. (1992). Using vulnerability indicators to compare conceptual models of genetic heterogeneity in schizophrenia. *The Journal of Nervous and Mental Disease, 180,* 141–152.

Lachner, G., & Engel, R. (1994). Differentiation of dementia and depression by memory test: A meta-analysis. *Journal of Nervous and Mental Disease, 182,* 34–39.

Lanyon, R. (1985). Review of Millon Behavioral Health Inventory. In J. V. Mitchell, Jr. (Ed.), *The ninth mental measurements yearbook* (Vol. 1). Lincoln: University of Nebraska Press.

Lee-Riordan, D., & Sweet, J. (1995). Relationship between the Millon Behavioral Health Inventory and the MMPI in low back pain patients. *Journal of Clinical Psychology in Medical Settings, 1,* 387–398.

Lees-Haley, P. (1992). Efficacy of MMPI-2 validity scales and MCMI-II modifier scales for detecting spurious PTSD claims: F, F-K, Fake Bad Scale, Ego Strength, Subtle–Obvious subscales, DIS, and DEB. *Journal of Clinical Psychology, 48,* 681–689.

Leventhal, D., Schuck, J., Clemons, T., & Cox, M. (1982). Proprioception in schizophrenia. *The Journal of Nervous and Mental Disease, 170,* 21–26.

Levin, S., Yurgelun-Todd, D., & Craft, S. (1989). Contributions of clinical neuropsychology to the study of schizophrenia. *Journal of Abnormal Psychology, 98,* 341–356.

Levy, D., Holzman, P., Matthysse, S., & Mendell, N. (1994). Eye tracking and schizophrenia: A selective review. *Schizophrenia Bulletin, 20,* 47–62.

Libb, J., Murray, J., Thurstin, H., & Alarcon, R. (1992). Concordance of the MCMI-II, the MMPI, and axis II discharge diagnosis in psychiatric inpatients. *Journal of Personality Assessment, 58,* 580–590.

Lipton, R., Levy, D., Holzman, P., & Levin, S. (1983). Eye movement dysfunctions in psychiatric patients: A review. *Schizophrenia Bulletin, 9,* 13–32.

Lucas, J., Telch, M., & Bigler, E. (1991). Memory functioning in panic disorder: A neuropsychological perspective. *Journal of Anxiety Disorders, 5,* 1–20.

Malloy, P., Noel, N., Longabough, R., & Beattie, M. (1990). Determinants of neuropsychological impairment in antisocial substance abusers. *Addictive Behaviors, 15,* 431–438.

Manschreck, T. (1986). Motor abnormalities in schizophrenia. In H. Nasrallah & D. Weinberger (Eds.), *Handbook of schizophrenia: Vol. 1 The neurology of schizophrenia* (pp. 65–96). New York: Elsevier.

Manschreck, T., Keuthen, N., Schneyer, M., Celada, M., Laughery, J., & Collins, P. (1990). Abnormal involuntary movements and chronic schizophrenic disorders. *Biological Psychiatry, 27,* 150–158.

Marquart, P. (1935). Some signs of organic disorder in schizophrenia. *Archives of Neurology and Psychiatry, 34,* 280–288.

Marsden, C. (1982). Motor disorders in schizophrenia. *Psychological Medicine, 12,* 13–15.

Mather, J. A., & Putchat, C. (1984). Motor control of schizophrenics—II. Manual control and tracking: Sensory and motor deficits. *Journal of Psychiatric Research, 18,* 287–298.

May, J. V. (1931). The dementia praecox–schizophrenia problem. *American Journal of Psychiatry, 11,* 401–446.

McCann, J. (1991). Convergent and discriminant validity of the MCMI-II and MMPI personality disorder scales. *Psychological Assessment: A Journal of Consulting and Clinical Psychology, 3,* 9–18.

McCann, J., Flynn, P., & Gersh, D. (1992). MCMI-II diagnosis of borderline personality disorder: Base rates versus prototypic items. *Journal of Personality Assessment, 58,* 105–114.

McNeil, T., Harty, B., Blennow, G., & Cantor-Graae, E. (1993). Neuromotor deviation in offspring of psychotic mothers: A selective developmental deficiency in two groups of children at heightened psychiatric risk? *Journal of Psychiatric Research, 27,* 39–54.

Meehl, P. (1990). Toward an integrated theory of schizotaxia, schizotypy, and schizophrenia. *Journal of Personality Disorders, 4,* 1–99.

Meltzer, H. (1976). Neuromuscular dysfunction in schizophrenia. *Schizophrenia Bulletin, 2,* 106–135.

Meltzer, H. (1987). Biological studies in schizophrenia. *Schizophrenia Bulletin, 13,* 77–111.

Miller, M., Chapman, J., Chapman, L., & Collins, J. (1995). Task difficulty and cognitive deficits in schizophrenia. *Journal of Abnormal Psychology, 104,* 251–258.

Miller, H., Goldberg, J., & Streiner, D. (1993). The effects of the modifier and correction indices on MCMI-II profiles. *Journal of Personality Assessment, 60,* 477–485.

Millon, T., Green, C., & Meagher, R. (1979). The MBHI: A new inventory for the psychodiagnostician in medical settings. *Professional Psychology, 10,* 529–539.

Millon, T., Green, C., & Meagher, R. (1982). *Millon Behavioral Health Inventory manual* (3rd ed.). Minneapolis, MN: National Computer Systems.

Millon, T., Millon, C., & Davis, R. (1994). *Millon Clinical Multiaxial Inventory—III manual.* Minneapolis, MN: National Computer Systems.

Mittenberg, W., Azrin, R., Millsaps, C., & Heilbronner, R. (1993). Identification of malingered head injury on the Wechsler Memory Scale—Revised. *Psychological Assessment, 5,* 34–40.

Morey, L. (1991). *Personality Assessment Inventory: Professional manual.* Odessa, FL: Psychological Assessment Resources.

Morrison-Stewart, S., Williamson, P., Corning, W., Kutcher, S., Snow, W., & Merskey, H. (1992). Frontal and non-frontal lobe neuropsychological test performance and clinical symptomatology in schizophrenia. *Psychological Medicine, 22,* 353–359.

Moses, J., Jr. (1984). The effect of presence or absence of neuroleptic medication treatment on Luria–Nebraska neuropsychological battery performance in a schizophrenic population. *The International Journal of Clinical Neuropsychology, 6,* 249–251.

Moses, J., Jr., & Maruish, M. (1988). A critical review of the Luria–Nebraska Neuropsychological Battery literature: IV. Cognitive deficit in schizophrenia and related disorders. *International Journal of Clinical Neuropsychology, 10,* 51–62.

Murphy, K., & Davidshofer, C. (1994). *Psychological testing: Principles and applications* (3rd ed.). Englewood Cliffs, NJ: Prentice-Hall.

Murray, R., O'Callaghan, E., Castle, D., & Lewis, S. (1992). A neurodevelopmental approach to the classification of schizophrenia. *Schizophrenia Bulletin, 18,* 319–332.

Nasrallah, H. (1993). Neurodevelopmental pathogenesis of schizophrenia. *Psychiatric Clinics of North America, 16,* 269–280.

Newman, P., & Sweet, J. (1986). The effects of clinical depression on the Luria–Nebraska Neuropsychological Battery. *International Journal of Clinical Neuropsychology, 7,* 109–114.

Newman, P., & Sweet, J. (1992). Depressive disorders. In A. Puente & R. McCaffrey (Eds.), *Handbook of neuropsychological assessment: A biopsychosocial perspective* (pp. 263–307). New York: Plenum Press.

Nies, K., & Sweet, J. (1994). Neuropsychological assessment and malingering: A critical review of past and present strategies. *Archives of Clinical Neuropsychology, 9,* 501–552.

Nuechterlein, K. (1987). Vulnerability models for schizophrenia: State of the art. In H. Hafner, W. F. Gattaz, & W. Janzarik (Eds.), *Search for the causes of schizophrenia* (pp. 297–316). Berlin: Springer-Verlag.

Nuechterlein, K., & Dawson, M. (1984). Information processing and attentional functioning in the developmental course of schizophrenic disorders. *Schizophrenia Bulletin, 10,* 160–203.

Otto, M. (1992). Normal and abnormal information processing: A neuropsychological perspective on obsessive–compulsive disorder. *Psychiatric Clinics of North America, 15,* 825–848.

Owens, D., Johnstone, E., & Frith, C. (1982). Spontaneous involuntary disorders of movement: Their prevalence, severity, and distribution in chronic schizophrenics with and without treatment with neuroleptics. *Archives of General Psychiatry, 39,* 452–461.

Piersma, H. (1991). The MCMI-II depression scales: Do they assist in the differential prediction of depressive disorders? *Journal of Personality Assessment, 56,* 478–486.

Prescott, C., & Gottesman, I. (1993). Genetically mediated vulnerability to schizophrenia. *Psychiatric Clinics of North America, 16,* 245–267.

Puente, A., Rodenbough, J., & Orrell. T. (1993). Neuropsychological differentiation of chronic schizophrenia. *International Journal of Neuroscience, 82,* 193–200.

Purish, A., Golden, C., & Hammeke, T. (1978). Discrimination of schizophrenic and brain injured patients by a standardized version of Luria's neuropsychological test. *Journal of Consulting Clinical Psychology, 46,* 1266–1273.

Randolph, C., Goldberg, T., & Weinberger, D. (1993). The neuropsychology of schizophrenia. In K. Heilman & E. Valenstein (Eds.), *Clinical neuropsychology* (3rd ed., pp. 499–522). New York: Oxford Press.

Rasmussen, S., & Eisen, J. (1990). Epidemiology of obsessive compulsive disorder. *Journal of Clinical Psychiatry, 51,* 10–13.

Rawling, P., & Brooks, N. (1990). Simulation index: A method for detecting factitious errors on the WAIS-R and WMS. *Neuropsychology, 4,* 223–238.

Raz, S. (1993). Structural cerebral pathology in schizophrenia: Regional or diffuse? *Journal of Abnormal Psychology, 102,* 445–452.

Raz, S. (1994). Gross brain morphology in schizophrenia: A regional analysis of traditional diagnostic subtypes. *Journal of Consulting and Clinical Psychology, 62,* 640–644.

Raz, S., & Raz, N. (1990). Structural brain abnormalities in the major psychoses: A quantitative review of the evidence from computerized imaging. *Psychological Bulletin, 108,* 93–108.

Reiter, P. (1925). *Extrapyramidal motor-disturbances in dementia praecox.* Paper presented at the meeting of the Neurological Society, Copenhagen.

Retzlaff, P., Lorr, M., Hyer, L., & Ofman, P. (1991). An MCMI-II item-level component analysis: Personality and clinical factors. *Journal of Personality Assessment, 57,* 323–334.

Retzlaff, P., Ofman, P., Hyer, L., & Matheson, S. (1994). MCMI-II high point codes: Severe personality disorder and clinical syndrome extensions. *Journal of Clinical Psychology, 50,* 228–234.

Retzlaff, P., Sheehan, E., & Fiel, A. (1991). MCMI-II report style and bias: Profile and validity scales analyses. *Journal of Personality Assessment, 58,* 466–477.

Robinson, R., & Starkstein, S. (1990). Current research in affective disorders following stroke. *Journal of Neuropsychiatry and Clinical Neurosciences, 2,* 1–14.

Rogers, R., Bagby, M., & Dickens, S. (1992). *Structured interview of reported symptoms professional manual.* Odessa, FL: Psychological Assessment Resources.

Rogers, R., Ornduff, S., & Sewell, K. (1993). Feigning specific disorders: A study of the Personality Assessment Inventory (PAI). *Journal of Personality Assessment, 60,* 554–560.

Rosen, A., Lockhart, J., Gants, E., & Westergaard, C. K. (1991). Maintenance of grip-induced muscle tension: A behavioral marker of schizophrenia. *Journal of Abnormal psychology, 100,* 583–593.

Rossi, A., Galderisi, S., Di Michele, V., Stratta, P., Ceccoli, S., Maj, M., & Casacchia, M. (1990). Dementia in schizophrenia: Magnetic resonance and clinical correlates. *The Journal of Nervous and Mental Disease, 178,* 521–524.

Rosofsky, L., Levin, S., & Holzman, P. (1982). Psychomotility in the functional psychoses. *Journal of Abnormal Psychology, 91,* 71–74.

Rothke, S., Friedman, A., Dahlstrom, W., Greene, R., Arredondo, R., & Mann, A. (1994). MMPI-2 Normative data for the F-K Index: Implications for clinical. neuropsychological, and forensic practice. *Assessment, 1,* 1–15.

Roxborough, H., Muir, W., Blackwood, D., Walker, M., & Blackburn, I. (1993). Neuropsychological and P300 abnormalities in schizophrenics and their relatives. *Psychological Medicine, 23,* 305–314.

Rozensky, Sweet, & Tovian, (1997). *Psychological Assessment in Medical Settings.* New York: Plenum Press.

Saykin, A., Gur, R. C., Gur, R. E., Mozley, P., Mozley, L., Resnick, S., Kester, D., & Stafiniak, P. (1991). Neuropsychological function in schizophrenia: Selective impairment in memory and learning. *Archives of General Psychiatry, 4,* 618–624.

Saykin, A., Shtasel, D., Gur, R. E., Kester, D., Mozley, L., Stafiniak, P., & Gur, R. C. (1994). Neuropsychological deficits in neuroleptic naive patients with first-episode schizophrenia. *Archives of General Psychiatry, 51,* 124–131.

Schaffer, C., Davidson, R., & Saron, C. (1983). Frontal and parietal electroencephalogram asymmetry in depressed and nondepressed subjects. *Biological Psychiatry, 18,* 753–762.

Schneider, R., & Grossi, V. (1979). Differences in muscle activity before, during, and after responding in a simple reaction time task: Schizophrenics vs. normals. *Psychiatry Research, 1,* 141–145.

Schwartz, F., Carr, A., Munich, R., Bartuch, E., Lesser, B., Rescigno, D., & Viegener, B. (1990). Voluntary motor performance in psychotic disorders: A replication study. *Psychological Reports, 66,* 1223–1234.

Schwartz, F., Carr, A., Munich, R., Glauber, S., Lesser, B., & Murray, J. (1989). Reaction time impairment in schizophrenia and affective illnesses: The role of attention. *Biological Psychiatry, 25,* 540–548.

Schwartz, J., Martin, K., & Baxter, L. (1992). Neuroimaging and cognitive–behavioral self-treatment for obsessive compulsive disorder: Practical and philosophical considerations. In I. Hand, W. Goodman, & U. Evers (Eds.), *Obsessive–compulsive disorders: New research results* (pp. 82–101) New York: Springer-Verlag.

Seeman, P., & Niznik, H. (1990). Dopamine receptors and transporters in Parkinson's disease and schizophrenia. *The FASEB Journal, 4,* 2737–2744.

Seeman, P., Ulpian, C., Bergeron, C., Riederer, P., Jellinger, K., Gabriel, E., Reynolds, G., & Tourtellote, W. (1984). Biomodal distribution of dopamine receptor densities in brains of schizophrenics. *Science, 225,* 728–731.

Seidman, L., Cassens, G., Kremen, W., & Pepple, J. (1992). Neuropsychology of schizophrenia. In R. F. White (Ed.), *Clinical syndromes in adult neuropsychology: The practitioner's handbook* (pp. 381–449). New York: Elsevier.

Seidman, L., Yurgelun-Todd, D., Kremen, W., Woods, B., Goldstein, J., Faraone, S., & Tsuang, M. (1994). Relationship of prefrontal and temporal lobe MRI measures to neuropsychological performance in chronic schizophrenia. *Biological Psychiatry, 35,* 235–246.

Sharif, Z., Gewirtz, G., & Iqbal, N. (1993). Brain imaging in schizophrenia: A review. *Psychiatric Annals, 23,* 123–134.

Soldz, S., Budman, S., Demby, A., & Merry J. (1993). Diagnostic agreement between the Personality Disorder Examination and the MCMI-II. *Journal of Personality Assessment, 60,* 486–499.

Southard, E. (1919). On the focality of microscopic brain lesions found in dementia praecox. *Archives of Neurology and Psychiatry, 1,* 172–192.

Spielberger, C. (1983). *Manual for the State–Trait Anxiety Inventory.* Palo Alto, CA: Consulting Psychologists Press.

Spielberger, C. (1988). *State–Trait Anger Expression Inventory professional manual.* Odessa, FL: Psychological Assessment Resources.

Spitzer, R., Williams, J., Gibbon, M., & First, M. (1990). *Structured clinical interview for DSM-III-R user's guide.* Washington, DC: American Psychiatric Press.

Starkstein, S., & Robinson, R. (1988). Lateralized emotional response following stroke. In M. Kinsbourne (Ed.), *Cerebral hemisphere function in depression* (pp. 25–47.). Washington, DC: American Psychiatric Press.

Stein, D., Hollander, E., Cohen, L., Frenkel, M., Saoud, J., DeCaria, C., Aronowitz, B., Levin, A., Liebowitz, M., & Cohen, L. (1993). Neuropsychiatric impairment in impulsive personality disorders. *Psychiatry Research, 48,* 257–266.

Stevens, J. R. (1992) Abnormal reinnervation as a basis for schizophrenia: A hypothesis. *Archives of General Psychiatry, 49,* 238–243.

Strack, S. (1991). Factor analysis of MCMI-II and PACL basic personality scales in a college sample. *Journal of Personality Assessment, 57,* 345–355.

Strack, S., Lorr, M., Campbell, L., & Lamnin, A. (1992). Personality disorder and clinical syndrome factors of MCMI-II scales. *Journal of Personality Disorders, 6,* 40–52.

Strauss, J., & Ryan, R. (1988). Cognitive dysfunction in eating disorders. *International Journal of Eating Disorders, 7,* 19–28.

Strauss, M. (1993). Relations of symptoms to cognitive deficits in schizophrenia. *Schizophrenia Bulletin, 19,* 215–231.

Streiner, D., Goldberg, J., & Miller, H. (1993). MCMI-II item weights: Their lack of effectiveness. *Journal of Personality Disorders, 60,* 471–476.

Streiner, D., & Miller, H. (1989). The MCMI-II: How much better than the MCMI? *Journal of Personality Assessment, 53,* 81–84.

Sweeney, J., Haas, G., & Clementz, B. (1993). Schizophrenia: Etiology. In A. Bellack & M. Hersen (Eds.), *Psychopathology in adulthood* (pp. 195–215). Boston: Allyn and Bacon.

Sweet, J. (1991). Psychological evaluation and testing services in medical settings. In J. Sweet, R. Rozensky, & S. Tovian (Eds.), *Handbook of clinical psychology in medical settings* (pp. 291–313). New York: Plenum Press.

Sweet, J. (1997). Neuropsychological assessment in rehabilitation, neurology, and psychiatry. In R. Rozensky, J. Sweet, & S. Tovian (Eds.), *Psychological assessment in medical settings.* New York: Plenum Press.

Sweet, J., Breuer, S., Hazelwood, L., Toye, R., & Pawl, R. (1985). The Millon Behavioral Health Inventory: Concurrent and predictive validity in a pain treatment center. *Journal of Behavioral Medicine, 8,* 215–226.

Sweet, J., & Moberg, P. (1990). A survey of practices and beliefs among ABPP and non-ABPP clinical neuropsychologists. *The Clinical Neuropsychologist, 4,* 101–120.

Sweet, J., Moberg, P., & Westergaard, C. (1996). Five year follow-up survey of practices and beliefs of clinical neuropsychologists. *The Clinical Neuropsychologist, 10,* 202–221.

Sweet, J., Newman, P., & Bell, B. (1992). Significance of depression in clinical neuropsychological assessment. *Clinical Psychology Review, 12,* 21–45.

Tenhula, W., & Sweet, J. (1996). Double-cross validation of the Booklet Category Test in detecting malingered traumatic brain injury. *The Clinical Neuropsychologist, 10,* 104–116.

Touyz, S., Beumont, P., & Johnstone, L. (1986). Neuropsychological correlates of dieting disorders. *International Journal of Eating Disorders, 5,* 1025–1034.

Tucker, D. (1988). Neuropsychological mechanisms of affective self-regulation. In M. Kinsbourne (Ed.), *Cerebral hemisphere dysfunction in depression* (pp. 101–131). Washington, DC: American Psychiatric Press.

Turner, T. (1989). Rich and mad in Victorian England. *Psychological Medicine, 19,* 29–44.

Vaughn C., & Leff, J. (1976). The measurement of expressed emotion in the families of psychiatric patients. *British Journal of Social & Clinical Psychology, 15,* 157–165.

Verdoux, H., Magnin, E., & Bourgeois, M. (1995). Neuroleptic effects on neuropsychological test performance in schizophrenia. *Schizophrenia Research, 14,* 133–139.

Vrtunski, P., Simpson, D., & Meltzer, H. (1989). Voluntary movement dysfunction in schizophrenics. *Biological Psychiatry, 25,* 529–539.

Waddington, J., & Crow, T. (1988). Abnormal involuntary movements and psychosis in the pre-neuroleptic era and in unmedicated patients: Implications for the concept of tardive dyskinesia. In M. E. Wolf & A. D. Mosnaim (Eds.), *Tardive dyskinesia: Biological mechanisms and clinical aspects.* (pp. 51–66). Washington, DC: American Psychiatric Press.

Waddington, J., & Youssef, H. (1990). The lifetime outcome and involuntary movements of schizophrenia never treated with neuroleptic drugs: Four rare cases in Ireland. *British Journal of Psychiatry, 156,* 106–108.

Walker, E. (1994). Developmentally moderated expressions of the neuropathology underlying schizophrenia. *Schizophrenia Bulletin, 20,* 453–480.

Walker, E., Savoie, T., & Davis, D. (1994). Neuromotor precursors of schizophrenia. *Schizophrenia Bulletin, 20,* 441–451.

Walker, E., & Shaye, J. (1982). Familial schizophrenia: A predictor of neuromotor and attentional abnormalities in schizophrenia. *Archives of General Psychiatry, 39,* 1153–1156.

Walsh, W., & Betz, N. (1990). *Tests and measurements* (2nd ed.). Englewood Cliffs, NJ: Prentice-Hall.

Warren, W. (1994). *Revised Hamilton Rating Scale for Depression manual.* Los Angeles: Western Psychological Services.

Weinberger, D. (1987). Implications of normal brain development for the pathogenesis of schizophrenia. *Archives of General Psychiatry, 4,* 660–669.

Weinberger, D., Berman, K., & Illowsky, B. (1988). Physiological dysfunction of dorsolateral prefrontal cortex in schizophrenia. *Archives of General Psychiatry, 45,* 609–615.

Weinberger, D., Berman, K., & Zec, R. (1986). Physiological dysfunction of dorsolateral prefrontal cortex in schizophrenia: I. Regional cerebral blood flow evidence. *Archives of General Psychiatry, 43,* 114–124.

Westergaard, C. K. (1994). *Maintenance of grip induced muscle tension: Understanding a motor dysfunction in schizophrenia.* Unpublished doctoral dissertation, University of Illinois at Chicago.

White, W. (1921). Some considerations bearing on the diagnosis and treatment of dementia praecox. *American Journal of Psychiatry, 1,* 191–198.

Wilcoxson, M., Zook, A., & Zarski, J. (1988). Predicting behavioral outcomes with two psychological assessment methods in a outpatient pain management program. *Psychology and Health, 2,* 319–333.

Wolkin, A., Sanfilipo, M., Wolf, A., Angrist, B., Brodie, J., & Rotrosen, J. (1992). Negative symptoms and hypofrontality in chronic schizophrenia. *Archives of General Psychiatry, 49,* 959–965.

Wyatt, R. J. (1986). The dopamine hypothesis: Variations on a theme. *Psychopharmacology Bulletin, 22,* 923–927.

Wyatt, R. J. (1991). Neuroleptics and the natural course of schizophrenia. *Schizophrenia Bulletin, 17,* 325–351.

Young, D., Davila, R., & Scher, H. (1993). Unawareness of illness and neuropsychological performance in chronic schizophrenia, *Schizophrenia Research, 10,* 117–124.

Zielinski, C., Taylor, M., & Juzwin, K. (1991). Neuropsychological deficits in obsessive compulsive disorder. *Neuropsychiatry, Neuropsychology, & Behavioral Neurology, 4,* 110–126.

Zubin, J. (1988). Chronicity versus vulnerability. In H. A. Nasrallah (Ed.), *Handbook of schizophrenia: Vol 3. Nosology, epidemiology, and genetics of schizophrenia.* New York: Elsevier.

Zuckerman, M., & Lubin, B. (1985). *Manual for the Multiple Affect Adjective Check List—Revised.* San Diego, CA: Educational and Industrial Testing Service.

11

Computer Applications in Neuropsychological Assessment

ROBERT L. KANE AND GARY G. KAY

The microcomputer has opened up a potential new era in neuropsychological assessment. The clinical use of computerized assessment is still in its early stages, and current hardware and software do not address all needs of clinicians and patients. Nevertheless, the potential contribution of the computer to neuropsychological assessment is large and the continued development of these procedures is inevitable.

In this chapter, we focus on the clinical use of computerized tests and batteries. First, we discuss general advantages and limitations of this form of assessment. Second, we review issues specific to computerized assessment that clinicians and test publishers should appreciate in using and developing these instruments. Third, we present a brief review of available tests and batteries. This review is not intended to be comprehensive. From available instruments, we have selected tests and batteries that: (1) are available from and supported by test authors or publishers; (2) have a current or developing normative base; (3) have been used in clinical settings or in published clinical research; and (4) are not simply automated adaptations of frequently used clinical or laboratory procedures. While such adaptations can be useful and valuable, our purpose is to acquaint the reader with tests and batteries specifically developed for the microcomputer with which they may be less familiar. Fourth, we close with a discussion of future needs and directions in computerized assessment.

ROBERT L. KANE • Baltimore Department of Veterans Affairs Medical Center, Baltimore, Maryland 21201   GARY G. KAY • Department of Neurology, Georgetown University Hospital, Washington, DC 20007

ADVANTAGES AND CAVEATS OF COMPUTERIZED ASSESSMENT

Advantages of Computerized Assessment

Computerized testing offers many advantages over conventional neuropsychological testing with respect to test administration, response monitoring, and scoring. The computer is able to provide precise control over the presentation of test stimuli. In a computerized test, software controls the visual and auditory stimulus characteristics. These include stimulus intensity, frequency, location, and color. The software also controls the order of stimuli. Specifically, programs can employ fixed sequences of test stimuli, completely randomized stimuli, or non-fixed sequences that are contingent on a subject's performance. Programs can adaptively control the order, number, presentation rate, and/or complexity of items. The computer is also capable of controlling contrast intensity. There is also the option of presenting degraded auditory and visual stimuli. Many of these stimulus control advantages simply cannot be achieved by conventional testing.

The exact timing that is provided by computerization impacts stimulus presentation as well as the scoring and recording of the examinee's behavior. Computer programs are capable of presenting stimuli for very specific durations, of controlling the intervals between test stimuli, of defining the intervals during which an examinee can respond, and of controlling the total time of a test. At the same time that the computer is controlling the presentation of test stimuli, it can simultaneously record the time of each aspect of a subject's response. This gives the psychologist the capability of measuring a number of separate elements of behavior, including response latency, the time required to complete a response, and the variability of response times within and between tasks.

This ability to measure "process" dimensions of a subject's response was one of the first benefits of computerization to be described in the literature. Elithorn developed a version of the Perceptual Maze Test for the PDP-8, a popular mini-computer two decades ago. The Perceptual Maze Test is a measure of cognitive style and executive functions. Elithorn used this test to study a group of patients with Parkinson's disease (Elithorn, Lunzer & Weinman, 1975). He found that the computer allowed him to measure separately the time that subjects spent preparing their response (i.e., latency to response), the time spent responding to each step of the test, and the time spent checking or verifying the response. He reported that the response initiation time was the best marker of Parkinson's disease and was also the most sensitive indicator of successful treatment with L-dopa.

In conventional neuropsychological testing, many of the most sensitive test indices are obtained by measuring the time taken to complete a test (e.g., the Trail Making Tests, the time scores on the Tactual Performance Test, and the Finger Tapping Test). A number of the other tests considered highly sensitive to brain dysfunction are presented for a fixed amount of time. For these measures, the test is scored by counting the number of items correctly completed during a set time interval (e.g., Seashore Rhythm Test, Paced Auditory Serial Addition Test, and digit substitution tests). A quick review of neuropsychological measures will show that speed scores are among the most sensitive indices in neuropsychology. However, because of timing limitations inherent in the human test administrator, we are generally not able to record such things as the response intervals between individual items on a test or the variability of response speed.

There are relatively few neuropsychological tests that present items at a fixed rate. Some notable exceptions are the Paced Auditory Serial Addition Test (PASAT), various adaptations of continuous performance tests (CPTs), and the Continuous Visual Memory Test (CVMT). The PASAT is one of the only tests where the rate of item presentation is varied in order to study the examinee's information-processing speed. It is also a sensitive test of brain dysfunction and one of the best predictors of recovery following head trauma (Gronwall, 1977).

Computer-based tests can present items in either a subject-paced or a computer-paced mode. For example, on a visual matching to sample test, the pattern to be remembered by the examinee can be presented for a fixed period of time (i.e., computer paced) or it can be presented for as long as the subject desires to have it shown (i.e., subject paced). In the latter case, subjects can be instructed to press a key when they feel they can remember the visual stimulus. On subject-paced tests, response accuracy is generally very high, if the items are of reasonable difficulty. In contrast, on computer-paced tests, response accuracy can be quite variable and reflects the examinees' processing speed and tendency to "trade speed for accuracy" or vice versa.

In contrast to the computer, the human test examiner is very limited in administering tests that require divided attention or the simultaneous performance of more than one task. Even for testing simple or choice reaction time, a stopwatch is inadequate. The inadequacy of the stopwatch is compounded in the case of tests that involve divided attention or multitasking. These tests require the subject to simultaneously perform two (or more) different tasks at the same time (e.g., tracking and working memory). Computers, unlike humans with stopwatches, are very well suited for presenting simultaneous tasks and for simultaneously measuring response characteristics on two or more tasks. The ability of the computer to assess divided attention is probably one of the most significant contributions of computer-based testing to the assessment process.

Measures of divided attention or multitasking are known to be especially sensitive to subtle brain dysfunction. Furthermore, these measures provide the practitioner with the ability to assess a domain of attention and executive functioning that, prior to the advent of computerized testing, was neglected. This is in spite of the relevance of these skill to everyday life and to many job settings. For example, studies of pilot performance derived from analysis of flight data recorders have shown that tests of multitasking proficiency are highly correlated with pilot performance (Kay, 1994).

Computers are also especially well suited for repeated testing in both clinical and research settings. Neuropsychologists frequently encounter patients who are referred for "follow-up testing." The follow-up evaluation is generally requested to help the treating physician gauge the patient's response to surgical or medical treatment or the progression of disease. Follow-up testing is especially important in cases where the medical treatment is highly toxic and/or is associated with a significant risk of morbidity. Another group of patients who require reevaluation are individuals who are referred for assessment of their fitness to return to cognitively demanding occupations, such as flying airplanes. Also, for those psychologists who perform forensic evaluations, there is frequently a need to retest individuals who are undergoing an "independent neuropsychological examination." In addition to these clinical and forensic applications, repeated testing is often required in research studies of environmental agents, drug effects, or other treatment effects.

Unfortunately, most of our conventional tests were not designed for readministration. These tests tend to show substantial practice effects that markedly diminish their sensitivity to changes in brain functioning and render them less effective tools for monitoring changes in performance.

In contrast, the computer can actually generate multiple forms of a test. This is important not only in producing parallel forms, but also in generating a stable baseline against which to evaluate change. Algorithms can specify the nature and form of the test stimuli. Computer programs typically use the "session number" as a "seed" number in the equation that generates the test items. This method assures that all subjects taking session 1 will be administered the same items, and likewise, that all subjects taking session 2 will receive the same items but different from those administered in session 1. These techniques ensure that examinee's will not be administered the same items across different sessions. For those tests where the computer can not generate the test items (e.g., word lists), software programs typically are designed to select from among different groups of stored test items, again based on the session number. For example, CogScreen-Aeromedical Edition contains 12 "forms." In the entire battery, only two tests have "stored" items. The items for the other tests are automatically generated by the program. This approach to alternate-form production has been shown to be a highly sensitive method of monitoring changes in performance resulting from disease, recovery of function, treatment effects, or responses to various stressors. This is especially important since an increasing number of referrals are oriented toward questions related to the progression of neurocognitive changes occurring over time. Traditional test instruments were not designed for this type of application.

This feature of repeatability has led to the inclusion of computerized tests in specialized clinical applications that require that test batteries be repeated following very short time intervals. For example, at Georgetown University Medical Center, the neurocognitive functioning of patients undergoing embolization of pathological arteries in the brain is monitored by repeatedly testing lateralized brain functions (i.e., a letter sequence comparison test and a spatial rotation test) while the vessel is being occluded. A similar procedure is followed in cases where the internal carotid artery is occluded by the temporary inflation of a balloon at the end of a catheter inserted into the artery (Spector, Kay, Geyer, Deveikas & Sullivan, 1991).

In addition to being a skillful test administrator, the computer is a superb accountant. The computer is capable of scoring and recording the accuracy and speed of each and every response. At the completion of a test, the program can calculate the relevant statistics for the test and then report the results in a variety of different formats. The computer's accuracy in recording and scoring the examinee's responses cannot be matched by the human test administrator.

The output from computerized tests is easily incorporated into most spreadsheet and database programs. This greatly facilitates research and further statistical analysis. Data can be readily stored for future research studies. The improved standardization of test administration, subject–examinee interaction, and scoring also facilitate neuropsychological research and the combining of data obtained at different research sites.

Many of the potential benefits of computerized assessment have yet to be realized. The popularity and decreasing price of CD-ROM devices make it likely that this technology will be used in the near future for automated assessment. CD-ROM technology will allow for true multimedia presentation of test stimuli and will permit simulation of a wide range of environments. Current sound technology and CDs also allow for presentation of sophisticated verbal and other auditory test items. Auditory instructions can be presented to the subject as if read by an examiner, which will hopefully avoid problems caused by examinees' failing to read instructions. The potential of virtual reality to expand the domain of neurocognitive testing, presently a gleam in the examiner's eye, has revolutionary implications.

In these days of shrinking health care dollars and rapidly shrinking reimbursement for all kinds of psychological testing services, computerized testing may offer an efficient and cost-effective solution. Multiple patients can be tested simultaneously, and there is likely to be a decreased need for examiners. For example, in a study recently conducted for a pharmaceutical company under the direction of Georgetown University, 58 subjects were simultaneously administered a 75-minute computerized cognitive test battery. Another advantage of computerized testing is that the clinician can perform other activities while the patient is completing the test.

The computer is not only free from examiner bias and halo effects, it continues to administer tests exactly according to standardization procedures without looking for abbreviations or short forms. These improvements in standardization allow for easier comparison of data obtained from different sites and by different examiners.

Caveats and Limitations

In spite of the compelling features and advantages of computerized testing, this type of assessment has its limitations and drawbacks. Among the most serious deficiencies of some existing test software has been the use of inaccurate timing procedures, the use of poorly designed human–computer interfaces, the lack of usable reports and data sets, and the failure to meet established testing standards (American Psychological Association, 1986). Even for well-designed and innovative programs with accurate timing, at present the computer has only limited capability for assessing expressive language skills. Although the computer is capable of providing verbal instructions and can even record the human voice, the technology for voice recognition, handwriting recognition and analysis, and natural language comprehension is not yet sufficiently sophisticated to allow for testing of visual confrontation naming, expressive speech, oral reading, or repetition. In short, many clinicians are sensitive to the fact that the computer is not yet capable of assessing all aspects of neurocognitive functioning that may be both clinically and theoretically relevant.

Another drawback of computerized testing is that it may result in a reduction in the amount of interaction taking place between the examiner and the examinee. A skilled examiner is often capable of coaxing the examinee to complete testing and to stay motivated. The skilled examiner also knows when the subject is ignoring or only partially reading test instructions. Furthermore, unlike the human test administrator, the computer is deficient in the sincere expression of compliments, criticisms, and encouraging comments.

A number of the drawbacks of computerized testing are the result of poorly designed applications rather than problems with the technology per se. Subjects may fail to read instructions if they are poorly written. Some programs use the computer as a high-tech workbook or automated slide projector. This noninnovative use of computer technology, while useful in some ways, demonstrates a lack of creativity and understanding of computers.

In addition to our list of drawbacks and limitations, clinicians frequently identify cost as a significant drawback of computerized testing. They also express reservations about *the computer.* Although clinicians have become familiar with word-processing and financial packages, there are many clinicians who have at least a mild degree of computer phobia.

A serious but rarely mentioned drawback of computerized testing is the ease with which this technology could be exploited by naive or unscrupulous individuals to provide incomplete or unnecessary neuropsychological evaluations. Clinicians who fail to take the time to carefully evaluate the reliability and validity of the computerized tests that they employ are especially likely to misuse this technology. Since the computer can function as tester, it is vulnerable to unethical misuse by individuals without sufficient training to provide thoughtful and appropriate neuropsychological evaluations.

SPECIAL ISSUES IN COMPUTERIZED ASSESSMENT

Basic test development principles relating to standardizations, reliability, and validity apply to all tests, traditional or computerized. In addition, a number of other factors must be addressed in the development and evaluation of computerized neuropsychological instruments. These issues include: (1) the method by which the patient interacts with the computer; (2) the procedures used for stimulus and response timing; (3) the effects of different displays on the appearance of test stimuli; (4) the impact of prior computer experience on test performance; and (5) the patient's acceptance of the computer as a test platform (Kane & Kay, 1992).

Contrary to the initial fears of some examiners, experience has taught that patients appear to accept computers. While previous computer experience may influence test results, the effect of prior experience can be made manageable by interfacing the subject with the computer in ways that are simplified and intuitive. In general, it is advisable to bypass the keyboard as an input device when possible. Tests employing the keyboard as a response device generally attempt to limit the subject to pressing a limited number of select keys when making responses.

Computers are popularly regarded as devices that process information both rapidly and accurately. Consequently, individuals not familiar with technical aspects of computer operations fail to appreciate the difficulties of obtaining accurate stimulus and response timing with computers. Timing at the millisecond level is difficult to accomplish with computers, despite their speed. This is true of programs written for the Macintosh and for those running under DOS. It is especially true for programs running under Windows. Fortunately, there are ways around timing problems. In the early stages of computerized testing, precise timing was obtained using timers on add-in boards that were plugged into the computer. By writing the program to use the add-in card timer, test authors were able to obtain precise control over stimulus presentation and to more accurately measure response speed. The disadvantages to this method were that some boards were expensive, companies producing these boards would occasionally go out of business, and add-in boards did not solve the problem of test administration using portable or notebook computers. Within the last several years, software developers have implemented special software timers to overcome the inherent timing problems with microcomputers. Software timers have permitted near-millisecond timing. With the implementation of software timers, impediments to accurate response timing are a function of the input devices employed for different measures. The use of the keyboard as a response device complicates timing. Timing accuracy is enhanced by using alternative response devices such as a mouse or newer lightpens. In essence, the user must be aware of the method of timing used by a test program, have an appreciation for the realistic limits that the method of timing imposes, and select measures appropriate for their clinical and research objectives.

In addition to technical issues related to event timing, the method by which the subject interacts with the computer can significantly affect test scores. Subjects vary in their experience with keyboards and numeric key pads. Lack of familiarity with these response devices can affect both response time and the stability of test scores with repeated test administration (Banderet et al., 1988). Response device characteristics and configurations can substantially impact the accuracy with which responses are measured (Kane & Kay, 1992). The most accurate way to interface a joystick with a computer is through the use of an analog-to-digital converter. Tests designed to assess fine motor movement but which attach the joystick to a game port sacrifice both sensitivity and accuracy. Further, with continued use there is significant deterioration in the performance of most joysticks.

The type of video display used to present stimuli may affect a subject's performance. Displays differ in resolution and contrast. A figure that appears circular on one screen may appear as an oval on another. Flat screen monitors produce less peripheral field distortion than curved monitors. Flat screens are preferable when stimuli are presented in the periphery. Display clarity has improved over the years with more advanced graphic standards. Software using earlier standards produced characters and figures with poorer resolution. With the continued advancement in graphics standards, accuracy of the display has become less of an issue.

All video monitors will introduce ± 14 to 20-millisecond error variance in reaction time measures. However, this problem can be controlled with appropriate programming techniques. Specifically, programs have to be written to disable the video, wait for retrace, enable the video, and then start or restart timing. This problem is more complicated when test software is run on earlier laptop and notebook computers using monochrome liquid crystal displays (LCD). The frame rates for these computer screens were seldom documented. It was not possible for test developers to synchronize timing precisely with the visual display of the stimulus. Inaccuracies in timing were also introduced by the character decay time of most inexpensive monochrome monitors. The on–off time of LCD elements introduce inaccuracies in response time measurements and prevent tachistoscopic presentations. Presently, when employing portable computers for testing, best results are achieved with color or fast phosphor monitors. Active matrix color displays, presently available on most notebook computers, are recommended for use if a portable system is employed for patient assessment (D. Thorne, personal communication, May 15, 1995). Clinicians and researchers should be cognizant of the fact that response time norms collected using high-resolution displays may not apply if an equivalent system is not used during data collection.

In addition to problems with subject familiarity, the use of the keyboard as a response device interjects additional problems in response timing. With the keyboard, subject responses are not recorded instantaneously. The computer registers keyboard responses by scanning each key, looking for input. When the computer's central processing unit (CPU) detects that a key has been pressed, it rescans for verification. The CPU also checks for other information that may affect its handling of the key press. For example, it checks to see if the "Caps-Lock" key is in the up or down position and if other keys, such as the shift or alternate key, have also been pressed. Keyboards differ with respect to their scan and check rates. Typically, these rates are undocumented, and test developers are not able to calculate the precise error rates associated with different keyboards. In addition, most manufacturers do not permit easy control over the auto-repeat function. This last point can be especially troublesome when testing patients with poor motor control or who hold keys down far longer than necessary.

Obtaining precise timing with computers is challenging, but it can be accomplished with proper attention to programming and the selection of input devices. In addition, it is important to keep the nature of the timing problem in perspective. A computer at its worst is a more accurate and reliable timekeeper than a psychologist holding a stopwatch in one hand and attempting to manipulate test stimuli with the other. Since not all computerized batteries produce the same level of timing accuracy, it is important for the neuropsychologist to know the limitations of available batteries and to select instruments appropriate for his or her clinical and research needs. For example, if the purpose is to screen for dementia in a lower-functioning patient, millisecond accuracy may be unnecessary. If a drug intervention is planned with such a patient, then it may be necessary to employ a test battery that provides both finer time resolution and the capacity for repeated measures.

COMPUTER TESTS AND BATTERIES: A SELECTIVE REVIEW

Some Early Test Batteries

Computerized assessment has varied roots. Its developers came from diverse but related traditions of clinical neuropsychology, toxicology, and performance assessment. There were early attempts to bring the computer into the clinic as an assessment tool. These will be discussed briefly under headings consistent with their original intent.

Clinical Batteries

One of the first automated neuropsychological batteries was the SAINT-II (Swiercinsky, 1984). The SAINT-II consisted of 10 computerized tests, many of which were based on Swiercinsky's experience with the Halstead–Reitan Battery. The SAINT-II assessed domains including spatial orientation, motor persistence, verbal and visual memory, visual search speed, vocabulary, sequencing, rhythm discrimination, numerical skill, and set shifting. The SAINT-II never achieved widespread use or substantially impacted clinical practice.

The Bexley–Maudsley was developed in England (Acker & Acker, 1982). It was intended to be a time-efficient and cost-effective way to screen alcoholics and other individuals who may suffer from mild brain impairment. The Bexley–Maudsley saw some limited use in the United States. Only a few research studies were published making use of this battery.

The Alzheimer's Disease Assessment Battery was designed for the assessment of dementia (Branconnier, 1986). It was developed for the Apple II computer with the patient and examiner making use of separate terminals. Branconnier (1986) reported initial data regarding the battery's sensitivity to dementia. However, the battery's development appears to have been limited and its reliance on older technology will undoubtedly affect its use for both clinical and research purposes.

The Sbordone–Hall Memory Battery (SHMB) became available (Sbordone, 1990) in the mid-1980s. It was designed specifically to bring the advantages of the computer to memory assessment and specifically to capture different facets of memory. The SHMB was a serious effort to make use of the computer to control stimulus presentation and to analyze various aspects of a subject's responses. However, it never saw wide clinical use.

Neurotoxicology Batteries

There also was an interest in automated assessment on the part of psychologists studying the effects of environmental toxins. The Neurobehavioral Evaluation System was one of the first standardized computer batteries designed for environmental hazards research (Baker et al., 1985). It was eventually translated into eight languages and has been administered to well over 5000 individuals (Letz, Mahoney, Hershman, Woskie & Smith, 1990).

The Microcomputer-Based Testing System (MTS) is an Apple II-based system developed in cooperation with the US Environmental Protection Agency (EPA) to assess basic cognitive skills (Eckerman et al., 1985). The battery uses a touch screen to provide an intuitive interface and an add-in clock to facilitate recording of reaction time. Initial data demonstrated that the MTS was sensitive to the toxic effects of alcohol and carbon monoxide (Eckerman et al., 1985)

Performance Assessment Batteries

The greatest boost to development of computerized assessment has came from the Department of Defense, which had a need to assess changes in performance in nonclinical populations resulting from personal or environmental stressors. Typically, the focus was on individuals functioning in high-demand occupations. Consequently, tests used to assess performance had to measure efficiency as well as accuracy and had to be designed so that subjects could be tested on multiple occasions. The specific demands of performance assessment both fostered and necessitated the development of computerized testing.

The Walter Reed Army Institute of Research Performance Assessment Battery (WRPAB) (Thorne, Genser, Sing, & Hegge, 1985) and the Navy's Performance Evaluation Tests for Environmental Research (PETER) Battery (Bittner, Carter, Kennedy, Harbeson, & Krause, 1986) were two of the earlier performance assessment batteries. The WRPAB was designed to assess performance changes in sustained/continuous performance paradigms, as well as the efficacy of countermeasures to inhibit performance degradation (Thorne et al., 1985). According to the test's author (Thorne et al., 1985), tasks were selected: (1) to represent samples of basic skills presumed to underlie real-world tasks; (2) for brevity and repeatability; (3) for their ability to be implemented on the computer; and (4) for their demonstrated or presumed sensitivity to physiological, psychological, or environmental variables. The original WRPAB contained 21 tests. It contained tests assessing various aspects of attention, working memory, spatial processing, grammatical reasoning, performance efficiency, and mood.

Although it was an early entry into the performance assessment arena, the WRPAB continues to be used worldwide. It is available through Dr. David Thorne at the Walter Reed Army Institute of Research. Additional tasks are presently being developed for inclusion into the WRPAB. The WRPAB also influenced the development of other computerized batteries to be discussed more fully in this chapter. Specifically, CogScreen—Aeromedical Edition and the Automated Neuropsychological Assessment Metrics trace their early origins to the WRPAB.

The initial work leading to the development of the PETER Battery began in 1977 (Bittner et al., 1986). The program began as a effort to identify traditional cognitive measures that were suitable for repeated administration. Over 150 tests were reviewed, and from these a subset of tests that stabilize quickly and appeared suitable for repeated administrations was selected. Subsequently, many of these tests were implemented on the computer, resulting in the automated version of PETER Battery (Irons & Rose, 1985). The PETER Battery did not see continued development within the Navy. However, a commercial version, the Automated Portable Test System (APTS) later became available through the Essex Corporation on a proprietary bases. The latest modification of the APTS, called Delta, is also available through the Essex Corporation.

Current Clinical Neuropsychological Test Batteries

CogScreen—Aeromedical Edition

The CogScreen—Aeromedical Edition (CogScreen-AE) (Kay, 1995) was the result of a Federal Aviation Administration (FAA) sponsored project to develop a test battery to detect changes in "cognitive function, which left unnoticed may result in poor pilot judgment or slow reaction time in critical operational situations" (Engelberg, Gibbons & Doege, 1986). A literature review of available test procedures was conducted along with a comparison study of various neuropsychological measures. The results of these investigations suggested that computer-based performance tests, in addition to their other advantages, had adequate levels of sensitivity and specificity to be used to screen for brain impairment (Kane & Kay, 1992). As a result of these initial investigations, the FAA sponsored the development of a relatively brief and fully automated cognitive screening examination. The resulting test battery, CogScreen-AE was developed to meet FAA specifications.

CogScreen-AE works with an IBM-compatible computer equipped with an 80286 (or later) microprocessor with a clock speed of 10 megahertz or faster. It employs sophisticated software timers and uses an intuitive lightpen interface. Subjects respond to all tasks using the lightpen except on the tracking component of the Dual-task Test, which also requires the use of the left and right arrow keys. Eleven tasks are included in the aeromedical edition of CogScreen. They include:

1. Backward Digit Span
2. Mental Arithmetic
3. A Number/Letter Sequence Comparison Test
4. A Symbol-Digit or Code Substitution Test (with Immediate and Delayed Paired Associate Recall)
5. Matching to Sample (Pattern Memory)
6. Manikin
7. Combined Visual Monitoring and Sequence Comparison
8. Auditory Sequence Comparison
9. Pathfinder (Analogue to Trail Making Tests)
10. A Shifting Attention Test
11. Dual Task (Combined Tracking and Previous Number)

All tasks begin with instructions and practice items. CogScreen-AE is a standardized battery with tasks presented in a fixed order. Alternate forms are produced by randomizing test items using the session number as a random number seed. Repeated administrations are unique, but each like-numbered session contains identical items. CogScreen tasks are scored for accuracy, mean response time, and throughput (computed score based on number of correct responses per minute). Scores are produced for each task, which include the mean response time, standard deviation of response time, the number of correct and incorrect responses, and lapses in responding. Accuracy, response time, and throughput scores are also presented graphically. CogScreen-AE exploits the advantages of the computer by including tests involving the simultaneous performance of two tasks. For these exercises, tasks are presented in both single and combined modes and separate scores are obtained for both the single and combined presentations.

CogScreen has been normed extensively on an aviator population (Kay, 1995). The United States aviator normative sample was based on 584 pilots. A Russian version of CogScreen was also developed. In an initial validation study employing an earlier version (phase B) of CogScreen, 40 pilots, 40 age- and IQ-matched nonpilot normals, and 40 age- and IQ-matched patients with mild brain dysfunction were administered the battery along with a group of traditional neuropsychological measures. The traditional measures included a partial Wechsler Adult Intelligence Scale—Revised (WAIS-R), the Paced Auditory Serial Addition Test, the Trail Making Test, and the Symbol Digit Modalities Test. Pilots and nonpilot normals performed significantly better than patients on 38 of the 50 dependent measures derived from CogScreen. Adopting a seven-variable cutoff rule, CogScreen was able to correctly classify 35 of 40 patients with brain dysfunction. Using this same rule, only four pilots were misclassified. Twenty of the 40 patients were correctly classified using the traditional neuropsychological measures employing the standard cutoff scores. Only two pilots were misclassified using these traditional tests.

The CogScreen-AE test manual (Kay, 1995) presents construct validity data derived from comparing scores obtained from the battery with those from traditional tests putatively assessing similar consructs. A number of CogScreen tests correlated in expected ways with related paper-and-pencil measures. At the same time, it was also apparent that CogScreen measures contributed unique variance and that they were not simply assessing psychometric intelligence.

Twenty-eight measures from 13 CogScreen-AE subtests were placed into a principal-components factor analysis with varimax rotation. This was an initial exploratory analysis that employed some overlapping measures. A nine-factor solution resulted. These factors were: (1) visual scanning and sequencing, (2) attribute identification, (3) visual perceptual and spatial processing, (4) motor coordination, (5) choice visual reaction time, (6) visual associative memory, (7) tracking, (8) working memory, and (9) numerical operations. The initial factor structure was derived from only a partial sample of American and Russian aviator data. This permitted the analysis to be repeated on a second independent aviator sample. This second analysis again produced a nine-factor solution as did a factor analysis limited to 475 US pilots. While the second factor analysis produced the same factors as the first, there was some alteration in the order in which factors were extracted.

CogScreen-AE is being employed in a number of biomedical research studies to track changes in cognitive functioning associated with eosinophilic myalgia syndrome, human immunodeficiency virus (HIV) infection, and head trauma rehabilitation. The battery is also being used in the United States and Russia to investigate the effects of antihypertension drugs on cognition under normal and hypoxic conditions.

During the normative processes, 120 pilots were also administered the WAIS-R and a modified Halstead–Reitan Battery. When Halstead and WAIS-R data were scored using the Heaton norms (Heaton, Grant, & Matthews, 1991), pilots on average scored within expected ranges. The pilots performed normally when compared to their age- and education-matched peers. This finding was noteworthy, and suggests that CogScreen-AE may be an appropriate screening instrument for individuals other than aviators, provided they are comparable to the normative groups in age and education.

At present, extant norms area being augmented by additional samples of normal pilots and nonpilot normals. Data on pathological groups are being collected from a variety of sources. These sources are from pilots undergoing fitness evaluations, from patients enrolled in a head injury rehabilitation program, from a longitudinal study of patients with HIV infection, and from patients recovering from alcoholism.

CogScreen-AE is available through Psychological Assessment Resources. At this writing, an expanded version of the test battery is under development and will be called CogScreen—Investigators Toolkit (IT). CogScreen-IT is being designed as a flexible shell that will incorporate a number of computerized tests. Initially, it will run the standard CogScreen menu, the Nonverbal Selective Reminding Test, and tests from the Automated Neuropsychological Assessment Metrics system to be discussed later in this chapter. The shell will permit the addition of new tests as they are developed and will allow investigators to modify test parameters.

MicroCog

MicroCog is published by the Psychological Corporation (Powell et al., 1993). Initially, the battery was named the Assessment of Cognitive Skills (ACS) and was funded through the Risk Management Foundation of the Harvard Medical Institutions (Powell et al., 1993). The ACS was designed to assess cognitive status changes that might impede job performance in physicians and other professionals. It was targeted to assess individuals over the age of 65. Later in its development, the ACS was renamed MicroCog and normed as a general neurocognitive screening instrument.

MicroCog runs on MS-DOS-compatible computers. It uses the computer's keyboard as its subject interface. To simplify the task of responding, subjects respond by pressing the 0–9 keys on the numeric key pad, the <enter> key, and the <backspace> key. MicroCog begins by presenting subjects with a brief introduction to the keyboard, specifically reviewing the keys that will be used during testing. While MicroCog suffers the inherent limitations that come from using the keyboard as the subject interface, the test appears manageable for the majority of patients likely to be seen for screening in clinical settings.

There is both a short and long form of MicroCog. Tasks found in the battery are listed below. Asterisks indicate tasks included in the short form.

1. Timers 1 & 2* (simple reaction time)
   This test is presented both at the beginning and the end of the test battery, except in the short form during which it is given only once.
2. Address* (memory for a name and address—initial learning phase)
3. Clocks* (telling time: multiple choice)

4. Story 1,* with immediate recall
5. Math* (arithmetic computation)
6. Tic Tac (visual working memory)
7. Analogies* (verbal)
8. Numbers Forward* (forward visual digit span)
9. Story 2,* with immediate recall
10. Wordlist 1* (selection by category)
    Wordlist 2* (list recognition—incidental memory)
11. Numbers Backwards (backward visual digit span)
12. Address* (delayed recognition of name and address)
13. Object Match (abstract reasoning using visual stimuli)
14. Story 1* (delayed recognition)
15. Alphabet (continuous performance test)
16. Tic Tac 2 (visual working memory)
    Same task as Tic Tac 1, but with different items.
17. Story 2* (delayed recognition)

Each MicroCog test is preceded by an instruction screen. Administration time is usually 60 minutes for the long form and 30 minutes for the short form. Tests are presented in a fixed order with fixed parameters. MicroCog employs a fixed-item set and has no alternate forms. The method of response timing improved with the batteries' continued development. Timing on the original ACS was imprecise and was accomplished by software calls to the system clock. MicroCog now uses more sophisticated software timing. Nevertheless, some inaccuracies in timing will result, since the keyboard is used as the input device, as was noted in the earlier discussion on timing in this chapter. MicroCog norm tables were developed from data using both versions of the battery: the original (ACS) and the newer version with software timers. Of the 810 subjects used in the standardization, 500 were tested using the ACS with the old timers and 310 using the newer version of the program with the more accurate timers.

MicroCog yields both accuracy and response proficiency scores for each of its subtests. The proficiency score is computed to reflect both response latency and accuracy. The longer the latency of a correct response, the less response time contributes to the proficiency score. Hence, the proficiency score is a weighted score.

MicroCog also combines subtests into five performance dimensions including: attention/mental control, memory, reasoning/calculation, spatial processing, and reaction time. Separate scores are computed that assess general information processing speed, accuracy, and proficiency for each dimension. The battery prints out scores with confidence bands based on the standard error of measurement. T scores or percentile scores are not provided. Rather, subject's test scores are categorized as above average, average, low average, or below average. MicroCog proficiency scores are based on the standardization sample's mean response time for correct responses. Response times were computed for each item.

MicroCog was normed on a sample of 810 individuals. They ranged in age from 18 to 89. The normative sample is composed of 90 individuals (45 male, 45 female) in nine age groups. African Americans, Hispanics, and Caucasians were included in proportions based on the 1988 US Census. Subjects were selected to represent proportionally four broad geographic regions of the United States and were stratified across three broad education levels: less than high school, high school, and greater than high school.

Subtest reliabilities were computed using split-half measures of consistency when appropriate. Otherwise, generalizability coefficients were employed. Reliability coefficients ranged from .43 to .99. The reliability of some subtests varied as a function of age. Reliability coefficients for index scores and global measures tend to be well within acceptable ranges.

The manual presents test–retest reliability data in terms of means and standard deviations for individual scores and global indices for each test episode within the three broad age groups. Specific reliability coefficients are presented based on the consistency of classification. These calculations were based on the frequency with which a test score fell into one of the four general classification ranges (i.e., below average, low average, average, or above average), rather than on actual correlations between test scores. For the most part, consistency scores were moderate to high across age groups.

An initial exploratory factor analysis of the individual subtests produced two factors reflecting information-processing accuracy and speed. MicroCog's Information Processing Accuracy Index and General Cognitive Proficiency Index both correlate .54 with the WAIS-R Full Scale IQ score.

MicroCog's five index scores were placed in discriminant functions to assess the batteries' ability to detect pathology in various clinical groups. The groups included individuals with the following diagnoses: dementia, depression, lobectomy, lupus, schizophrenia, and mixed psychiatric/neurological disturbances. Classification accuracies varied by disorder. Dementia patients were separated from controls with a high (>90%) degree of accuracy. More moderate classification rates were obtained with both lobectomy (78.75%) and lupus (64.71%) patients. A different group of dementia patients were also given the Mattis Dementia Rating Scale. They scored in the mild-to-moderate (110–135) range of impairment. MicroCog was able to identify 88.9% of these patients as impaired. Additional studies of MicroCog's effectiveness as a screening or triage battery are needed and would be most useful given present-day demands to make health care more cost effective.

Automated Neuropsychological Assessment Metrics

The Automated Neuropsychological Assessment Metrics (ANAM) project began formally in 1990. It was the outgrowth of a program to develop tests of processing efficiency that could also be used to evaluate subjects on multiple occasions (Reeves, Kane, Winter, & Goldstone, 1995). The project's main objective was to adapt a subset of automated tests, developed through the Office of Military Performance Assessment Technology (OMPAT), for use in clinical settings (Kane & Kay, 1992). A number of clinical procedures require patients to be evaluated serially. These include: (1) monitoring effects of medication on mental functioning; (2) assessing the effects of medical interventions such as serial spinal taps or ventricular shunts; (3) tracking the progression of a disease; and (4) assessing the effects of behavioral and environmental treatment interventions in brain-injured patients. Traditional neuropsychological tests had not been developed for repeated-measures assessment. OMPAT tests, initially developed to assess changes in performance over time, appeared an obvious choice for assessing changes serially in clinical settings.

ANAM tests were derived from the OMPAT-sponsored Tester's WorkBenc h (TWB). TWB is a library of automated tests constructed to assess cognitive-processing efficiency in performance assessment applications. Thirty-one independent tests were included in TWB. ANAM is comprised of a specified set of batteries derived from the TWB test library configured for a variety of clinical applications and populations. Currently there are batteries within the ANAM system designed to: (1) screen for brain impairment in higher-functioning patients; (2) screen for impairment and monitor medication effects in the more severely impaired patient; (3) be employed in neurotoxicology investigations; and (4) facilitate the assessment of attention deficit disorders. The current standard ANAM V3.11 also contains abbreviated modules that include a Continuous Performance Test, a Modified Galveston Orientation and Amnesia Test (MOAT), and an automated version of the Tower of Hanoi. The following TWB tests are included in ANAM V3.11:

1. Subject Information Form (demographics)
2. Stanford Sleepiness Scale (modified for lower-functioning individuals)
3. Walter Reed Mood Scale 2 (a Profile of Mood States)
4. Simple Reaction Time
5. Two-Choice Reaction Time
6. Sternberg Memory Search Tasks
7. Running Memory Continuous Performance Task
8. Mathematical Processing Task
9. Digit Set Comparison Task
10. Logical Reasoning (symbolic)
11. Tower of Hanoi (tower puzzle)
12. Stroop Color/Word Interference Task
13. Code Substitution (letter/symbol comparison)
14. Code Substitution (immediate and delayed recall)
15. Spatial Processing Task (simultaneous)
16. Matching to Sample
17. Tapping (left and right index finger)
18. Modified Orientation and Amnesia Test

ANAM was designed especially for repeated and/or continuous measurement for both clinical and research applications. Each ANAM test uses either a large pool of items or computer-generated stimuli to create multiple alternate forms. ANAM uses the test session number in an algorithm to select or generate items through pseudorandomization. Although ANAM consists of a series of preconfigured batteries, an investigator can modify tests or reconfigure batteries to fit their individual needs. Test instructions are written as independent ASCII text files and can be rewritten in different languages or modified for multicultural administration.

Two types of data files are generated by each test module. A file with summary statistics provides scores that include percent accuracy, mean and median response time, number of response omissions, and throughput. A second file provides an item-by-item summary of the entire test. ANAM comes with two data presentation support modules. One module summarizes data for easy inspection and retrieval. The other provides more detailed presentation of test data. Data can also be summarized in a file formatted for easy export to spreadsheet or statistical packages and which also provides a graphic presentation of repeated-measures data.

ANAM has been modified through clinical experience with the battery obtained at various medical centers, including the National Rehabilitation Hospital, Walter Reed Army Medical Center, the National Naval Medical Center, and the Baltimore VA Medical Center. These modifications have been guided by patients' limitations and examiners' needs for flexibility in administration and data management (Reeves, Bleiberg, & Spector, 1993). Specific modifications included larger stimulus displays, forced-pacing of responses, the addition of simplified response devices such as the mouse, and a more flexible executive menuing system. Final configuration of the standard ANAM batteries has only recently been completed. However, a review of available data and a summary of studies currently underway is presented below.

Pertinent ANAM Studies

Walter Reed Army Medical Center. ANAM is presently being used in a seven-center Department of Defense–Veterans Administration joint head injury project. Select subtests are being employed to assess the effectiveness of short-term interventions (Spector, Reeves, & Lewandowski, 1993).

National Institutes of Health. Goel and Grafman (1995) used the ANAM implementation of the Tower of Hanoi Puzzle to examine errors in planning made by head injury patients. Based on results obtained from the Tower Puzzle, they concluded that patients' impaired performances were not a result of failing to plan but rather resulted from goal–subgoal conflict.

National Naval Medical Center. ANAM batteries are being used to track recovery of function in mild head injury patients and have been used to monitor the efficacy of electroconvulsive shock treatment for depression (Reeves, Dutka, Nadler, Kane, & Bleiberg, 1995; Reeves, Nadler, Kane, Bleiberg, & Damis, 1994).

National Rehabilitation Hospital (NRH). Research conducted at NRH is directed at assessing performance variability in premorbidly high-functioning brain injury patients. Bleiberg et al. (1994) reported that ANAM's cognitive efficiency measures revealed subtle but significant effects of mild head trauma that were not demonstrated with traditional neuropsychological measures. Bleiberg, Garmoe, Cederquist, Reeves, and Lux (1993) demonstrated that ANAM was sensitive to the effects of pharmaceutical interventions in a patient following closed head injury.

Baltimore VAMC. ANAM is being used at the Department of Veterans Affairs Medical Center in Baltimore as part of a study of the effects of depleted uranium shrapnel on soldiers wounded during Operation Desert Storm. Initial results suggest that ANAM was more sensitive to the presence of urine uranium than traditional neuropsychological measures (Kane, Kaup, Keogh, Hooper, & DiPino, 1996). The effects of Alzheimer's dementia on performance consistency are also being investigated (Kane, Loreck, May, DiPino, & Reeves, 1996).

Defense Nuclear Agency. Data are presently being collected at Chernobyl, Ukraine in a longitudinal study of chronic exposure to various levels of ionizing radiation sponsored by the Defense Nuclear Agency (G. Gamache, personal communication, April 5, 1996). In this study, ANAM is being administered to individuals working as eliminators at the former nuclear plant, forestry workers outside the plant, farmers living approximately 200 kilometers from the plant, and control subjects living approximately 450 kilometers from the plant in a noncontaminated area.

NASA. ANAM has been used to study the effects of adverse conditions on cognitive status. Wood and Holland (Reeves, Kane, & Wood, 1992) studied three divers who lived for 30 days in an undersea habitat in LaChalupa near Key Largo, FL. This study was designed to look at extended duration performance in a remote environment similar to that anticipated for International Space Station-Alpha. The divers took a practice and test version ANAM daily during their prolonged undersea mission. Performance on a number of ANAM tests stabilized quickly. The divers performed their undersea tasks well and their performance mirrored the divers' job performance. However, there was also evidence that the ANAM tests were sensitive to stress-producing factors.

The UpJohn Company. A considerable amount of data related to using ANAM in clinical trials have been collected at the UpJohn Company's clinical laboratories in Kalamazoo, MI. Primarily under the direction of Dr. Alan Lewandowski, methodologies for using ANAM in pharmaceutical research have been developed.

Normative Studies. Funding for the development of single-administration clinical norms was not part of the Department of Defense effort to develop performance assessment batteries. However, norms for ANAM are presently being collected at various sites. Currently, normative data are being collected on normal healthy adults (Benedetto, Harris, & Goernert, 1995; Dennis & McCroskey, 1995), clinical populations such as elderly stroke victims (Goldstone, Reeves, Levinson,

& Pelham, 1995), traumatic brain injury patients (Levinson & Reeves, 1994), and on Marine recruits (Reeves, Levinson, Batsinger, Winger, & Gastaldo, 1995). Further, normative studies are planned and a national database is being developed by the National Cognitive Recovery Foundation for use on the Internet.

Neurobehavioral Evaluation System—2

Test selection for the Neurobehavioral Evaluation System—2 (NES2) was developed primarily for studies in neurotoxicology (Letz & Baker, 1988). Tests were selected to assess psychomotor skill, memory, visuospatial skills, verbal skills, and mood. Examiners have the option of administering the entire battery or of selecting specific tests.

The NES2 runs on IBM-compatible computers, and requires a color graphics adapter. Subjects respond either by using the keyboard or by pressing response keys located on a joystick. Templates and key markers are available to simplify the use of the keyboard as an input device. However, timing is more precise using joystick keys. The NES2 has a Hand–Eye Coordination test that requires the use of a joystick. The joystick is interfaced with the computer through the game port rather than through an analog-to-digital converter. This interface method results in some loss in accuracy when assessing motor movements. The NES2 uses different timing methods for different tasks. Stimulus presentation is controlled through delay loops written into the software, and the program calibrates different delay frequencies for different microprocessors. Timing for reaction time is accomplished by bypassing the time-of-day clock and going directly to a timing chip.

The following tests are included in the NES2:

1. Finger Tapping
2. Visual Motor Tracking
3. Simple Reaction Time
4. Continuous Performance Test
5. Symbol-Digit/Code Substitution
6. Digit Recall
7. Switch/Shift Attention
8. Pattern Comparison
9. Serial Digit Learning
10. Associate Learning
11. Pattern Matching
12. Arithmetic Computation
13. Grammatical/Logical Reasoning
14. Vocabulary

Instructions precede each test. Some measures include practice trials. Examiners can modify the test parameters. Possible variations include: (1) the length of the interstimulus interval for the reaction time tests; (2) pattern changes for the Pattern Comparison and Pattern Matching Tests; and (3) sequence changes for the Symbol–Digit and Digit Span tests. Alternate forms are available for selected subtests using the session number to seed a random number generator.

The NES2 produces summary scores for each test which include: (1) the time the test began, the time it ended, and elapsed time; (2) test results; (3) the specific test parameters that were used; and (4) an indication of any incidents in which the subject was prompted to call the examiner or the examiner was forced to interrupt the test. Data are saved in ASCII format and the NES2 contains a data-formatting program to facilitate transfer to other programs.

The NES2 was developed for epidemiological research in the area of neurotoxicology. Normative data have not been published. However, NES2 measures have been used in a large number of studies where it has been shown to be sensitive to the effects of environmental toxins (cf. Kane & Kay, 1992). Although the battery was developed primarily for epidemiological research, it contains a number of interesting tasks and has potential as a general clinical tool should norms become available.

Automated Portable Test System: Delta

The Automated Portable Test System (APTS) is a commercial battery developed by the Essex Corporation. It is an outgrowth of the Navy's Performance Evaluation Tests for Environmental Research (PETER) program (Kennedy, Jones, Dunlap, Wilkes, & Bittner, 1985). The PETER program began in 1977 (Bittner et al., 1986). Its objective was to identify tests suitable for repeated administration. Initially, over 150 tests were reviewed and analyzed with respect to their stability over multiple administrations. Computer versions of promising measures followed. Data from the PETER program were used to select measures for the APTS.

The APTS was designed to be portable for administration outside the laboratory. Initially, it ran on the NEC model PC8201A, which weighed less than 4 pounds. Latter, the APTS was adapted to run on an IBM-compatible computer. The latest adaptation of the battery is called Delta. Delta employs a special keypad to replace the keyboard as the subject interface.

Both APTS and Delta were designed as repeated-measures batteries. Traditional single-administration norms are not provided. In developing these batteries, emphasis was placed on the stability of the tests over repeated administrations, factor diversity, and the sensitivity of the measures to environmental stressors. Studies pertaining to the development of the APTS are reviewed in Kane and Kay (1992).

Automated Psychological Test Battery

The Automated Psychological Test Battery (APT) is a computerized neuropsychological test battery developed in Sweden by Levander (1987). It was originally programmed for the Apple II series of computers, then subsequently re-programmed to work with IBM-compatible computers. The APT is a multilingual battery with instructions in six languages (Swedish, Danish, Norwegian, German, English, and Dutch). The APT comes as a package that includes the test software, a special response box, and timing card. Tasks on the IBM version of the test are similar to those used in the earlier Apple II version. Tasks were kept similar to enhance the comparability of results obtained with the earlier and later version of the APT.

The APT extensive library of tests presently include:

1. Associative Learning
2. Continuous Performance
3. Digit Span
4. Maze Exit
5. Finger Tapping
6. Grammatical Reasoning
7. Hemispheric Test
8. K-Test of selective attention
9. Maze Test
10. Numerical Skill
11. Long-term Memory
12. Perspective Reversals
13. Reaction Time Tests
14. Simultaneous Capacity
15. Trail Making
16. Word Recognition

Some tests are implemented in various versions. For example, there are four subtests to assess reaction time: simple auditory, simple visual, two-choice visual, and two-choice visual requiring response inhibition if an auditory signal is presented along with the visual stimulus. Also, there are five modules to the tapping test. These include: (1) right index finger tapping, (2) left index finger tapping, (3) alternate tapping with the right index and middle fingers, (4) alternate tapping with the left index and middle fingers, and (5) alternate tapping with the right and left index fingers.

The APT also contains a questionnaire and visual analogue module that can be used for presenting instructions, recording responses in fixed response categories, or for implementing visual analogue scales with or without anchor points. Scales that have already been implemented include the: (1) Karolinska Scales of Personality, (2) Eysenk Personality Questionnaire, and (3) and "Aggravation test" based on memory for numbers. However, the module is flexible and allows other questionnaires to be adapted and integrated into the test battery.

The APT is a flexible system that allows the examiner to select an individual test or groups of tests. The examiner can also select the appropriate language for the presentation of instructions. Initially, test results are stored in a raw data file. Raw data files are processed by an "evaluate" option, which can output results to the monitor, a printer, a screen copy file for integration with a word processor, or a final data file for export to a statistical or database package.

The APT also contains a meta-analyses option. This option looks at the relationship among different test indices. The only meta-analysis presently implemented in the APT focuses on speed. Test indices are presented based on the processing demands of the tests. Subjects can be compared to themselves and to their peers on tests of varying difficulty.

The APT has been used in studies to assess the affects of various drugs (King, Bell, Bratty, & McEntegrat, 1991; Klinteberg, Levander, Oreland, Sberg, & Schalling, 1987; Levander, 1987; Levander & Farde, 1990; Reichard, Berglund, Birtz, Levander, & Rosenqvist, 1991). It has also been used to assess cognitive impairment in schizophrenia (Levander & Farade, 1990) and diabetes (Wirsn, Tallroth, Lindgren, & Agardh, 1992; Wredling, Levander, Adamson, & Lins, 1990).

California Computerized Assessment Package

The California Computerized Assessment Package (CalCAP) consists of 10 simple and choice reaction time measures. The battery was designed to assess specific facets of cognition, including: processing speed, language skills, rapid visual scanning, form discrimination, recognition memory, and divided attention (Miller, 1996). Instructions and stimulus materials for the CalCAP are available in English, Spanish, and Norwegian. The battery requires an IBM-compatible computer using an Intel 80286 microprocessor or better. It accommodates a variety of graphics standards including Color Graphics Adapter, Enhanced Graphics Adapter (EGA) and Video Graphics Array (VGA). Administration time for the entire battery is approximately 25 minutes. There is also an 8-10 minute abbreviated version of the battery. CalCAP tasks are listed below. Tasks on the abbreviated version are preceded by an asterisk. An additional measure of sequential reaction time is also added to the abbreviated version:

1. Simple Reaction Time* (dominant hand)—iteration #1
2. Simple Reaction Time (nondominant hand)
3. Choice Reaction Time for Single Digits*
4. Serial Pattern Matching/Sequential Reaction Time*
5. Lexical Discrimination
6. Simple Reaction Time (dominant hand)—iteration #2
7. Visual Selective Attention
8. Response Reversal and Rapid Visual Scanning
9. Form Discrimination
10. Simple Reaction Time (dominant hand)—iteration #3

Since CalCAP measures emphasize processing efficiency, response timing is critical. The CalCAP program adjusts to different computers with different processor speeds through the use of special software routines. These routines first check to see that no other programs are running in the background that could interfere with stimulus or response timing. Second, these routines compute the microprocessor's speed so that timing can be more accurately controlled. Tasks are preceded by instructions and practice trials. CalCAP does not permit the examiner to preconfigure different batteries. However, the examiner does have the option of choosing between preconfigured versions of the battery and of skipping individual tests during the administration of the battery.

CalCAP provides three forms of printed data output. The standard printout provides an individual's mean, median, and range of scores on each task. An alternate printout provides a subject's score along with normative ranges. The third printout displays subject performance data graphically. CalCAP also contains a data management program called "shorten." This program arranges test data in a fixed format suitable for export to statistical and database packages.

The CalCAP was normed on 641 HIV-1 seronegative gay men. This sample was obtained from the Multicenter AIDS Cohort Study. The mean age of the sample was 36.0 (SD = 6.97). The mean education level was 16.4 years (SD = 2.26). Ninety-three percent of the sample were Caucasian, 2% were African American, 4% were Hispanic, and 1% were Asian or from another ethnic group.

Both test–retest and internal consistency reliability coefficients are reported in the test manual. Simple reaction time measures tended to show high internal consistency but low test–retest reliability. Within-session correlations for simple reaction time tasks that are readministered in the course of a testing episode are modest (.41–.68). Reported 6-month test–retest reliability measures for choice reaction time tasks ranged from .43 to .68. Internal consistency coefficients for the CalCAP choice reaction time measures were high and ranged from .81 to .96.

CalCAP simple and choice reaction time measures were placed into a factor analysis along with selected conventional neuropsychological tests. Conventional measures included: (1) Digits Forwards and Backwards, (2) Symbol–Digit Substitution, (3) Rey Auditory Verbal Learning Test, (4) Verbal Fluency, (5) Parts A and B of the Trail Making Tests, and (6) Grooved Pegboard. Results of the analysis indicated that both simple and choice reaction time measures formed independent factors that were also distinct from factors formed by the conventional measures. Hence, CalCAP measures appeared to add unique information to the neuropsychological examination.

The CalCAP has been employed in a number studies of patients with HIV-related neurocognitive deficits. Miller, Satz, and Visscher (1991) demonstrated that both the CalCAP and conventional neuropsychological measures were sensitive to cognitive impairments in symptomatic HIV-1-positive homosexual males. Miller (1995) reported data suggesting that simple and choice reaction time measures could supplement traditional neuropsychological measures in assessing the effects of early brain disease. Specifically, CalCAP reaction time measures appeared useful in screening for HIV-related neurocognitive impairment (Miller, Satz, VanGorp, Visscher, & Dudley, 1989; Worth, Savage, Baer, Esty, & Navia, 1993).

The CalCAP was specifically designed to permit the assessment of various components of reaction time as part of the neuropsychological examination. Hence, it does not offer the same range of tasks as some other batteries. Nevertheless, it is an example of how automated assessment can be used effectively to augment the traditional neuropsychological examination.

Individual Computer Tests

The Nonverbal Selective-Reminding Tests

One problem in assessing material-specific learning is that verbal and nonverbal memory assessment frequently employ nonparallel procedures. A second problem has been that, in factor studies, methods of assessing nonverbal memory frequently load more highly on an spatial factor than on a memory factor (Larrabee, Kane, Schuck & Francis, 1985). In an effort to address these difficulties, Kane, Perrine, and Kay (cf. Kane & Perrine, 1988) developed computerized verbal and figural selective-reminding tests. As their names imply, these tests follow the selective-reminding procedure for stimulus presentation developed by Buschke (Buschke, 1973; Buschke & Fuld, 1974). Both the verbal and nonverbal selective reminding tests produce scores typically associated with the selective-reminding procedures.

Both the Verbal and Nonverbal Selective Reminding tests have three independent forms. They have the same "look and feel." They employ similar instructions, a recognition format, and use a lightpen interface, with subjects making their responses on the computer screen. The Selective Reminding Tests will be part of the Investigators Toolkit version of CogScreen (CogScreen-IT).

The Nonverbal Selective Reminding Test (NSRT) uses three sets of 21 abstract designs: 7 targets and 14 distractors. During the learning phase, the computer presents the designs individually for 2.5 seconds. The computer then presents 21 designs including the 7 targets. The subject's task is to identify the seven target designs. The figures change screen positions for each recognition trail. Subjects have 3 minutes per trial to complete their selections, and a countdown clock is provided at the bottom right of the screen. A second counter at the bottom left of the screen keeps track of the number of designs selected. The NSRT also includes a 20-minute delayed recognition trial.

The Verbal Selective Reminding Test (VSRT) follows the same format as the NSRT. However, for the VSRT, the 3 sets of 21 designs are replaced by 3 sets of 42 words. All 126 words are concrete nouns with a Thorndike–Lorge rating of AA or AAA. The subject's task is to learn a 14-word list. For each target word, there are two distractors beginning with the same letter, having the same number of letters, and having an identical Thorndike–Lorge rating.

A number of studies were accomplished with an earlier Apple II version of the NSRT. These studies explored the NSRT's construct validity, sensitivity to brain impairment, vulnerability to practice effects, and alternate form comparability. Results demonstrated that the NSRT: (1) was sensitive to effects of mild head trauma, (2) appeared to measure nonverbal memory independent of verbal memory and spatial ability, and (3) had three alternate forms that appeared equivalent in difficulty (Kane & Kay, 1992).

SYNWORK

SYNWORK is a unique measure designed to simulate the demands of the work environment (Elsmore, 1994). It was developed as a demonstration program to show how the computer could be used to create a test employing multiple tasks that operate simultaneously and require subjects to systematically allocate their resources among tasks. SYNWORK requires subjects to perform four tasks concurrently. SYNWORK was designed as a laboratory task emulating a work setting in which an operator had to attend to multiple tasks of different complexity and with different consequences associated with performance or failure to perform. SYNWORK was not developed to simulate a specific real-world job. However, tasks were selected to sample relevant job related skills.

SYNWORK runs on an IBM PC-AT-compatible computer. It requires a color monitor (EGA or better) and a mouse. SYNWORK divides the computer screen into four quadrants. A different task runs in each quadrant. The tasks include: (1) a Sternberg memory task, (2) a self-paced three-column addition task, (3) a visual monitoring task, and (4) an auditory monitoring task. A composite score is displayed in a small window located in the center of the screen. The composite score reflects the subject's performance of all four tasks. Subjects receive 2 minutes of training on each task individually prior to the beginning of the test. Typically, the test runs for 15 minutes and subjects are instructed to maximize their composite score.

SYNWORK allows investigators flexibility when running the program. Parameters for all tasks can be modified. The experimenter can shift priorities among the tasks by assigning different values to the four tasks. Individual task parameters are also modifiable for each test. The session number seeds a random number generator for production of test items for a given session and thus provides automatic generation of alternate forms. SYNWORK produces summary statistics for all tasks, spreadsheet-compatible data files, and a graphic display of performance within a session.

SYNWORK was developed as a repeated-measures instrument in the classic performance assessment tradition. Consequently, there are no established norms for this measure. SYNWORK has been used by the Navy in sleep deprivation studies. Performance decrements appeared following the first night of sleep deprivation and became more severe following the second sleepless night (Kane & Kay, 1992). SYNWORK was deployed in Operation Desert Storm. The data obtained in this study demonstrated that stable performance on SYNWORK can be achieved within 8–10 sessions under field conditions (Elsmore, Leu, Popp, & Mays, 1991).

Computer-Based Continuous Performance Tests

A number of microprocessor-based continuous performance tests (CPTs) have been developed, and this paradigm was incorporated into some of the batteries already reviewed. While a number of CPTs are available, we limit our review to two tests that are in current use and that demonstrate different implementations of this assessment paradigm.

Test of Variables of Attention

The Test of Variables of Attention (TOVA) (McCarney & Greenberg, 1990) was developed to assess attention deficit hyperactive disorder (ADHD) and also to study medication effects when treating this disorder. Stimuli consist of a colored square containing a small inner square. The inner square is either adjacent to the top or bottom edge of the larger square. Stimuli with the inner square adjacent to the top of the larger square are targets. Subjects are instructed to press a microswitch whenever a target appears. The TOVA is a fixed-interval test. It uses a stimulus duration of 100 msec and an interstimulus interval of 2 seconds. The frequency with which targets appear varies throughout the 23 minutes of the test. At present, norms are available based on 2800 individuals ranging in age from 4 to over 80. An auditory version of the TOVA, presently called the TOVA-A, is scheduled to be available by April, 1996 (S. Lobe, personal communication, November 12, 1995). The TOVA-A was normed on 2550 individuals ranging in age from 6 to 19. The auditory version follows the visual version in design. The test runs for 22 minutes. In the first half of the test, the target tone occurs infrequently. In the second half it becomes a frequently recurring event and the subject has to inhibit response to the nontarget tone.

The TOVA produces summary scores for the entire test and for performance during each quarter of the test. Scores include: (1) omission errors, (2) commission errors, (3) mean response time for correct responses to targets, (4) standard deviations of mean correct response times, (5) incidents of multiple responses, and (6) frequency of anticipatory responses.

The TOVA has been employed to screen for the presence of an attention deficit disorder, as part of a general attention deficit disorder assessment, and to monitor the effects of medication. Greenberg (1987) noted improvements in TOVA performance for 44 children who appeared to respond positively to methylphenidate but not for 6 children who showed a poor response to the drug. McCarney (cf. McCarney & Greenberg, 1990) used the TOVA along with the Conners' Parent–Teacher Questionnaire to discriminate children with attention deficit disorders from age- and sex-matched controls. Using a discriminant function, the author was able to identify 87% of the normal controls and 90% of the attention deficit disorder with hyperactivity children. Greenberg (cf. McCarney & Greenberg, 1990) demonstrated that changes in TOVA performance in response to a challenge dose of methylphenidate correlated with improvement during a 6-week clinical trial with this medication.

Conners' Continuous Performance Test

CPTs were developed to assess sustained attention or vigilance. Typically, they use the paradigm of requiring the subject to respond to an occasional or rare event. The subject monitors the computer screen and responds only when a specific target or target sequence occurs. The Conners' CPT offers the user this option. The test can be set so that the subject is required to respond to the appearance of either an "X" or an X when preceded immediately by an A ("AX^2"). However, the Standard Conners' CPT uses a variation of the more typical paradigm. In the standard version, the subject responds to all letters *except* the letter "X." Hence, the occurrence of the infrequent event requires response inhibition.

If the examiner selects the default settings, the standard version of the Conners' has six sections or blocks. Each section has three subsections or subblocks. Each subblock consists of 20 stimulus presentations. The subblocks differ with respect to their interstimulus intervals (ISIs). The subblocks employ ISIs of 1, 2, or 4 seconds, with the order varying among blocks. Display time is a constant 250 milliseconds for all stimuli. Although the Conner's CPT is preset with default parameters, the program permits customization. Researchers may alter the number of trials, ISIs, and display time. Data output can be directed to the screen and/or be made available in a printed report. Data can also be sent to an ASCII file for archiving and exportation for later analysis. Data output include the total number of stimuli presented, number correct, omission errors, commission errors, and reaction times. Other scores important in assessing CPT results, including d' (sensitivity) and beta, are also provided. The data output includes raw scores, T scores, and percentile scores. T scores are adjusted so that high scores represent a more problematic performance. To facilitate the assessment of performance during various portions of the test, tables provide detailed report statistics by block.

Norms for the Conners' are based on a sample of 520 general population controls and 670 individuals who were clinical referrals. Data were obtained from individuals aged 4 to over 18. Not unexpectedly, Conners (1995) found that subjects improve with age on key CPT measures. The test manual lists studies in which the Conners' CPT was sensitive to drug effects for individuals being treated for ADHD.

CURRENT STATUS AND FUTURE DIRECTIONS

The use of automated assessment in clinical neuropsychology has experienced slow growth. In some ways, this slow growth is surprising. Neuropsychologists in clinical practice are increasingly feeling the pressure for cost-effective assessment with a rapid turnaround of findings and results. The computer appears to be a potentially powerful tool to assist neuropsychologists to adapt to the changing health care market. In addition, the computer yields important clinical information not easily available from traditional assessment approaches. Response time, performance efficiency, and variability are aspects of performance important for diagnosis, monitoring the effects of treatment, and for making judgments about the implications of test data to real-world performance. The computer makes the assessment of response time, efficiency, and consistency an integrated part of neuropsychological assessment. Why then have neuropsychologists been slow to employ the computer as an important patient assessment device? There appears to be several reasons for this reluctance and clear areas in which computerized assessment needs further development.

The clinical or forensic use of any assessment instrument requires that the instrument have an adequate normative base. The dearth of age, education, and culturally based norms for neuropsychological tests has been problematic in the field. This problem persists for automated procedures. While the Aeromedical edition of CogScreen is well normed, the standardization sample was composed of healthy functioning pilots. The normative base permits CogScreen-AE to be used for assessing pilots and for assessing individuals with similar levels of education. However, the norms are not applicable for individuals with lower levels of education, and many CogScreen-AE tasks are too difficult for the more severely impaired. MicroCog has a more generally applicable normative base. However, these norms were collected using two different versions of the test with timers of different accuracy. Also, MicroCog tasks do not fully exploit the power of the computer, and more data are required to judge its use as a screening instrument with different clinical populations. Limited norms are now being collected for ANAM. A larger and more diverse normative sample is needed before ANAM can be employed in screening. Clearly, further normative development and basic validation work are needed before computers will make their full impact in clinical settings.

A second issue that may have slowed the clinical implementation of computerized assessment is that current computerized batteries do not cover all cognitive domains that are traditionally assessed during a clinical evaluation. Neuropsychologists typically include measures of language and memory as part of their assessment. Traditionally, aphasic disorders are assessed and classified by evaluating language characteristics including fluency, repetition, and comprehension. The assessment of memory requires the evaluation of rate of learning, the stability of recall, and recognition. Language is not well assessed with today's computers and most computerized batteries are limited in their assessment of memory. These limitations are especially problematic if the clinician approaches computerized assessment with an "all-or-none" attitude. While current computerized tests do some things less well than standard testing methods, they do other things better. While tests like CogScreen-AE and ANAM do not assess learning as well as traditional verbal learning measures, they do assess working memory more thoroughly than is usually done during a standard clinical examination. Hence, clinicians need to direct their attention as to how best to use computerized measures to augment the traditional neuropsychological examination.

A third issue that appears to be slowing down the clinical implementation of computerized testing is cost. Before computerized testing becomes widely accepted as *a standard* in cognitive assessment, the costs of hardware and software must drop. Although users prefer to purchase test materials at a low cost and then duplicate (appropriately or otherwise) forms when their original supply runs short, the publishers of computerized test programs do not appear to be willing to give away their programs after investing in software development, normative data collection, and the publication of APA-quality manuals. As a result, currently available programs are generally available with "test-use" fees. This system appears to be highly aversive to many practitioners.

A fourth issue impeding the implementation of computerized assessment is the clinicians' lack of familiarity and training in these procedures. It will be important for publishers and test authors to demonstrate clearly the superiority of computerized assessment methods over conventional methods. Computerized assessment will need to become part of graduate student education. The software will need to become intuitive and "user friendly." Even more importantly, research findings using computerized tests will need to be published in peer-reviewed journals as opposed to technical reports and test manuals. An informal survey of recently published articles showed that very few neuropsychological studies employed computerized testing. In contrast, a review of the experimental cognitive psychology literature, and especially the psychopharmacology literature, indicates that computerization has led to significant advances. Cognitive psychology studies frequently employ computerized testing. The acceptance of this methodology in experimental cognitive psychology is probably attributable to the superiority of stimulus control and data recording that are afforded by computerized tests.

If test developers and publishers respond to the criticisms stated above, then computerized testing should be expected to become more of a standard with clinicians. This will be especially true for neuropsychologists involved in treatment studies, in the investigation of processes underlying recovery of brain functioning, and in studies designed to detect subtle effects of various toxins on health conditions.

During this growth period of computerized testing, both test developers and test users will need to adhere to professional testing standards. Users need to determine if instruments meet professional guidelines (American Psychological Association, 1986). For example, computerized tests should only be used if the author/publisher provides an adequate manual and preferably one that meets APA test standards. Normative data should be made available and equivalence studies should be conducted for computer analogs of conventional tests.

Despite the fact that the clinical use of computerized tests is still in an early developmental stage, the potential power and advantages of this form of assessment are already apparent. Further hardware and software development is needed before computers will become the principal means for performing refined neuro-cognitive assessment. However, even today, computers provide a potent adjunct to traditional techniques by permitting the assessment of performance efficiency and consistency in a way not possible with standard measures, increasing the range of tasks that can be implemented during an examination, and permitting an assessment of domains (e.g., divided attention) not possible with standard metrics.

REFERENCES

Acker, W., & Acker, C. (1982). *Bexley Maudsley Automated Psychological Screening and Bexley Maudsley Category Sorting Test manual*. Windsor, Great Britain: NFER-Nelson.

American Psychological Association (1986). *Guidelines for computer-based tests and interpretations*. Washington, DC: American Psychological Association.

Baker, E. L., Letz, R. E., Fidler, A. T., Shalat, S., Plantamura, D., & Lyndon, M. (1985). A computer-based neurobehavioral evaluation system for occupational and environmental epidemiology: Methodology and validation studies. *Neurobehavioral Toxicology and Teratology, 7*, 369–377.

Banderet, L. E., Shukitt, B. L., Walthers, M. A., Kennedy, R. S., Bittner, A. C., & Kay, G. G. (1988, November). *Psychometric properties of three addition tasks with different response requirements*. Paper presented at the 30th Annual Meeting of the Military Testing Association, Arlington, VA.

Benedetto, J., Harris, W., & Goernert, P. (1995). *Automated Neuropsychological Assessment Metrics (ANAM) performance stability during repeated cognitive assessments* (Technical Report EPRL-TR-95-02). Mankato State University, Mankato, Michigan.

Bittner, A. C., Carter, R. C., Kennedy, R. S., Harbeson, M. M., & Krause, M. (1986). Performance evaluation tests for environmental research (PETER): Evaluation of 114 measures. *Perceptual and Motor Skills, 63*, 683–708.

Bleiberg, J., Garmoe, W., Cederquist, J., Reeves, D., & Lux, W. (1993). Effects of dexedrine on performance consistency following brain injury. *Neuropsychiatry, Neuropsychology, and Behavioral Neurology, 6*(4), 245–248.

Bleiberg, J., Nadler, J., Reeves, D., Garmoe, W., Lux, W., & Kane, R. (1994, February). *Inconsistency as a marker of mild head injury*. Paper presented at the Twenty-second Annual Meeting of the International Neuropsychological Society, Cincinnati, OH.

Branconnier, R. J. (1986). A computerized battery for behavioral assessment in Alzheimer's disease. In L. W. Poon, T. Crook, K. L. Davis, B. J. Eisdorfer, A. W. Gurland, A. W. Kaszniak, & L. W. Thompson (Eds.), *Handbook for clinical memory assessment of older adults* (pp. 189–196). Washington, DC: American Psychological Association.

Buschke, H. (1973). Selective reminding for analysis of memory and learning. *Journal of Verbal Learning and Verbal Behavior, 12*, 543–549.

Buschke, H., & Fuld, P. A. (1974). Evaluating storage, retention, and retrieval in disordered memory and learning. *Neurology, 11*, 1091–1105.

Conners, K. C. (1995). *Conners' Continuous Performance Test computer program 3.0: User's manual*. Toronto: Multi-Health Systems.

Dennis, K., & McCroskey, B. (1995). Automated Neuro-Psychological Assessment Metrics (ANAM) in vocational evaluation: Study #6. *Journal of Vocationology, 1*(1), 50–55.

Eckerman, D. A., Carroll, J. B., Foree, D., Gullion, C. M., Lansman, M., Long, E. R., Waller, M. B., & Wallsten, T. S. (1985). An approach to brief field testing for neurotoxicity. *Neurobehavioral Toxicology and Teratology, 7*, 387–393.

Elithorn, A., Lunzer, M., & Weinman, J. J. (1975). Cognitive deficits associated with chronic hepatic encephalopathy and their responses to levadopa. *Journal of Neurology, Neurosurgery, and Psychiatry, 38*, 794–798.

Elsmore, T. (1994). SYNWORK 1: A pc-based tool for assessment of performance in a simulated work environment. *Behavioral Research Methods, Instruments, and Computers, 26,* 421–426.

Elsmore, T. F., Leu, J. L., Popp, K., & Mays, M. Z. (1991). *Performance assessment under operational conditions using a computer-based synthetic work task.* US Army Research Institute of Environmental Medicine, Natick, MA.

Engelberg, A. C., Gibbons, H. L., & Doege, T. C. (1986). A review of the medical standards for civilian airmen: Synopsis of a two-year study. *Journal of the American Medical Association, 225*(12), 1589–1599.

Goel, V., & Grafman, J. (1995). Are the frontal lobes implicated in "planning" functions? Interpreting data from the Tower of Hanoi. *Neuropsychology, 33*(5), 623–642.

Goldstone, A., Reeves, D., Levinson, D., & Pelham, M. (1995). *ANAM V3.11 geriatric normative and CVA data* (Scientific Report NCRF-SR-95-01). Irvine, CA: National Cognitive Recovery Foundation.

Greenberg, L. (1987). An objective measure of methylphenidate response: Clinical use of the MCA. *Psychopharmocology Bulletin, 23,* 279–282.

Gronwall, D. (1977). Paced Auditory Serial Addition task: A measure of recovery from concussion. *Perceptual and Motor Skills, 44,* 367–373.

Heaton, R. K., Grant, I., & Matthews, C. G. (1991). *Comprehensive norms for an expanded Halstead–Reitan Battery: Demographic corrections, research fundings, and clinical applications.* Odessa, FL: Psychological Assessment Resources.

Irons, R., & Rose, P. (1985). Naval biodynamics laboratory computerized cognitive testing. *Neurobehavioral Toxicology and Teratology, 7,* 395–397.

Kane, R. L., Loreck, D., May, C., DiPino, R. K., & Reeves, D. L. (1996). Metrics for assessing treatment efficacy in dementia: A new perspective regarding speed and accuracy measures [Abstract]. *Archives of Clinical Neuropsychology,*

Kane, R. L., Kaup, B., Keogh, J., Hooper, F., & DiPino, R. K. (1996, February). *Neuropsychological and psychiatric findings in Gulf War participants exposed to depleted uranium.* Paper presented at the 23rd Annual Meeting of the International Neuropsychological Society, Chicago.

Kane, R. L., & Kay, G. G. (1992). Computerized assessment in neuropsychology: A review of tests and test batteries. *Neuropsychology Review, 3*(1), 1–117.

Kane, R. L., & Perrine, K. R. (1988, February). *Construct validity of a nonverbal analogue to the selective reminding verbal learning test.* Paper presented at the meeting of the International Neuropsychological Society, New Orleans, LA.

Kay, G. G. (1994). *Phase C Cognitive Function Test Development: Final report.* (Technical Report No. DTFA-02-90-C-90118). Oklahoma City: Federal Aviation Administration, Civil Aeronautical Medical Institute.

Kay, G. G. (1995). *CogScreen—Aeromedical Edition: Professional manual.* Odessa, FL: Psychological Assessment Resources.

Kennedy, R. S., Jones, M. B., Dunlap, W. P., Wilkes, R. L., & Bittner, A. C. (1985). *Automated Portable Test System (APTS): A performance assessment tool* (Technical Report 81775). SEA Technical Paper Series (Abstract).

King, D. J., Bell, P., Bratty, J. R., & McEntegrat, D. J. (1991). A preliminary study of the effects of Flosequinan on psychomotor function in health volunteers. *International Clinical Psychopharmacology, 6,* 155–168.

Klinteberg, A. F., Levander, S., Oreland, L., Sberg, M., & Schalling, D. (1987). Neuropsychological correlates of platelet MAO activity in female and male subjects. *Biological Psychology, 24,* 237–252.

Larrabee, G. J., Kane, R. L., Schuck, J. R., & Francis, D. J. (1985). Construct validity of various memory testing procedures. *Journal of Clinical and Experimental Neuropsychology, 7,* 239–250.

Letz, R., & Baker, E. L. (1988). *Neurobehavioral Evaluation System 2: Users manual (version 4.2).* Winchester, MA: Neurobehavioral Systems.

Letz, R., Mahoney, F. C., Hershman, D. L., Woskie, S., & Smith, T. J. (1990). Neurobehavioral effects of acute styrene exposure in fiberglass boatbuilders. *Neurotoxicology and Teratology, 12,* 665–668.

Levander, S. (1987). Evaluation of cognitive impairment using a computerized neuropsychological test battery. *Nordic Journal of Psychiatry, 41,* 417–422.

Levander, S., & Farde, L. (1990). *Complex neuropsychological effects of a D2-specific dopamine antagonist.* Lund, Sweden: Department of Psychiatry, University of Lund.

Levinson, D., & Reeves, D. L. (1994). *Automated Neuropsychological Assessment Metrics: ANAM V1.0 TBI data.* (Scientific Report NCRF-SR-94-02). Irvine, CA: National Cognitive Recovery Foundation.

McCarney, D., & Greenberg, L. M. (1990). *Test of variables of attention computer program, version 5.01 for IBM PC or IBM compatibles: TOVA manual.* Minneapolis: University of Minnesota.

Miller, E. N. (1995). Cognitive testing using reaction time and traditional neuropsychological procedures. *Journal of the International Neuropsychological Society, 1,* 393.

Miller, E. N. (1996). *California Computerized Assessment Package: Manual.* Los Angeles: Norland Software.

Miller, E. N., Satz, P., VanGorp, W., Visscher, B., & Dudley, J. (1989). Computerized screening for HIV-related cognitive decline in gay men: Cross-sectional analyses and one-year follow-up [Abstract]. *International Conference on AIDS, 5,* 465.

Miller, E. N., Satz, P., & Visscher, B. (1991). Computerized and conventional neuropsychological assessment of HIV-1-infected homosexual men. *Neurology, 41,* 1608–1616.

Powell, D. H., Kaplan, E. F., Whitla, D., Weintraub, S., Catlin, R., & Funkenstein, H. H. (1993). *Microcog: Assessment of cognitive functioning—Manual.* San Antonio, TX: The Psychological Corporation.

Reeves, D. L., Bleiberg, J., & Spector, J. (1993). Validation of the ANAM battery in multi-center head injury rehabilitation studies [Abstract]. *Archives of Clinical Neuropsychology, 8*(3), 262.

Reeves, D. L., Dutka, A., Nadler, J., Kane, R. L., & Bleiberg, J. (1995). Verbal memory deficits and functional recovery following a left thalamic infarction [Abstract]. *Archives of Clinical Neuropsychology, 10*(4), 382.

Reeves, D., Kane, R. L., Winter, K. P., & Goldstone, A. (1995). *Automated Neuropsychological Assessment Metrics (ANAM V3.11): Clinical and neurotoxicology subsets* (Scientific Report NCRF-SR-95-01). San Diego, CA: National Cognitive Recovery Foundation.

Reeves, D. L., Kane, R. L., & Wood, J. (1992). Adapting computerized tests for neuropsychological assessment [Abstract]. *The Clinical Neuropsychologist, 6*(3), 356.

Reeves, D. L., Levinson, D., Batsinger, K., Winger, B., & Gastaldo, E. (1995). *ANAM-USMC normative data* (Scientific Report NCRF-SR-95-05). San Diego, CA: National Cognitive Recovery Foundation.

Reeves, D. L., Nadler, J., Kane, R. L., Bleiberg, J., & Damis, L. (1994, July). *Depression, cognitive efficiency, and ECT.* Paper presented at the American Neuropsychiatric Association Annual Meeting and Scientific Program, Providence, RI.

Reichard, P., Berglund, B., Britz, A., Levander, S., & Rosenqvist, U. (1991). Hypoglycemic episodes during intensified insulin treatment: Increased frequency but no effect on cognitive function. *Journal of Internal Medicine, 229,* 9–16.

Sbordone, R. J. (1990). *Sbordone–Hall Memory Battery Version 2.0: User's manual.* Unpublished manuscript, Orange County Neuropsychology Group, Irvine, CA.

Spector, J., Kay, G. G., Geyer, C. A., Deveikas, J. P., & Sullivan, R. A. (1991). Neuropsychological screening during trial balloon occlusion of the internal carotid artery [Abstract]. *Archives of Clinical Neuropsychology, 6,* 229.

Spector, J., Reeves, D. L., & Lewandowski, A. (1993, May). *Automated neuropsychological assessment: DoD contributions.* Paper presented at the Proceedings of the 1993 AMEDD Clinical Psychology Short Course, Washington, DC.

Swiercinsky, D. (1984, February). *Computerized neuropsychological assessment.* Paper presented at the Annual Meeting of the International Neuropsychological Association, Houston, TX.

Thorne, D., Genser, S., Sing, H., & Hegge, F. (1985). The Walter Reed Performance Assessment Battery. *Neurobehavioral Toxicology and Teratology, 7,* 415–418.

Wirsn, A., Tallroth, G., Lindgren, M., & Agardh, C. D. (1992). Neuropsychological performance differs between type I diabetic patients and normal men during insulin-induced hypoglycaemia. *Diabetic Medicine, 9,* 156–165.

Worth, J. L., Savage, C. R., Baer, L., Esty, E. K., & Navia, B. A. (1993). Computer-based neuropsychological screening for AIDS dementia complex. *AIDS, 7,* 677–681.

Wredling, R., Levander, S., Adamson, U., & Lins, P. E. (1990). Permanent neuropsychological impairment after recurrent episodes of severe hypoglycemia. *Diabetes Research and Clinical Practice, 5,* 625.

12

Concluding Remarks

THERESA INCAGNOLI AND GERALD GOLDSTEIN

It has been 10 years at this writing since the appearance of the volume by Incagnoli, Goldstein, and Golden (1986) in which an overview was provided of developments in clinical neuropsychological assessment at that time. The chapters in that volume reflected several major trends that were then current. There was a major interest in the standard comprehensive test batteries, an interest in specialized tests assessing various cognitive domains, specifically language, memory, and visual–spatial abilities, and there were the beginnings of a conceptual model utilizing a so-called flexible battery that has become known as the "process approach."

The contents of this volume clearly reflect stable and changing trends in the field. While there is still great interest in all of these topics, it would probably be fair to say that there have been major changes in emphasis. In our view these changes are a reduced interest in standard, comprehensive batteries, an increased interest in special populations, notably children and the elderly, and important advances in process and cognitive approaches to neuropsychological assessment. A topic not even discussed 10 years ago but currently of great interest is the use of computers in neuropsychological assessment. Those that remain advocates of standard batteries have become increasingly concerned with issues related to computerization, scaling, and other psychometric issues, as clearly indicated in the chapters by Kane and Kay (Chapter 11) and by Russell (Chapter 2). Another trend of major significance is an extension of neuropsychological assessment to the field of psychopathology and general medical illness. Exclusive interest in patients with classic neurological disorders appears to be a thing of the past. These concluding comments will be made as brief discussions of these changing trends.

THERESA INCAGNOLI • School of Medicine, State University of New York, Stony Brook, New York 11790   GERALD GOLDSTEIN • Pittsburgh VA Health Care System, and University of Pittsburgh, Pittsburgh, Pennsylvania 15260

THE STANDARD COMPREHENSIVE BATTERIES

This volume, as in Incagnoli et al. (1986), has chapters on the Halstead–Reitan and Luria–Nebraska standard batteries. However, in 1986, there was an atmosphere of controversy concerning these two procedures, and extensive efforts were made to compare one with the other, basically in order to determine which one was better. Both batteries survive as sound, valid, and reliable assessment procedures. We have better norms now, more sophisticated scaling, and a better understanding of their psychometric properties. Elegant computerized scoring systems have become available, and some of the tests may be computer administered. Extensive normative systems for the Halstead–Reitan Battery have been provided by Reitan (1991), Heaton, Grant, and Matthews (1991), and Russell and Starkey (1993). Russell compared these three systems in Chapter 2. In addition, the MAYO group has published norms for the elderly for the Wechsler Adult Intelligence Scale—Revised (WAIS-R), the Wechsler Memory Scale—Revised (WMS-R), and the Rey Auditory Verbal Learning Test (Ivnik et al., 1992a–c).

The chapter on the process approach by White and Rose (Chapter 6) and the chapter on cognitive neuropsychology by Ritter and Morrow (Chapter 7) reflect perhaps an increasing tendency toward less reliance by practitioners on the standard batteries. It would probably be fair to say that many, if not most, practitioners utilize a combination of at least some portions of standard batteries and individual tests developed within the framework of cognitive or process approaches.

SPECIAL POPULATIONS

During recent years, a large literature has appeared in the areas of child neuropsychology (e.g., Reitan & Wolfson, 1993) and the neuropsychology of aging (e.g., Goldstein & Nussbaum, 1996). These areas in essence have become subspecialties of neuropsychology, each having its own procedures and scientific basis.

Research in child neuropsychological assessment has expanded in several areas including the development of many new tests, the extension of neuropsychological assessment to children with general medical disorders, extensive research in the areas of specific and pervasive developmental disorders, and the use of various neuroimaging procedures in conjunction with neuropsychological tests. Significant advances have been made in our understanding of various neurodevelopmental disorders such as autism, children with low birth weight, and attention deficit hyperactivity disorder. The fields of cognitive and developmental psychology now have an important influence on child clinical neuropsychology, as illustrated in the chapter by Williams and Boll (Chapter 8).

Within the area of aging, there has been increased interest in normal aging, particularly with regard to two matters, both of which are controversial. There is the issue of the status of age-associated memory impairment (Crook et al., 1986) and the matter of utilization of age-corrected scores in neuropsychological assessment (Reitan & Wolfson, 1995). Extensive study of the dementias of the elderly has provided much enhanced sophistication to assessment of individuals with these disorders. Much has been learned about the distinctive features of the various disorders, such as Alzheimer's disease and vascular dementia (Cummings, Miller, Hill, & Neshkes, 1987), and there is much increased understanding of the status of the various cognitive domains in dementia, notably memory (Bondi, Salmon, & Butters, 1994). Extensive work has been done in differentiating the cortical (e.g., Alzheimer's disease) from the subcortical (e.g., Parkinson's disease) dementias (Cummings, 1990). Some of this work has been done with standard psychometric instruments through the development of psychometric test profile formulas (Fuld, 1984; Russell & Polakoff, 1993), some with systematic clinical observation, such as a study of the "closing-in" phenomenon (Gainotti, Parlato, Monteleone, & Carlomagno (1992), and some with experimental studies (e.g., Jacobs, Salmon, Troster, & Butters, 1990).

PROCESS AND COGNITIVE APPROACHES

In 1986, clinical neuropsychology appeared to be characterized by a dichotomy between assessment, as performed by practicing clinicians, and experimental neuropsychology, as accomplished in academic settings. Assessment of neurobehavioral function was done in different ways by behavioral neurologists and by psychologists, most of whom had received their training in clinical psychology. There now seems to be a confluence among these three branches of the field, stimulated to a large extent by Nelson Butters (Butters, 1986), and reflected largely in process and cognitive approaches to assessment. These approaches, while utilizing standard psychometric tests to some extent, have also incorporated methods developed by behavioral neurology and in the experimental laboratory into assessment of individual patients. As Ritter and Morrow point out in their chapter (Chapter 7), the application of findings from the cognitive psychology laboratory can substantially help to identify underlying functions disrupted by brain damage. Similarly, White and Rose (Chapter 6) mention the collaboration between behavioral neurologists and psychologists in the development of the Boston process approach.

To some extent, the editors of this volume have replaced the chapters on the domains of language, memory, and visual–spatial abilities with the chapters on cognitive and process approaches. There are several possible reasons underlying this shift. Perhaps most significantly, the scientific study of these domains has become highly influenced by cognitive psychology. The neuropsychology of language is now heavily oriented toward neurolinguistics and is strongly influenced by experimental developmental studies of language in normal and language-disabled children (e.g., Tallal, Stark, & Mellits, 1985). Similarly, the neuropsychology of the amnesic disorders is now largely based on research models coming from the experimental psychology of memory and attention. Ritter and Morrow (Chapter 7) provide an account of the impact of cognitive psychology on visual cognition.

It also is apparent that the new and newly modified tests developed within the framework of the process approach have become extraordinarily popular. The Boston Naming Test, the Boston Diagnostic Aphasia Examination, the California Verbal Learning Test, and the WAIS-R/NI are all in widespread use. Even users of the standard batteries have incorporated some of these tests into their assessments. Additionally, the new refined scoring methods for standard tests described by White and Rose (Chapter 6) are commonly used.

PSYCHOPATHOLOGY

The chapter by Sweet and Westergaard (Chapter 10) reflects the establishment of a clear role for neuropsychology in experimental and clinical psychopathology. As these authors point out, many referrals for neuropsychological testing come from psychiatrists, who have diagnostic and other questions concerning their patients with psychiatric disorders. These referrals are not restricted to the dementias and related disorders with clear structural, neurological bases, but actually run the gamut of child and adult psychopathology. In current practice, numerous referrals are made in the child area for individuals with specific and pervasive developmental disorders, attention deficit hyperactivity disorder, and eating disorders. With regard to adults, referrals are commonly made for individuals with mood disorders, schizophrenia, and obsessive–compulsive disorder. Evaluation for depression has become a standard part of neuropsychological assessment of the elderly.

At a more basic level, the extension of neuropsychology into psychopathology reflects a paradigm shift associated with the biological revolution in psychiatry. Traditionally as neuropsychologists, we commonly evaluated patients with alcoholism, mental retardation, and the progressive dementias because the association between these disorders and brain function was patent. Now, it has become clear that schizophrenia, several forms of mood disorder, and some of the anxiety disorders have neurobiological bases and are not specifically produced by environmental agents. Sophisticated explanatory constructs, such as vulnerability or stress–diathesis theories, have offered explanations of how some forms of psychopathology develop from an interaction between biological and environmental influences (Zubin & Spring, 1977). In children, it is now clear that attention deficit hyperactivity disorder and autism are developmental neurobiological illnesses, although the etiologies and pathophysiologies are not fully understood.

This new model of mental illness has produced a substantial body of brain–behavior research in psychopathology, often involving extensive interdisciplinary collaboration. Neuroimaging, neuropathology, pharmacology, immunology, neurophysiology, and neurochemistry, often in association with neuropsychology, are some of the specialties concerned with brain function in schizophrenia, the mood disorders, autism, obsessive–compulsive disorder, and other forms of psychopathology. A review of research of this type forms the major portion of Chapter 10, by Sweet and Westergaard. We now have various theories concerning the neuropsychology of schizophrenia (Steinhauer, Gruzelier, & Zubin, 1991), autism (Minshew, Goldstein, & Siegel, in press), obsessive–compulsive disorder (Cummings & Frankel, 1985), and mood disorder (Kinsbourne, 1988), all postulating some form of brain dysfunction. We do not have complete answers to how the brain creates any of these illnesses, but there has been clear progress and articulation of directions for future research. One important methodology in that regard is the seeking of correlations between neuropsychological test results with data from structural and functional neuroimaging, or other biological procedures (e.g., Minshew, Goldstein, Dombrowski, Panchaligam, & Pettegrew, 1993).

MEDICAL DISORDERS

In a compelling presentation, Tarter (1996) has shown how various organs and organ systems can impact on cognitive function. While the brain may be the organ of behavior, it does not exist in isolation but interacts with and is influenced by the rest of the body. During the past 10 years, this relationship between the brain and the rest of the body has been reflected in numerous studies of neuropsychological function in a wide variety of illnesses involving organs and organ systems other than the brain. A brief list of disorders studied includes chronic obstructive pulmonary disease (Grant, Heaton, McSweeny, Adams, & Timms, 1982), hypertension (King & Miller, 1990), cardiovascular disease (Farmer, 1994), leukemia (Stebbins et al., 1991), diabetes (Ryan & Williams, 1993), systemic lupus erythematosus (Denburg, Carbotte & Denburg, 1987), human immunodeficiency virus (HIV) infection (Grant & Martin, 1994), liver disease (Tarter, Edwards, & Van Thiel, 1988), and various endocrinological disorders (Gordon, Lee, & Tamres, 1988). A related developing area is neuropsychological toxicology (Hartman, 1988, 1995). This subspecialty focuses on the effects of environmental toxins on behavior and has close associations with the fields of environmental toxicology and occupational medicine. Studies of specific agents such as paint, lead, mercury, organophosphates, and radioactive materials have appeared in the literature and are reviewed in Hartman (1988, 1995). Neuropsychological studies of these systemic and environmentally induced disorders have produced varying findings characterized by specific deficit profiles or more generalized cognitive impairment. These findings have encouraged an alliance with health psychology and preventive medicine efforts in general, since numerous prevention and treatment issues relate to these disorders and the possible role neuropsychology may play.

COMPUTERIZATION

The chapter by Kane and Kay (Chapter 11) reflects remarkable advancement in computerized assessment over the past decade. Numerous individual tests and full test batteries can now be administered and scored by computer. A major issue relates to whether it is best to adapt available clinical tests for computer administration and scoring, or to develop analogous tests that are developed specifically for computers. Kane and Kay have emphasized the latter option, probably wisely so, particularly since our own experience with the early adaptations of standard tests indicated that they were often unsatisfactory substitutes for the original procedures.

Computerized testing is not yet commonly used in office practice, but we would predict that its use will be quite common before the turn of the century. The technology is available, and as Kane and Kay point out, we have all of the advantages of uniformity of administration, precise timing, and detailed monitoring of responses. Precise measurement of response under standard and systematically variable stimulus conditions (e.g., control of speed of presentation) may reflect the future of our field. Extensive efforts are now being made to develop computerized batteries that are suitable for clinical, scientific, and industrial applications.

SUMMARY

In these brief concluding remarks, we have commented on what we see as the important changes in the field of clinical neuropsychology over the past 10 years. We have emphasized the increased balance between use of comprehensive and specialized testing procedures, growing emphasis on the neuropsychology of children and the elderly, expansion of the field into application to patients with mental and general medical illness, gains in the influence of cognitive and process approaches to neuropsychology, and perhaps the beginnings of widespread conversion to computerized assessment.

As suggested, the field has become increasingly specialized, particularly with regard to the differing knowledge bases needed for child and adult practice. Geriatric neuropsychology has also become a somewhat specialized area. With regard to child neuropsychology, we now know a great deal more about the development of various cognitive functions, and normative expectations related to age can now be considered on the basis of empirical data. Furthermore, we have greatly expanded our knowledge base concerning developmental disorders, notably learning disability, autism, and attention deficit hyperactivity disorder. In the geriatric area, we now have further clarification of the cognitive effects of normal aging, which has been achieved through various means such as combined cross-sectional and longitudinal studies, improved diagnostic evaluation of subjects, and an increased appreciation of sociocultural influences. There has been a huge amount of dementia research accomplished over the past 10 years, and we can now characterize cognitive function in dementia, differences among different kinds of dementia, and the varying courses of the dementing illnesses much more precisely than we could in the past.

In view of these recent developments, it behooves practicing neuropsychologists to pay particular attention to maintenance of continuing education and to modify practice patterns and clinical assessment in accordance with the admittedly rapidly occurring changes in the field. Issues of credentialing, peer evaluation of competency, and restriction of practice to one's areas of competence are becoming increasingly important matters in the field. This matter is one of particular significance at present because, as we have seen in several places in this volume, many formerly held views are outdated or are, in fact, incorrect. For example, it is apparently not true, as formerly believed, that memory is spared in schizophrenia. Individuals with schizophrenia have been shown to have significant working memory deficits (Gold, Randolph, Carpenter, Goldberg, & Weinberger, 1992). Autism is not a psychogenic disorder produced by "refrigerator parents" (Minshew et al., 1993). It is not true that "pseudodementia" in the elderly is what the term implies, but rather has a documentable anatomical substrate (Nussbaum, 1994). Misconceptions of this type could lead to instances of diagnostic and prognostic error that might be avoidable through keeping up with our rapidly growing profession.

REFERENCES

Bondi, M., Salmon, D., & Butters, N. (1994). Neuropsychological features of memory disorders in Alzheimer's disease. In R. D. Terry, R. Katzman, & K. Bick (Eds.), *Alzheimer disease* (pp. 41–63). New York: Raven Press.

Butters, N. (1986). The clinical aspects of memory disorders: Contributions from experimental studies of amnesia and dementia. In T. Incagnoli, G. Goldstein, & C. J. Golden (Eds.), *Clinical application of neuropsychological test batteries* (pp. 361–382). New York: Plenum Press.

Crook, T., Bartus, R. T., Ferris, S. H., Whitehouse, P., Cohen, G. D., & Gershon, S. (1986). Age-associated memory impairment: Proposed diagnostic criteria and measures of clinical change—Report of a National Institute of Mental Health work group. *Developmental Neuropsychology, 2,* 261–276.

Cummings, J. L. (Ed.). (1990). *Subcortical dementia.* New York: Oxford University Press.

Cummings, J. L., & Frankel, M. (1985). Gilles de la Tourette syndrome and the neurological basis for obsessions and compulsions. *Biological Psychiatry, 20,* 1117–1126.

Cummings, J. L., Miller, B., Hill, M. A., & Neshkes, R. (1987). Neuropsychiatric aspects of multi-infarct dementia and dementia of the Alzheimer's type. *Archives of Neurology, 44,* 389–393.

Denburg, S. D., Carbotte, R. M., & Denburg, J. A. (1987). Cognitive impairment in systemic lupus erythematosus: A neuropsychological study of individual and group deficits. *Journal of Clinical and Experimental Neuropsychology, 4,* 323–339.

Farmer, M. E. (1994). Cognitive deficits related to major organ failure: The potential role of neuropsychological testing. *Neuropsychology Review, 4,* 117–160.

Fuld, P. A. (1984). Test profile of cholinergic dysfunction and of Alzheimer-type dementia. *Journal of Clinical Neuropsychology, 6,* 380–392.

Gainotti, G., Parlato, V., Monteleone, D., & Carlomagno, S. (1992). Neuropsychological markers of dementia on visual–spatial tasks: A comparison between Alzheimer's disease and vascular forms of dementia. *Journal of Clinical and Experimental Neuropsychology, 14,* 239–252.

Gold, J. M., Randolph, C., Carpenter, C. J., Goldberg, T. E., & Weinberger, D. R. (1992). Forms of memory failure in schizophrenia. *Journal of Abnormal Psychology, 101,* 487–494.

Goldstein, G., & Nussbaum, P. D. (1996). The neuropsychology of aging. In J. G. Beaumont & J. Segent (Eds.), *The Blackwell dictionary of neuropsychology.* London: Wiley.

Gordon, H. W., Lee, P. A., & Tamres, L. K. (1988). The pituitary axis: Behavioral correlates. In R. E. Tarter, D. H. Van Thiel, & K. L. Edwards (Eds.). *Medical neuropsychology: The impact of disease on behavior* (pp. 159 –196). New York: Plenum.

Grant, I., Heaton, R. K., McSweeny, A. J., Adams, K. M., & Timms, R. M. (1982). Neuropsychologic findings in hypoxemic chronic obstructive pulmonary disease. *Archives of Internal Medicine, 142,* 1470–1476.

Grant, I., & Martin, A. (1994). *Neuropsychology of HIV infection.* New York: Oxford University Press.

Hartman, D. E. (1988). *Neuropsychological toxicology: Identification and assessment of human neurotoxic syndromes.* New York: Pergamon Press.

Hartman, D. E. (1995). *Neuropsychological toxicology. Identification and assessment of human neurotoxic syndromes.* (2nd ed.). New York: Plenum Press.

Heaton, R. K., Grant, I., & Matthews, C. G. (1991). *Comprehensive norms for an expanded Halstead–Reitan Battery. Norms manual and computer program.* Odessa, FL: Psychological Assessment Resources

Incagnoli, T., Goldstein, G., & Golden, C. J. (1986). *Clinical application of neuropsychological test batteries.* New York: Plenum Press.

Ivnik, R. J., Malec, J. F., Smith, G. E., Tangalos, E. G., Petersen, R. C., Kokmen, E., & Kurland, L. T. (1992a). Mayo's older normative studies: WAIS-R norms for ages 56–97. *The Clinical Neuropsychologist, 6 (Suppl.),* 1 –30.

Ivnik, R. J., Malec, J. F., Smith, G. E., Tangalos, E. G., Petersen, R. C., Kokmen, E., & Kurland, L. T. (1992b). Mayo's older normative studies: WMS-R norms for ages 56–97. *The Clinical Neuropsychologist, 6 (Suppl.),* 49–82.

Ivnik, R. J., Malec, J. F., Smith, G. E., Tangalos, E. G., Petersen, R. C., Kokmen, E., & Kurland, L. T. (1992c). Mayo's older normative studies: Updated AVLT norms for ages 56–97. *The Clinical Neuropsychologist, 6 (Suppl.),* 83–104.

Jacobs, D., Salmon, D., Troster, A., & Butters, N. (1990). Intrusion errors in the figural memory of patients with Alzheimer's and Huntington's disease: A clinical and pathological entity. *Neurology, 40,* 1–8.

King, H. E., & Miller, R. E. (1990). Hypertension: Cognitive and behavioral consideration. *Neuropsychology Review, 1,* 31–73.

Kinsbourne, M. (1988). *Cerebral hemisphere function in depression.* Washington, DC: American Psychiatric Press.

Minshew, N. J., Goldstein, G., Dombrowski, S. N., Panchaligam, K., & Pettegrew, J. W. (1993). A preliminary ^{31}P-NMR study of autism: Evidence for undersynthesis and increased degradation of brain membranes. *Biological Psychiatry, 33,* 762–773.

Minshew, N. J., Goldstein, G., & Siegel, D. J. (in press). Neuropsychologic functioning in autism: Profile of a complex information processing disorder. *Journal of the International Neuropsychological Society.*

Nussbaum, P. D. (1994). Pseudodementia: A slow death. *Neuropsychology Review, 4,* 71–90.

Reitan, R. M. (1991). *The Neuropsychological Deficit Scale for Adults: Computer program and users manual.* Tucson, AZ: Neuropsychology Press.

Reitan, R. M., & Wolfson, D. (1993). *The Halstead–Reitan Neuropsychological Test Battery: Theory and clinical interpretation.* Tucson, AZ: Neuropsychology Press.

Reitan, R. M., & Wolfson, D. (1995). Influence of age and education on neuropsychological test results. *The Clinical Neuropsychologist, 9,* 151–158.

Russell, E. W., & Polakoff, D. (1993). Neuropsychological test patterns in men for Alzheimer's and multi-infarct dementia. *Archives of Clinical Neuropsychology, 8,* 327–343.

Russell, E. W., & Starkey, R. I. (1993). *Halstead, Russell Neuropsychological Evaluation System: Manual and computer program.* Los Angeles: Western Psychological Services.

Ryan, C., & Williams, T. (1993). Effects of insulin-dependent diabetes on learning and memory efficiency in adults. *Journal of Clinical and Experimental Neuropsychology, 15,* 685–700.

Stebbens, J. A., Kaleita, T. A., Noll, R. B., MacLean, Jr., W. E., O'Brien, R. T., Waskerwitz, M. J., & Hammond, G. D. (1991). CNS prophylaxis of childhood leukemia: What are the long-term neurological, neuropsychological, and behavioral effects? *Neuropsychology Review, 2,* 147–177.

Steinhauer, S. R., Gruzelier, J. H., & Zubin, J. (Eds.). (1991). *Handbook of schizophrenia: Vol. 5. Neuropsychology, psychophysiology, and information processing.* London: Elsevier.

Tallal, P., Stark, R. E., & Mellits, D. (1985). The relationship between auditory temporal analysis and receptive language development: Evidence from studies of developmental language disorder. *Neuropsychologia, 23,* 527–534.

Tarter, R. E. (1996, February). Herbert Birch Lecture presented at the meeting of the International Neuropsychological Society, Chicago, IL.

Tarter, R. E., Edwards, K. L., & Van Thiel, D. H. (1988). Neuropsychological dysfunction due to liver disease. In R. E. Tarter, D. H. Van Thiel, & K. L. Edwards (Eds.), *Medical neuropsychology: The impact of disease on behavior* (pp. 75–97). New York: Plenum Press.

Zubin, J., & Spring, B. (1977). Vulnerability—A new view of schizophrenia. *Journal of Abnormal Psychology, 86,* 103–126.

Index

Absolute scales, 22–23
Academic achievement tests, for brain-injured children, 259
ACAT: *see* Adaptive Category Test
Accommodation, 71
Achievement tests, for children, 242–244
Activities of daily living (ADLs), assessment scales for, 287, 308, 309–310, 314, 315
Adaptive Category Test, 23, 24
Affective disorders, Halstead–Reitan Neuropsychological Battery assessment of, 107
Aging
  cognitive effects of, 398–399
  normal, lack of definition of, 277–278
Agrammatism, 184
Albert, Marilyn, 174
Albert, Martin, 173
Alzheimer's disease, 6, 395
  cognitive decline in, 316
  cognitive reaction time in, 227–228
  neuropsychological assessment instruments for
    Alzheimer's Disease Assessment Battery, 368
    behavior rating scales, 297, 301, 302–304
    brief cognitive screening instruments, 283–284, 285, 286, 287–288
    cognitive ability tests, 306–309, 312
    computerized tests, 368
    Halstead–Reitan Neuropsychological Battery, 116
    intermediate-length tests, 289, 290, 291
    for language deficits, 197, 198, 199
    Luria–Nebraska Neuropsychological Battery, 154–155
    process approach of, 174, 188, 195, 196, 198, 200, 201, 204–205

Alzheimer's disease (*cont.*)
  neuropsychological assessment instruments for (*cont.*)
    proverb interpretation, 196
    for visuospatial dysfunction assessment, 200, 201
  phonemic distortions in, 182
Alzheimer's disease patients, care level for, 287
Alzheimer's Disease Assessment Battery, 368
American Board of Clinical Neuropsychology, diplomate examination of, 122
Amnesia, 395–396
  memory deficits in, 71
  retrograde, 205
Analogies test, 33
ANAM: *see* Automated Neuropsychological Assessment Metrics
Anxiety disorders, neurobiological basis of, 396
Aphasia
  anomic, 198
  Broca's, 197, 198
  conduction, 197, 198
  construction, 94
  fixed versus flexible battery assessment of, 85
  language deficit assessment in, 197, 198–200
  mood assessment in, 189
  process appproach assessment of, 172, 173, 183–185, 197, 198–200
  skull fracture-related, 199–200
  traumatic brain injury-related, 199–200, 257
  Wernicke's, 197, 198
Aphasia Screening Test, 237
Apprehension span, 249
Apraxia, 94
APT: *see* Automated Psychological Test Battery
APTS: *see* Automated Portable Test System
Area coverage, 20
Arithmetic learning disorder, 260

ISBN 0-306-45521-8

90000

9 780306 455216